AF520951

Progress in Diabetes

Progress in Diabetes

Editor-in-Chief

Anuj Maheshwari

MD FICP FIACM FIMSA FRSSDI FACP(USA) FACE(USA) FRCP(London, Edinburgh)

Diabetologist and Metabolic Physician

Hind Institute of Medical Sciences (HIMS)

Lucknow, Uttar Pradesh, India

Executive Editor

Shambo Samrat Samajdar

MD DM(Clinical Pharmacology) PG Diploma in Endocrinology and Diabetes(RCP) Diploma in Allergy Asthma and Immunology Fellowship in Respiratory and Critical Care(WBUHS) Fellow Diabetes India

Independent Clinical Pharmacologist and Consultant

Diabetes and Allergy-Asthma Therapeutics Specialty Clinic

Kolkata, West Bengal, India

Foreword

Kamalakar Tripathi

JAYPEE

JAYPEE BROTHERS MEDICAL PUBLISHERS

The Health Sciences Publisher

New Delhi | London

Jaypee Brothers Medical Publishers (P) Ltd

Headquarters
EMCA House, 23/23-B
Ansari Road, Daryaganj
New Delhi 110 002, India
Landline: +91-11-23272143, +91-11-23272703
+91-11-23282021, +91-11-23245672
e-mail: jaypee@jaypeebrothers.com

Corporate Office
4838/24, Ansari Road, Daryaganj
New Delhi 110 002, India
Phone: +91-11-43574357
Fax: +91-11-43574314
e-mail: jaypee@jaypeebrothers.com

Overseas Office
JP Medical Ltd.
83, Victoria Street, London
SW1H 0HW (UK)
Phone: +44-20 3170 8910
e-mail: info@jpmedpub.com

EU GPSR Authorised Representative
Logos Europe, 9 rue Nicolas Poussin
17000, La Rochelle, France
Phone: +33 (0) 6 67 93 73 78
e-mail: contact@logoseurope.eu

Website: www.jaypeebrothers.com
Website: www.jaypeedigital.com

© 2026, Jaypee Brothers Medical Publishers

The views and opinions expressed in this book are solely those of the original contributor(s)/author(s) and do not necessarily represent those of editor(s) or publisher of the book.

All rights reserved. No part of this publication may be reproduced, stored or transmitted in any form or by any means, electronic, mechanical, photocopying, recording or otherwise, without the prior permission in writing of the publishers.

All brand names and product names used in this book are trade names, service marks, trademarks or registered trademarks of their respective owners. The publisher is not associated with any product or vendor mentioned in this book.

Medical knowledge and practice change constantly. This book is designed to provide accurate, authoritative information about the subject matter in question. However, readers are advised to check the most current information available on procedures included and check information from the manufacturer of each product to be administered, to verify the recommended dose, formula, method and duration of administration, adverse effects and contraindications. It is the responsibility of the practitioner to take all appropriate safety precautions. Neither the publisher nor the author(s)/editor(s) assume any liability for any injury and/or damage to persons or property arising from or related to use of material in this book.

This book is sold on the understanding that the publisher is not engaged in providing professional medical services. If such advice or services are required, the services of a competent medical professional should be sought.

Every effort has been made where necessary to contact holders of copyright to obtain permission to reproduce copyright material. If any have been inadvertently overlooked, the publisher will be pleased to make the necessary arrangements at the first opportunity.

Inquiries for bulk sales may be solicited at: jaypee@jaypeebrothers.com

Progress in Diabetes* / *Anuj Maheshwari

First Edition: **2026**

ISBN: 978-93-7202-499-9

Printed at: Samrat Offset Pvt. Ltd.

Govt. Issued Document; Copying is an Illegal Act.

प्रारूप आरजी - 2
Form RG - 2

सत्यमेव जयते

INTELLECTUAL PROPERTY INDIA
Patents | Designs | Trademarks Geographical Indications

भारत सरकार
Government of India
व्यापार चिन्ह रजिस्ट्री
Trade Marks Registry
व्यापार चिन्ह अधिनियम, 1999

Trade Marks Act, 1999

व्यापार चिन्ह के रजिस्ट्रीकरण का प्रमाणपत्र, धारा 23 (2), नियम 56 (1)

Certificate of Registration of Trade Mark, Section 23 (2), Rule 56 (1)

क्रमांक
No. 2442588

व्यापार चिन्ह संख्या / **Trade Mark No.** 3436251 दिनांक /**Date** 19/12/2016 ज. संख्या /**J. No.** 1930

यह प्रमाणित किया जाता है कि जिस प्रकार चिन्ह की समाकृति इसके साथ संलग्न है, वह ....
के बारे में दिनांक ....नाम से रजिस्ट्रीकृत हो चुका है।

Certified that Trade Mark / a representation is annexed hereto, has been registered in the name(s) of :-
JAYPEE BROTHERS MEDICAL PUBLISHERS PRIVATE LIMITED, 4838/24, ANSARI ROAD, DARYAGANJ, NEW DELHI-110002, Body Incorporate, Service Provider, (Body Incorporate)

In Class 41 Under No. 3436251 as of the date 19 December 2016 in respect of

PUBLICATION SERVICES RELATING TO BOOKS, NOTE-BOOKS, MAGAZINES, BROCHURES, PAMPHLETS, MANULAS, PUBLICATION OF PRINTED MATTERS, ELECTRONIC PUBLICATON INCLUDED IN CLASS-41

JAYPEE BROTHERS MEDICAL PUBLISHERS

मेरे निर्देश पर आज .... के .... मास के .... वे दिन को इस पर मुद्रा लगायी गई

Sealed at my direction, this 07th day of August , 2020

व्यापार चिन्ह रजिस्ट्री
Trade Marks Registry MUMBAI

व्यापार चिन्ह रजिस्ट्रार
Registrar of Trademarks

रजिस्ट्रीकरण आवेदन की तारीख से १० वर्ष के लिए है और तदोपरांत वह १० वर्ष की कालावधि के लिए और प्रत्येक १० वर्ष की कालावधि के अवसान पर भी नवीनीकृत किया जा सकेगा।

Registration is for 10 years from the date of application and may then be renewed for a period of 10 years and also at the expiration of each period of 10 years.

यह प्रमाणपत्र विधि कार्यवाहियों में प्रयोग के लिए या विदेश में रजिस्ट्रीकरण अभिप्राप्त करने के लिए नहीं है

This certificate is not for use in legal proceedings or for obtaining Registration abroad.

टिप्पणी - इस व्यापार चिन्ह के स्वामित्व में कोई परिवर्तन होने पर, या कारोबार के मुख्य स्थान के पते में या भारत में तामील के लिए पते में परिवर्तन होने पर परिवर्तन के लिए आवेदन तुरंत किया जाना चाहिए.

Note: Upon any change of ownership of this Trademark, or change in address, of the principal place of business or address for service in India a request should **AT ONCE** be made to register the change.

Govt. Issued Document; Copying is an Illegal Act.

INTELLECTUAL PROPERTY **INDIA**
PATENTS | DESIGNS | TRADE MARKS
GEOGRAPHICAL INDICATIONS

प्रारूप आरजी - 2
Form RG - 2
क्रमांक No. 3772319

व्यापार चिन्ह रजिस्ट्री, भारत सरकार Trade Marks Registry, Government Of India

व्यापार चिन्ह अधिनियम, 1999 Trade Marks Act, 1999

व्यापार चिन्ह के रजिस्ट्रीकरण का प्रमाणपत्र | Certificate of Registration of Trade Mark

(धारा 23 (2), नियम 56 (1)) | Section 23 (2), Rule 56 (1)

व्यापार चिन्ह संख्या / Trade Mark No. : 5191318
दिनांक / Date : 28-10-2021
ज. संख्या / J. No. : 2158

प्रमाणित किया जाता है कि व्यापार चिन्ह / जिसका प्रतिरूप इसके साथ संलग्न है, वह .... के नाम से .... वर्ग में .... संख्या के अधीन दिनांक .... को .... के संबंध में रजिस्ट्रीकृत किया गया है|

Certified that Trade Mark / a representation is annexed hereto, has been registered in the name(s) of :- JAYPEE BROTHERS MEDICAL PUBLISHERS PRIVATE LIMITED, 4838/24, ANSARI ROAD, DARYAGANJ, NEW DELHI-110002., Body Incorporate, (Body Incorporate)

In Class 41 Under No. 5191318 as of the date 28 October 2021 in respect of

Publication Services , Electronic Publication , Issue of Publications, Publication of Books and Textbooks, Publication of Booklets, Publication of Brochures, Publication of Journals, included Under Class-41.

Trade Mark as annexed

आज वर्ष 20.................... के .... माह के .... वें दिन को मेरे निर्देश पर मुद्रांकित किया गया

Sealed at my direction, this 19th day of October, 2024

उन्नत पी पंडित

व्यापार चिन्ह रजिस्ट्री मुंबई
Trade Marks Registry MUMBAI

व्यापार चिन्ह रजिस्ट्रार
Registrar of Trademarks

रजिस्ट्रीकरण आवेदन की तारीख से १० वर्ष के लिए है और तदोपरांत वह १० वर्ष की अवधि के लिए और प्रत्येक १० वर्ष की अवधि की समाप्ति पर भी नवीनीकृत किया जा सकेगा।
यह प्रमाणपत्र विधि कार्यवाहियों में प्रयोग के लिए या विदेश में रजिस्ट्रीकरण प्राप्त करने के लिए नहीं है
टिप्पणी : इस व्यापार चिन्ह के स्वामित्व में कोई परिवर्तन होने पर, या कारोबार के मुख्य स्थान के पते में या भारत में सेवा के लिए पते में परिवर्तन होने पर परिवर्तन को दर्ज करने के लिए एक बार अनुरोध किया जाना चाहिए.
Registration is for 10 years from the date of application and may then be renewed for a period of 10 years and also at the expiration of each period of 10 years.
This certificate is not for use in legal proceedings or for obtaining Registration abroad.
Note: Upon any change of ownership of this Trademark, or change in address, of the principal place of business or address for service in India a request should AT ONCE be made to register the change.

व्यापार चिन्ह के लिए अनुलग्नक / Annexure of Trade Mark Certificate

क्रमांक / No. **3772319**

व्यापार चिन्ह संख्या / Trade Mark No. **5191318**

दिनांक / Date **28-10-2021**

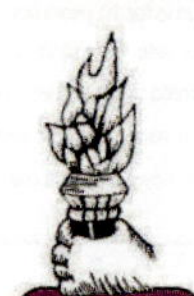

JAYPEE

DEDICATION

To our patients—
The silent teachers, the resilient warriors, and the unwavering souls
who entrust us with their stories, their struggles, and their strength.

Each heartbeat, each trial, and each triumph becomes a lesson—
A sacred whisper guiding our pursuit of knowledge, healing, and compassion.
In your courage, we find our calling.
In your perseverance, we find our purpose.
In your journey, we find the roadmap to progress.

This work is humbly dedicated to you—
from whom we are learning every day.

Editorial Committee

Editor-in-Chief

Anuj Maheshwari

Executive Editor

Shambo Samrat Samajdar

Advisors

Shashank R Joshi

Banshi Saboo

Ashok K Das

Kamlakar Tripathi

Editorial Board

Jothydev Kesavadev

Sunil S Gupta

Sanjay Agarwal

Jayanta Kumar Panda

Narsingh Verma

Ajoy K Tewari

Sajid Ansari

Veneeta Tewari

Nisha Maheshwari

Amit Gupta

Alok Modi

Shivangi Maheshwari

Sanjay Singla

Shubhashree Patil

Krishnadev Jothydev

Karthik Munichoodappa

Raghunath Dantu

Vanshika Arora

Banshi Saboo MD PhD FACE
Diabetologist and Metabolic Physician
Dia-Care
Ahmedabad, Gujarat, India

Bharat Saboo MBBS MSc(Endocrinology) Diploma in Diabetology Scope Certified - Obesity
Director
Prayas Diabetes Center
Indore, Madhya Pradesh, India

Bijay Patni FACP FDI FIDF FISH FISCM
Senior Physician (With Expertise in Cardiometabolic and Diabetes)
Scope Certified
Head
Diabetes Wellness Care
Kolkata, West Bengal, India

Brij Mohan Makker MD FRCP(Glasgow, Edinburgh) FACP FACE
Consulting Diabetes and Bariatric Physician
Diabetes and Obesity Centre
New Delhi, India

Dhruvi Hasnani MD(Medicine)
Co-founder Head
Department of Clinical Research
Rudraksha Institute of Medical Sciences
Ahmedabad, Gujarat, India

Hemant P Thacker MD(Bombay) MRSH(London) FACE(USA) FACP(USA) FRCP(Edinburgh)
Consultant Physician and CardioMetabolic Specialist
Director
Department of Medicine
Jaslok Hospital
Head, Department of Medicine
Bhatia Hospital
Senior Consultant Breach Candy and Reliance HN Hospitals
Mumbai, Maharashtra, India

Jayanta Kumar Panda MD(Internal Medicine) FACP(USA) FICP FIMAMS FRSSDI FRCP(London) Fellow Diabetes India
Consultant in Diabetes, Metabolic and Critical Care Medicine
Professor
PG Department of Internal Medicine
SCB Medical College
Cuttack, Odisha, India

Jayshree Swain DM(Endocrinology)
Professor and Unit Head
Department of Endocrinology
IMS and SUM Hospital
Bhubaneswar, Odisha, India

Jay Tewari MBBS
Clinical Observer
Department of Medicine
Washington Hospital
San Francisco, California, United States

Jothydev Kesavadev MD FRCP(London) FACE FRCP(Glasgow) FRCP(Edinburgh) FACP FRSSDI
Chairman and Managing Director
Jothydev's Diabetes Research Centre
Thiruvananthapuram, Kerala, India

Kenjom Ngomdir MBBS PGDSM(Sports Medicine)
Commandant (Medical)/Chief Medical Officer (SG)
I/C Sports Medicine and Sports Sciences Centre, CRPF, Delhi
ISSEM, IFSM, ISMN, IDTM, SDTI, IDCO (ITA), MCCP, FCCP
New Delhi, India

Krishnadev Jothydev MBBS 1st Year MD(General Medicine)
Resident, Department of Medicine
Sree Gokulam Medical College
Jothydev's Diabetes Research Centre
Thiruvananthapuram, Kerala, India

Krishna G Seshadri American Board Certified Endocrinologist
American Board Certified
Senior Consultant
Department of Endocrinology Diabetes and Metabolism
Chennai Diabetes and Endocrine Clinic
Chennai, Tamil Nadu, India

Manoj Chawla MBBS DDiab FRSSDI FRCP(Edinburgh)
Director and Consultant Diabetologist
Lina Diabetes Care and Mumbai Diabetes Research Centre, Andheri, Mumbai
Consultant Diabetologist
PD Hinduja Hospital, Khar
SL Raheja Fortis, Bharatiya Arogya Nidhi Hospital, BSES Municipal General Hospital
Mumbai, Maharashtra, India

Mohamed Abdul Khader M MSc(Biotechnology)
Scientific Project Coordinator
Jothydev's Diabetes Research Centre
Thiruvananthapuram, Kerala, India

M Shunmugavelu MD FICP FRCP(Glasgow) FRSSDI
Specialist in Internal Medicine
Diabetologist, Chairman
Managing Director
Trichy Diabetes Speciality Centre (P) Ltd
Tiruchirappalli, Tamil Nadu, India

Narsingh Verma MD FRCP(London) FRCP(Edinburgh) FACP(USA) FIACM FICN FAMS FIMSA FISC FIPF FRSSD
Principal and Dean
Hind Institute of Medical Sciences
Lucknow, Uttar Pradesh, India

Neeta Deshpande MD
FRCP(Edinburgh) PG Endo (London)
ASBP Obesity Cert (USA)
Diabetologist and Bariatric
Physician, Medical Director
Centre Care Institute of Diabetes,
Obesity and Metabolic Health
CentraCare Super Speciality
Hospital and MRC and Belgaum
Diabetes Centre
Belgaum, Karnataka, India

N Bhavatharini DDiab(MMC)
FRCP(London)
Diabetologist
SRC Diabetes Care Center
Erode, Tamil Nadu, India

NK Singh MD(Internal Medicine)
Director
Department of Diabetology
Diabetes and Heart Research
Centre
Dhanbad, Jharkhand, India

Praveen Gangadhara MBBS
FDiab (CMC Vellore)
Consultant
Dr Mohan's Diabetes Specialities
Centre
Bengaluru, Karnataka, India

Purvi Chawla MBBS
MS(Pharmaceutical Sciences)
PG Diploma Diabetology PG Diploma
Endocrinology
Consultation Diabetologist
Director Clinical Research
Lina Diabetes Care and Mumbai
Diabetes Research Centre
Andheri, Mumbai
Consultant Diabetologist
VLSR Clinic, Bharatiya Arogya
Nidhi Hospital, BSES Municipal
General Hospital
Mumbai, Maharashtra, India

Ranjit Mohan Anjana MD PhD
Managing Director and President
Dr Mohan's Diabetes Specialities
Centre and Madras Diabetes
Research Foundation
Chennai, Tamil Nadu, India

Reshma Mirshad MDS
Medical Associate
MV Hospital for Diabetes and
Professor M Viswanathan Diabetes
Research Centre
Chennai, Tamil Nadu, India

Rutul Gokalani MD
Consultant Diabetologist
Department of Diabetology
Diabetes and Metabolic Physician
AHC Diabetes Centre
Ahmedabad, Gujarat, India

Sabat Imran Ansari MSc
PhD(Nutrition)
Visiting Lecturer, Department for
Foods and Nutrition, The Maharaja
Sayajirao University of Baroda
Vadodara, Gujarat, India

Sanjay Agarwal MD FACE
Senior Consultant in Diabetes and
Medicine
Department of Diabetology
Jehangir Hospital and Apollo
Group of Hospital, Ruby Hall Clinic
Pune, Maharashtra, India

Shambo Samrat Samajdar MD
DM(Clinical Pharmacology) PG Diploma
in Endocrinology and Diabetes(RCP)
Diploma in Allergy Asthma and
Immunology Fellowship in Respiratory
and Critical Care(WBUHS) Fellow
Diabetes India
Independent Clinical
Pharmacologist and Consultant
Diabetes and Allergy-Asthma
Therapeutics Specialty Clinic
Kolkata, West Bengal, India

Shashank R Joshi MD DM
FICP FACP(USA) FACE(USA) Hon
DSc(Medicine) FRCP(London, Glasgow
and Edinburgh)
Consultant
Department of Endocrinology
Joshi Clinic
Lilavati Hospital and
Sir HN Reliance Foundation
Hospital
Mumbai, Maharashtra, India

Shivangi Maheshwari MBBS
PGY- 2, MD Pediatrics
Department of Pediatrics
IMS and SUM Hospital
Bhubaneswar, Odisha, India

Shonima Venugopal MSc
PhD(Nutrition)
Assistant Professor (CES)
Department for Foods and
Nutrition
The Maharaja Sayajirao University
of Baroda
Vadodara, Gujarat, India

Shubhashree Patil MBBS
DNB(General Medicine) Diploma
Diabetology
Consultant Physician and
Diabetologist
Department of Diabetology
Diabetes and Wellness Clinic
Seven Hills Hospital
Apollo Clinics
Criticare Asia Hospital
Mumbai, Maharashtra, India

Sidharth Shankar Panigrahi
DM Resident(Endocrinology)
MD(Medicine)
DM Resident
Department of Endocrinology
IMS and SUM Hospital
Bhubaneswar, Odisha, India

Soumyaranjan Mohanty MBBS PGDMCH FDIAB Fellow IDF Fellow Diabetes India FISC
Consultant Diabetologist
SRM's Complete Diabetes Care
Dhenkanal, Odisha, India

Sujoy Ghosh MD DM(Endocrinology)
Professor
Department of Endocrinology
IPGMER, Ayush Senior Resident
Kolkata, West Bengal, India

Sunil S Gupta MD FACE FRCP(London, Glasgow, and Edinburgh)
Diabetologist
MD, Sunil's Diabetes Care n' Research Centre Pvt Ltd
Nagpur, Maharashtra, India

Supratik Bhattacharya MD MRCP(UK) FRCP FACE
Director, SKN Diabetes and Endocrine Centre
Senior Consultant
Department of Endocrinology and Diabetes, Manipal Broadways Hospital and Apollo Sugar
Kolkata, West Bengal, India

TEO Boon Wee Jimmy MBBCh
Associate Professor, Senior Consultant, Division of Nephrology
Department of Medicine
Yong Loo Lin School of Medicine
National University of Singapore
Singapore

Vanisha S Nambiar MSc PhD(Nutrition) FIUNS
Professor and Head (I/C)
Department for Foods and Nutrition
The Maharaja Sayajirao University of Baroda
Vadodara, Gujarat, India

Vijay Viswanathan MD PhD FRCP(London) FRCP(Glasgow)
Head and Chief Diabetologist
MV Hospital for Diabetes and Professor M Viswanathan Diabetes Research Centre
Chennai, Tamil Nadu, India

Vinayak Hiremath MD MRCP(UK) MRCP(Endocrinology and Diabetes) Fellow in Immunology(HMX, USA) SCOPE(Obesity)
Medical Director
Metabolic and Endocrine Consultant
Director, Obesity Clinic
Executive Director, RDOC NGO
Department of Internal Medicine, Endocrinology and Diabetes
KMK Hospital
Cochin, Kerala, India

Veneeta Tewari MD
Professor and Head
Department of Anatomy
Era's Lucknow Medical College and Hospital (ELMCH)
Lucknow, Uttar Pradesh, India

Vipul Chavda MD(Medicine)
Founder Director
Rudraksha Institute of Medical Sciences
Ahmedabad, Gujarat, India

VK Sanjeev MD DNB(Cardiology)
Consultant Cardiologist
Gleneagles HealthCity
Chennai, Tamil Nadu, India

Viswanathan Mohan MD PhD DSc
Chairman
Dr Mohan's Diabetes Specialities Centre and Madras Diabetes Research Foundation
Chennai, Tamil Nadu, India

FOREWORD

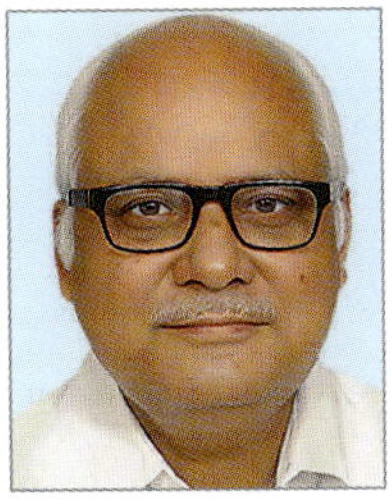

Kamalakar Tripathi MD DM DNB MNAMS(Nephrology) FRCP(Edinburgh) FACP
Padma Shri Awardee
Former Dean and Head
Department of Medicine
Institute of Medical Sciences, Banaras Hindu University
Vice Dean, Indian College of Physicians

It gives me immense pleasure to pen the foreword for *"Progress in Diabetes"*, a timely and forward-thinking contribution to the field of diabetology. As someone who has witnessed the evolving burden of diabetes over five decades—from its early epidemiological silence to its current place as a major public health challenge—I consider this volume not merely a compilation of chapters, but a reflection of India's intellectual and clinical leadership in this domain.

Diabetes today is no longer a singular metabolic disorder; it is an intricate web of multisystem involvement—impacting kidneys, heart, eyes, nerves, and, most importantly, the human experience. As a nephrologist, I have seen firsthand how diabetic kidney disease silently advances, often becoming the turning point in a patient's life journey. This makes books like Progress in Diabetes even more vital. They serve to educate, alert, and inspire all stakeholders—clinicians, researchers, policy architects, and caregivers.

Dr Anuj Maheshwari and Dr Shambo Samrat Samajdar have done a commendable job in assembling a panoramic view of diabetes care—from precision medicine and artificial intelligence to public health policy and traditional wisdom. What stands out is the blend of high science with grassroots relevance—chapters that resonate with both the researcher in a laboratory and the physician in a rural health center.

The breadth and depth of this book assure me that we are entering an era of hope—where diabetes may no longer mean a lifelong burden but a condition with potential for remission, even reversal. Let us not forget that science alone cannot win this war. It is compassion, equity, and continuous education that will eventually transform outcomes.

I wholeheartedly recommend this book to every medical student, resident, physician, and public health professional committed to the care of people with diabetes. May it serve as both a guiding light and a call to action.

PREFACE

The global landscape of diabetes is evolving rapidly, marked by scientific breakthroughs, digital transformation, and renewed hope for remission and prevention. "*Progress in Diabetes*" brings together distinguished voices from across the spectrum of diabetology—basic science, clinical care, public health, digital innovation, and patient-centered research. As editors, we envisioned this compendium as a forward-looking volume that reflects both the progress achieved and the challenges that lie ahead in combating diabetes. Each chapter in this book has been carefully curated to provide evidence-based insights, emerging paradigms, and future trajectories. From regenerative medicine and AI-driven diagnostics to psychosocial support and public health strategies, this collection offers a comprehensive, multidisciplinary exploration of diabetes care in the coming decade. We believe this work will serve as a valuable resource for clinicians, researchers, policy makers, and students, fostering a deeper understanding of how precision medicine, digital health, and systems-based approaches can converge to achieve better outcomes for people living with diabetes.

We are deeply grateful to the contributing authors—each a pioneer in their respective domains—for sharing their expertise, vision, and commitment to advancing diabetes science and care. This book stands as a testament to the collaborative spirit of the diabetes community, unified by a common goal: Transforming care, improving lives, and striving for a future where diabetes is not only better managed but prevented or reversed.

The Research Society for the Study of Diabetes in India (RSSDI) has played a pivotal role in advancing diabetes research and care across the country. As India's largest professional body dedicated to diabetes, RSSDI has tirelessly worked to bridge the urban–rural divide by extending education, awareness, and clinical support to peripheral regions. Through national guidelines, training programs, fellowships, and community outreach initiatives, RSSDI has empowered thousands of healthcare professionals and impacted millions of lives. Its commitment to indigenous research, context-specific solutions, and inclusive healthcare delivery has significantly strengthened India's fight against the diabetes epidemic.

Anuj Maheshwari
Shambo Samrat Samajdar

CONTENTS

1 The Global Diabetes Landscape in 2025: Epidemiology and Burden

Anuj Maheshwari, Shambo Samrat Samajdar

ABSTRACT

Background: Diabetes mellitus has emerged as a defining public health crisis of the 21st century. As of 2025, over 537 million adults globally are living with diabetes, with projections indicating a rise to 1.31 billion by 2050 if current trajectories continue. This rise is propelled by aging populations, urbanization, rising obesity, poor diets, physical inactivity, and environmental risk exposures, with low- and middle-income countries (LMICs) bearing the brunt of the burden.

Objective: To provide an evidence-based overview of global diabetes epidemiology, risk factors, regional disparities, and future projections, with a special focus on South Asia and India.

Methods: The chapter synthesizes data from the Global Burden of Disease (GBD) Study 2021, the IDF Diabetes Atlas (2025), and the ICMR–INDIAB study, covering prevalence trends, demographic profiles, and projections to 2050.

Findings: Type 2 diabetes accounts for over 96% of cases globally, with a growing prevalence in younger adults. The "South Asian phenotype"—characterized by early-onset diabetes, lower BMI thresholds, and insulin resistance—adds complexity in India, where 101 million people currently have diabetes and another 136 million have prediabetes. High BMI, sedentary behavior, and dietary transitions remain the primary modifiable drivers. Diabetes-related health expenditures are projected to exceed US $1.05 trillion by 2045. Disparities in access to diagnostics and care are especially acute in LMICs.

Conclusion: Urgent, multisectoral action is needed to stem the diabetes epidemic. Prevention strategies must address early-life risk, promote healthier environments, and expand access to affordable care—especially in high-burden regions such as South Asia. India stands both as a hotspot and as a potential global leader in diabetes innovation and control.

Keywords: Diabetes mellitus, Global burden of disease (GBD), South Asian phenotype, India, noncommunicable diseases (NCDs).

INTRODUCTION

Diabetes mellitus has become one of the most urgent global health challenges of the 21st century. As of *2025*, over *537 million* adults are living with diabetes worldwide, and projections indicate this number could rise to *1.31 billion by 2050* if current trends remain unmitigated.[1] This staggering growth is driven by population aging, urbanization, rising obesity, dietary transitions, physical inactivity, and exposure to environmental and social risk factors.

The burden of diabetes is multidimensional—impacting *health systems, economies, and societies* globally. It is a leading contributor to *premature mortality, disability, and chronic complications,* and places heavy demands on healthcare infrastructure, particularly in *low- and middle-income countries (LMICs),* where over *81%* of diabetes cases now occur.[1]

The global distribution of diabetes is highly unequal. Regions such as *Oceania, the Middle East, and Latin America* report significantly higher prevalence rates than the global average. Alarmingly, individuals aged *75–79 years* exhibit a *global prevalence exceeding 24%,* with some countries like *Qatar* reporting levels over *76%* in this age group.[1] Furthermore, the *age of onset* is decreasing—especially in LMICs—leading to longer disease duration and a higher likelihood of complications.

Type 2 diabetes (T2D) accounts for over *96%* of all cases and is closely linked to modifiable lifestyle factors such as obesity, diet, and sedentary behavior.[2] However, *type 1 diabetes (T1D)* remains a significant burden among children and adolescents, with rising incidence even in middle-income countries.

Of particular concern is the *South Asian region,* which is now the *epicenter of the diabetes epidemic.* Individuals from this region often present a distinct clinical profile—known as the *"South Asian phenotype"*—marked by early onset, diabetes at lower BMI, increased insulin resistance, and impaired β-cell function.[3] These features underscore the need for region-specific approaches to prevention, diagnosis, and management.

India, with *101 million people* currently living with diabetes and another *136 million with prediabetes,* illustrates the scale and complexity of the crisis.[4] The country also reflects how *urban-rural disparities, interstate variation,* and *socioeconomic inequalities* intensify chronic disease burdens in LMICs.

This chapter synthesizes the *global diabetes landscape as of 2025,* with a focus on *epidemiological trends, risk factors, regional disparities,* and *future projections.* Special emphasis is placed on *South Asia and India,* where demographic and metabolic transitions are reshaping the path of this epidemic. By highlighting current data and long-term projections, the aim is to guide *evidence-based, equitable,* and *scalable strategies* for diabetes prevention and control.

GLOBAL EPIDEMIOLOGICAL TRENDS

Prevalence and Distribution

As of *2021,* approximately *529 million people* globally were living with diabetes, corresponding to an *age-standardized global prevalence of 6.1%* [95% uncertainty interval (UI) 5.8–6.5%]. This number is projected to rise to *1.31 billion by 2050,* driven by demographic growth, rising obesity, and lifestyle transitions.

Regional prevalence highlights:

- *Oceania*: 12.3% (95% UI 11.5–13.0)
- *North Africa and the Middle East*: 9.3% (95% UI 8.7–9.9)
- *Latin America and the Caribbean*: 8.4% (95% UI 7.9–9.0)

At the national level, countries such as *Qatar* have already surpassed critical thresholds. In Qatar, diabetes prevalence among people aged *75–79 years* reached *76.1%* (95% UI 73.1–79.5%). Globally, prevalence *exceeds 20%* among people aged *65–95 years,* peaking at *24.4%* (22.3–26.2%) in the *75–79 age group.*

These patterns underscore a growing concentration of diabetes burden in *older populations and Global South countries,* many of which lack the health infrastructure to manage chronic metabolic disease effectively.

Type-specific Distribution

Diabetes is broadly categorized into:

Type 2 diabetes:

- Accounts for *96.0%* (95.1–96.8%) of all diabetes cases globally

- Responsible for *95.4%* (94.9–95.9%) of diabetes-related *DALYs*
- Linked to *obesity, sedentarism,* and *poor diet*
- Increasingly common in *younger adults* in LMICs

Type 1 diabetes:
- Less prevalent but *clinically significant* in *children and adolescents*
- Caused by *autoimmune destruction* of pancreatic β-cells
- Requires *lifelong insulin therapy*
- Incidence is *increasing* in several high-income and middle-income countries

Sex and Age Patterns

Global prevalence by sex:
- *Males*: *6.5%* (95% UI 6.2–7.0)
- *Females*: *5.8%* (95% UI 5.4–6.1)
- *Male-to-female ratio*: 1.14 (1.13–1.15)

This disparity varies regionally—some high-income regions show greater male prevalence, whereas, certain parts of *Latin America and the Caribbean* exhibit higher female prevalence.

Moreover, the *age of diabetes onset is trending younger*, particularly in *South Asia*, where diagnosis in the *30s and 40s* is increasingly common due to a combination of:
- Genetic predisposition
- Urban lifestyle transitions
- Early-life metabolic programming

REGIONAL BURDEN AND PROJECTIONS

South Asia: A High-burden Zone

South Asia—comprising India, Pakistan, Bangladesh, Sri Lanka, Nepal, Bhutan, Afghanistan, and the Maldives—has emerged as the global epicenter of the diabetes epidemic. The region is home to nearly *25% of the global population*, and its diabetes profile is distinct and deeply concerning.

One of the defining features of diabetes in South Asians is a unique constellation of clinical and metabolic traits, collectively termed the *"South Asian Phenotype"*. Key characteristics include:
- *Younger age at onset*: Diabetes is often diagnosed a decade earlier compared to Western populations, commonly affecting individuals in their 30s and 40s.
- *Lower BMI thresholds*: South Asians frequently develop T2D at BMIs below 25 kg/m^2, challenging conventional obesity definitions.
- *Excess insulin resistance and early β-cell dysfunction*: Even in the absence of obesity, South Asians exhibit high insulin resistance and a rapid decline in insulin secretory capacity.
- *Greater ectopic fat deposition*: Particularly in the liver and visceral areas, despite low total body fat

These pathophysiological features, shaped by *genetic predisposition, intrauterine programming, and rapid nutritional and lifestyle transitions*, contribute to the high and rising burden of diabetes in the region. The phenotype underscores the need for *ethnically tailored diagnostic criteria, screening thresholds, and intervention strategies* in South Asia.

India's Alarming Rise

India, now the most populous country globally, has emerged as one of the nations bearing the *heaviest burden of diabetes*. According to the nationally representative *ICMR-INDIAB Study*, which surveyed all *31 states and union territories*, the magnitude of the diabetes crisis is deeply concerning.[4,5]

Key findings (2021–2023):
- *101 million* individuals in India live with *diabetes*, corresponding to a *national prevalence of 11.4%* among adults aged >20 years.
- An additional *136 million individuals (15.3%)* have *prediabetes*, forming a critical pool at high risk of progression.

- *Urban centers* such as *Tamil Nadu, Goa, and Delhi* have recorded *prevalence rates exceeding 20–26%*, with *Goa peaking at 26.4%*.

The study revealed a *marked increase in diabetes starting from the 25–34-year age group*, a trend consistent across *urban and rural areas, and both sexes*. This shift toward *early-onset diabetes* raises significant concern due to *longer disease duration and higher lifetime complication risk*.

Interstate and Socioeconomic Disparities

The diabetes burden in India is not evenly distributed:

Southern and western states—such as *Tamil Nadu, Kerala, Maharashtra, and Gujarat*—report the *highest prevalence and DALY rates*. These trends are associated with:

- Greater *urbanization*
- Sedentary lifestyles
- Westernized dietary patterns

In contrast, *northern and northeastern states*—such as *Uttar Pradesh and Mizoram*—have *lower current prevalence* (e.g., *Uttar Pradesh: 4.8%*) but are *witnessing steep upward trends*, indicating an impending surge.

Higher diabetes-related *mortality and DALYs* are observed in *urban areas* and among individuals with *higher socioeconomic status*. This is partially due to:

- Increased diagnostic access
- Sedentary work profiles
- Higher consumption of processed foods

Future Projections

Using *time-series modeling*, the ICMR–INDIAB study estimates that by **2031**:[4]

- *Prevalence* will reach approximately *8,600 per 100,000 population*
- *Diabetes-related DALYs* will exceed *1,200 per 100,000 population*

These numbers underscore a steep and sustained rise unless *urgent and coordinated interventions* are adopted.

Implications and Call to Action

India's diabetes trajectory provides critical insights into the global NCD crisis. The country's *rapid economic development, urban migration, and nutrition transition have outpaced public health systems*, exposing millions to metabolic risk.

To curb the epidemic, *multi-tiered, life-course interventions* are essential:

- *Maternal nutrition* and *early-childhood interventions* to prevent intergenerational transmission of risk
- *Primary prevention programs* in schools, workplaces, and urban communities
- *Urban health infrastructure* enhancement, including screening at *150,000+ Health and Wellness Centers under Ayushman Bharat*
- *Community-based lifestyle interventions* for high-risk groups with prediabetes

With *more than 136 million Indians* currently classified as prediabetic, India holds a *window of opportunity* to avert further escalation by promoting *dietary change, physical activity, and public health awareness* at scale.[4,5]

Risk Factors and Drivers

The alarming global rise in diabetes prevalence is a consequence of complex interactions between behavioral, environmental, biological, and social determinants. While *genetic predisposition* plays a role, the current surge is primarily driven by *modifiable risk factors*, many of which have become more prevalent due to globalization, urbanization, and lifestyle transitions.

Obesity and Sedentarism

Among all modifiable risk factors, *high body-mass index (BMI)* is unequivocally the *most significant contributor* to the global burden of *T2D*.

According to the *Global Burden of Disease (GBD) 2021 Study*:[2]

- *High BMI accounted for 52.2% (95% UI 25.5–71.8%)* of all *T2D-related disability-adjusted life years (DALYs)* globally in 2021.

- Between *1990 and 2021*, the share of T2D DALYs attributable to high BMI *increased by 24.3%*, reflecting the growing impact of overweight and obesity across all populations and age groups.

This upward trend parallels the global spread of *overweight and obesity*, now prevalent in *both high- and low-income nations*. Sedentary behaviors—such as increased *screen time, automobile reliance, and low occupational energy expenditure*—are major contributors to the rising *inactivity levels*, especially in *urbanizing middle-income countries*.[6]

Notably, physical inactivity is strongly associated with early-onset T2D in younger adults, particularly in South Asia and Latin America.

Dietary Shifts and Urbanization

Nutritional transition is another major driver behind the diabetes epidemic. The global shift from traditional diets toward *energy-dense, nutrient-poor foods* has accelerated the progression of insulin resistance and obesity.[6] Key dietary contributors include:

- *Excessive consumption of refined carbohydrates*, especially *white rice and ultra-processed grains*, which have high glycemic indices and contribute to postprandial hyperglycemia.
- *Increased intake of sugar-sweetened beverages*, a trend most prominent among adolescents and young adults.
- *Low dietary fiber and protein content*, especially in South Asian populations, where carbohydrate intake often exceeds 65–70% of total caloric consumption

Urbanization amplifies these risks by fostering environments that promote *convenience eating*, reduce *opportunities for physical activity*, and increase *psychosocial stress*—all of which are known contributors to diabetes pathogenesis.

Environmental and Emerging Risks

Beyond traditional behavioral risk factors, recent evidence has identified *environmental and novel biological exposures* that may contribute to diabetes development and progression, especially in vulnerable populations:

- *Air pollution*—particularly *ambient particulate matter (PM2.5)*—has emerged as a significant risk factor in *South Asia*, where exposure levels are among the highest globally. Chronic inflammation and oxidative stress triggered by air pollution may impair insulin signaling and β-cell function.[7]
- *Micronutrient deficiencies*, especially *low intake of vitamin B12 and D*, are prevalent in India and may increase susceptibility to T2D through mechanisms involving mitochondrial dysfunction and impaired insulin secretion.[8]
- *Inadequate consumption of fruits, vegetables, and whole grains* further compounds the problem, particularly in low-income households.

Together, these risk factors form a *synergistic web* of influences that are fueling the global diabetes crisis. The situation calls for *multi-pronged prevention strategies* that go beyond individual behavior change and address *structural, environmental, and policy-level determinants* of health.

HEALTH SYSTEM AND ECONOMIC IMPLICATIONS

The escalating global burden of diabetes extends far beyond individual health outcomes. It places immense and growing pressure on health systems, particularly in countries with limited resources. The economic ramifications of diabetes—both direct and indirect—are profound, making it a central issue in health financing and public health planning worldwide.

GLOBAL HEALTHCARE COSTS

Diabetes imposes a *substantial economic burden* on individuals, families, and national health systems. According to the *International Diabetes Federation (IDF)*, the *global cost of diabetes in 2021* was approximately *US $966 billion*, representing >11% of global health expenditure. This figure includes direct medical costs such as insulin, medications, monitoring supplies, hospitalizations, and management of complications.[1]

Projections indicate that, without effective containment, global spending on diabetes is expected to *exceed US $1.05 trillion by 2045*, driven by rising prevalence, aging populations, and increasing use of advanced therapies.[1]

These expenditures are not evenly distributed. High-income countries account for a disproportionate share of global spending, while lower-income countries often spend far less per patient, even though their case numbers are growing more rapidly.

HEALTHCARE ACCESS INEQUITY

A striking feature of the global diabetes landscape is the *inequitable access to care*, especially in *LMICs*. Approximately *80% of people with diabetes now live in LMICs*, yet access to essential services remains *deeply inadequate:*[1]

- *Insulin and oral antidiabetic drugs* remain unaffordable or unavailable for large segments of the population.
- *Diagnostic services* such as HbA1c testing and glucometer access are limited, particularly in rural and underserved areas.
- Many LMICs face a *shortage of trained healthcare personnel*, as well as weak health infrastructure for chronic disease management.
- *Fragmented health insurance coverage* and out-of-pocket expenditure create barriers to early diagnosis, treatment adherence, and complication screening.

This mismatch between *disease burden and healthcare capacity* results in *delayed diagnosis, suboptimal glycemic control, and higher rates of preventable complications*, including diabetic foot, renal failure, and blindness. The situation underscores the urgent need to *strengthen primary care systems, integrate noncommunicable disease (NCD) services, and ensure equitable access to affordable diabetes care* worldwide.

Addressing the economic and systemic dimensions of diabetes requires *policy-level interventions*, including price regulation of insulin, national diabetes programs, and investment in universal health coverage. Without such efforts, the diabetes epidemic will continue to strain healthcare systems and contribute to avoidable morbidity and mortality, particularly in resource-constrained settings.

FORECASTING AND FUTURE OUTLOOK

2030 and Beyond

Looking ahead, the global diabetes burden is set to *escalate sharply*, with the majority of new cases emerging in *LMICs*. Projections from the *GBD Study 2021* and other authoritative sources outline a concerning trajectory:[2]

- By *2050*, the global number of people living with diabetes is projected to reach *1.31 billion*, more than *doubling* from *529 million* in 2021.
- The *age-standardized prevalence* of diabetes is expected to *exceed 10% in 89 of 204 countries and territories*, many of them in the *Global South*, including sub-Saharan Africa, Southeast Asia, and Latin America.
- *India*, due to its large population and already high prevalence, is expected to remain one of the *largest contributors* to the global diabetes burden, especially in *urban centers*, where rapid transitions in diet, activity, and obesity are accelerating disease risk.
- Although India-specific projections for 2031 are limited, existing national surveys and modeling studies indicate a *continuing upward trend* in both *diabetes prevalence and diabetes-related disability-adjusted life years (DALYs)*, particularly among younger adults and urban populations.

These trends underscore the urgent need for *comprehensive, multisectoral strategies* that include:

- Strengthening of *primary care and early detection* systems
- Promotion of *healthier food environments and physical activity*
- Long-term investment in *urban health infrastructure* and *community-based prevention*

Without bold and sustained action, diabetes threatens to overwhelm health systems, strain national economies, and reverse gains in global life expectancy—especially in the world's most vulnerable regions.[1,2]

URGENT POLICY PRIORITIES

To meaningfully curb the rise of diabetes, policy responses must shift from reactive treatment models to *proactive, preventive, and population-level strategies*. Key priorities include:

- *Primary prevention through lifestyle modification*:
  - Promote *balanced diets*, reduce *refined carbohydrate and sugar intake*, and increase *dietary fiber and protein*, particularly in carbohydrate-dominant diets common in South Asia.
  - Expand *community-level physical activity programs*, build walkable cities, and promote active transport to combat sedentarism.
- *Maternal and child health interventions*:
  - Address early-life risk through improved *maternal nutrition*, with a focus on *adequate vitamin B12 and folate intake.*
  - Tackle *intrauterine programming* effects that predispose children to insulin resistance and metabolic disorders later in life.
- *Localized, data-driven planning*:
  - In countries such as India, implement *state-level diabetes surveillance systems* to monitor risk factors, detect early cases, and identify high-burden zones.
  - Tailor interventions to local contexts, considering *urban-rural differentials, socioeconomic gradients, and cultural diversity.*
- *Policy integration and intersectoral collaboration*:
  - Embed diabetes prevention into broader *NCD* control frameworks, urban planning, education, agriculture, and environmental policy.
  - Ensure *universal access to affordable diagnostics, medications, and follow-up care*, particularly in rural and underserved areas.

The future trajectory of diabetes is not inevitable. With *evidence-informed, equity-focused, and scalable public health strategies*, the rising curve of the global diabetes epidemic can be flattened—protecting health systems, economies, and generations to come.

CONCLUSION

The global diabetes landscape in *2025* presents a critical inflection point for public health. The relentless rise in diabetes prevalence—fueled by demographic expansion, sedentary lifestyles, unhealthy diets, environmental exposures, and widening health inequities—reflects the cumulative impact of global transitions. While scientific understanding of the disease and its risk factors has advanced significantly, this knowledge has yet to translate into sufficient population-level control or prevention.

The forecasted *doubling of diabetes cases by 2050*, with nearly half of all countries projected to experience prevalence rates above 10%, highlights the inadequacy of current approaches. Urgent, coordinated efforts are required to shift from a reactive to a preventive paradigm. This includes scaling up *primary prevention strategies*, strengthening *health system capacity*, ensuring *universal access to affordable care*, and embedding *diabetes control into broader policy and development agendas*.

India exemplifies both the *urgency and complexity* of the diabetes crisis. As home to over 100 million people with diabetes, the country illustrates how *genetic predisposition, early onset, and diabetes at lower BMI*—hallmarks of the *South Asian phenotype*—interact with rapid urbanization and socioeconomic transitions. India's landscape is further complicated by *pronounced interstate disparities*, with southern and urban regions bearing a disproportionate burden, and many rural areas now catching up.

At the same time, India also offers a unique opportunity to lead in diabetes innovation—through *large-scale surveillance, community-based interventions, digital health tools, and intersectoral collaboration*. Lessons learned from India can inform strategies in other *low- and middle-income countries* navigating similar epidemiological transitions.

Ultimately, addressing diabetes in 2025 and beyond requires recognizing it not merely as a medical condition but as a *multidimensional societal challenge*. The path forward lies in building resilient health systems, designing inclusive policies, and empowering populations with the tools to lead healthier lives.

REFERENCES

1. International Diabetes Federation (IDF). IDF Diabetes Atlas, 11th edition. Brussels, Belgium: International Diabetes Federation; 2025. [online] Available from http://www. diabetesatlas.org. [Last accessed September, 2025].
2. GBD 2021 Diabetes Collaborators. Global, regional, and national burden of diabetes from 1990 to 2021, with projections of prevalence to 2050: a systematic analysis for the Global Burden of Disease Study 2021. Lancet. 2023;402:203-34.
3. Misra A, Sattar N, Ghosh A, Nassar M, Jayawardena R, Gupta R, et al. Type 2 diabetes in South Asians. BMJ. 2025;390:e079801.
4. Anjana RM, Unnikrishnan R, Deepa M, Pradeepa R, Tandon N, Das AK, et al.; ICMR-INDIAB Collaborative Study Group. Metabolic non-communicable disease health report of India: the ICMR-INDIAB national cross-sectional study (ICMR-INDIAB-17). Lancet Diabetes Endocrinol. 2023;11(7):474-89.
5. Mohan V, Anjana RM, Tandon N. Lessons learnt from the ICMR–INDIAB study. Natl Med J India. 2023;36: 137-9.
6. Mohan V. Lessons Learned From Epidemiology of Type 2 Diabetes in South Asians: Kelly West Award Lecture 2024. Diabetes Care. 2025;48(2):153-63.
7. Alderete TL, Chen Z, Toledo-Corral CM, Contreras ZA, Kim JS, Habre R, et al. Ambient and Traffic-Related Air Pollution Exposures as Novel Risk Factors for Metabolic Dysfunction and Type 2 Diabetes. Curr Epidemiol Rep. 2018;5(2):79-91.
8. Venkatesh U, Sharma A, Ananthan VA, Subbiah P, Durga R; CSIR Summer Research training team. Micronutrient's deficiency in India: a systematic review and meta-analysis. J Nutr Sci. 2021;10:e110.

2

Genetics and Epigenetics of Diabetes: Emerging Insights

Praveen Gangadhara, Shambo Samrat Samajdar

ABSTRACT

Type 2 diabetes mellitus (T2DM) represents a complex metabolic disorder influenced by both genetic and epigenetic mechanisms. Advances in genome-wide association studies (GWAS) have identified numerous susceptibility loci across diverse populations, highlighting the heterogeneity of diabetes risk. Epigenetic modifications—such as DNA methylation, histone acetylation, and microRNA regulation—serve as key mediators linking environmental exposures, including maternal nutrition and lifestyle factors, to altered gene expression and disease susceptibility. These insights enhance our understanding of how transgenerational and environmental factors shape metabolic phenotypes. Furthermore, pharmacogenomic research underscores the variability in antidiabetic drug responses driven by genetic polymorphisms, supporting the integration of genomic and epigenetic data in personalized diabetes management. Together, these emerging findings provide a foundation for predictive diagnostics, preventive strategies, and individualized therapeutic approaches in T2DM.

Keywords: Type 2 diabetes mellitus (T2DM), Epigenetic regulation, Genome-wide association studies (GWAS), Pharmacogenomics, Personalized medicine.

INTRODUCTION

Type 2 diabetes mellitus (T2DM), the most common form of diabetes, shows a rising incidence and widespread global prevalence, with numerous gene variants linked to glucose homeostasis, its complex pathogenesis, and associated complications.[1]

Epigenetics encompasses heritable modifications in gene expression that occur without alterations to the underlying DNA sequence. Over the past several decades, advancements in understanding the epigenetics of T2DM have elucidated previously unrecognized pathogenic mechanisms contributing to the disease's etiology. Concurrently, epigenetic research has provided insights into the influence of environmental factors, such as diet and physical activity, on T2DM pathogenesis. Furthermore, epigenetic modifications hold promise as biomarkers for assessing T2DM onset risk and predicting vascular complications.[2,3]

Genome-wide association studies (GWAS) have identified numerous gene variants associated with diabetes across various Indian subethnic populations, with population-specific risk alleles notably contributing to increased diabetes prevalence in South Asians.[4] The involvement of diverse gene loci in critical diabetic phenotypes, specifically insulin secretion, insulin resistance, obesity-associated diabetes, β-cell function, and complications underscores the potential of genomic data. These genomic insights are pivotal for developing proactive disease prevention strategies and implementation of personalized diabetic therapeutic regimens to attain optimal glycemic control, which is essential for preventing or delaying the diabetic complications[5] **(Flowchart 1)**.

EPIGENETICS AND TYPE 2 DIABETES MELLITUS

The role of epigenetics in the development of T2DM is highlighted by studies demonstrating a higher incidence of adult-onset diabetes in individuals whose mothers experienced either suboptimal nutrition or gestational diabetes during pregnancy. It is crucial to recognize that both maternal malnutrition and gestational diabetes independently elevate the offspring's risk of developing T2DM in later life.[6]

The "thrifty phenotype" hypothesis posits that an undernutritional intrauterine environment, particularly during early gestation, may induce epigenetic programming of fetal metabolic pathways. This is hypothesized to be an adaptive response, preparing the fetus for a potentially adverse nutritional environment in later life. However, when these individuals are subsequently exposed to abundant postnatal nutrition, this developmental programming can paradoxically increase their susceptibility to T2DM, obesity, and metabolic syndrome.[7] Yajnik et al. observed that specific maternal nutritional factors, including normal to high folate levels combined with vitamin B12 deficiency, were associated with increased adiposity and insulin resistance in Indian infants. This predisposition is hypothesized to be mediated by fetal epigenetic changes.[8]

The complex interactions of epigenetics in the evolution and progression of T2DM are summarized in **Figure 1**.

EPIGENETIC MODIFICATIONS IN TYPE 2 DIABETES PATHOGENESIS

Insulin resistance and impaired insulin secretion are two primary components in the pathogenesis of T2DM. Studies have demonstrated altered DNA methylation of genes, including *PPARG*, *KCNQ1*, *TCF7L2*, and insulin receptor substrate 1 (IRS1). These genes are implicated in insulin action within key metabolic tissues such as the liver, skeletal muscle, and adipose tissue. In

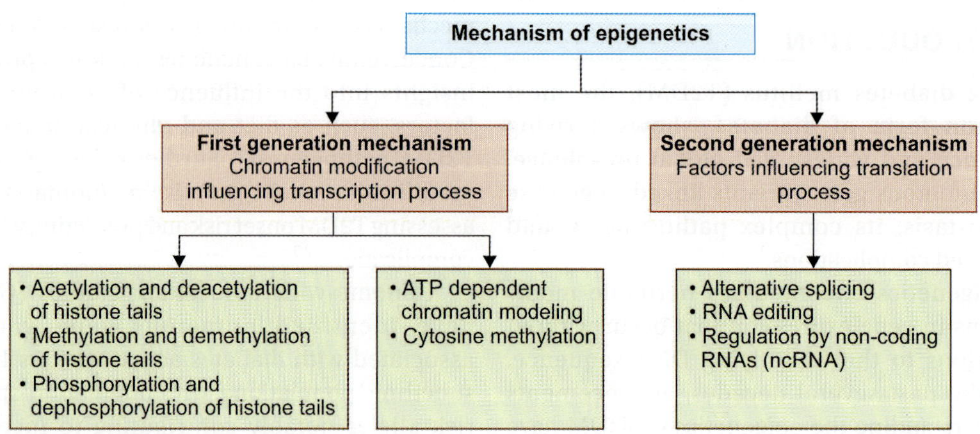

Flowchart 1: Mechanism of epigenetic changes.

Source: Adapted from Mannar V, Boro H, Patel D, Agstam S, Dalvi M, Bundela V. Epigenetics of the Pathogenesis and Complications of Type 2 Diabetes Mellitus. touchREV Endocrinol. 2023;19(1):46-53.

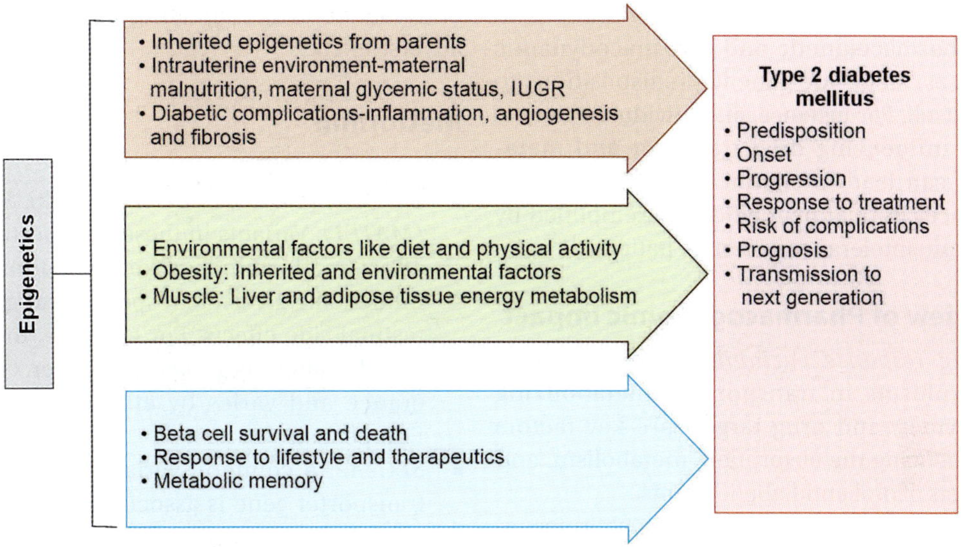

Fig. 1: Epigenetics and type 2 diabetes – complex interactions at various levels.

Source: Adapted from Mannar V, Boro H, Patel D, Agstam S, Dalvi M, Bundela V. Epigenetics of the Pathogenesis and Complications of Type 2 Diabetes Mellitus. touchREV Endocrinol. 2023;19(1):46-53.

individuals with T2DM, pancreatic islets exhibit decreased expression of genes critical for insulin secretion, including *PPARGC1A, INS*, and *PDX1*. This reduction in gene expression is attributed to increased methylation within these genetic loci.[9] The acetylation of the Forkhead box protein O1 *(FOXO1)* gene, a known regulator of pancreatic and duodenal homeobox 1 (PDX1), has significant implications for β-cell development and the maintenance of glucose homeostasis.[10] MiRNAs have been identified as significant regulators in both β-cell dysfunction and β-cell survival, processes that are pivotal in the pathogenesis of T2DM. They also contribute to the pathogenesis of insulin resistance by their action on the phosphoinositol-3 kinase (PI3K)/AKT and other insulin signaling pathways.[11,12]

ROLE OF PHARMACOGENOMICS AND DIABETES

Pharmacogenomics provides a framework for anticipating how an individual's genetic makeup influences their response to specific pharmacologic agents. This approach is central to realizing personalized medicine, as it enables the optimization of drug therapy by tailoring medications to achieve better efficacy and reduced risk.[13]

In the context of T2DM treatment, understanding the influence of genetic variation on drug response is paramount for tailoring effective therapies. These pharmacogenetic traits directly impact both the efficacy and safety of medications, thereby guiding personalized treatment approaches. Such genetic variations can be broadly classified based on their population frequency, the number of base pairs involved, their genomic location, and the resulting effects on the encoded protein. The variations in linkage disequilibrium patterns across populations highlight the need for population-specific studies to ensure the generalizability of pharmacogenomic applications in diabetes treatment. In order to fully leverage pharmacogenomics in T2DM management, a structured evaluative framework is essential for assessing its impact on therapeutic outcomes.

This framework should delineate variations in both pharmacokinetic and pharmacodynamic responses, alongside genetic predispositions to T2DM itself. For instance, an individual's genetic profile influencing drug transport and metabolism can lead to significant interindividual differences in treatment efficacy, exemplified by metformin intolerance in certain patients.[14,15]

Overview of Pharmacogenomic Impact

- *Drug response variability*: Genetic polymorphisms in transporters, metabolizing enzymes, and drug targets are key factors influencing the absorption, metabolism, and effects of oral antidiabetic agents.
- *Clinical relevance*: Incorporating pharmacogenomic data into clinical practice can improve drug selection, dosing accuracy, and risk stratification for adverse events, enabling a transition from the "one-size-fits-all" approach to individualized therapy.
- *Preemptive genotyping*: With technological advances and falling costs, genetic screening is increasingly feasible as a routine adjunct to diabetes management.

GENETIC VARIANTS AND RESPONSES TO COMMON ANTIDIABETIC DRUGS (TABLE 1)

Several genetic variants have been identified that influence patient responses to common antidiabetic drugs, affecting both efficacy and adverse effects:

Metformin

Key genes:

- *SLC22A1 (OCT1), SLC22A2 (OCT2), SLC47A1 (MATE1)*: Variants in these transporter genes affect metformin uptake and elimination, influencing glycemic response and gastrointestinal side effects. For example, the OCT1 420 del allele is linked to higher GI intolerance and varies by ethnicity (higher in Europeans).
- *SLC2A2*: A common variant in this glucose transporter gene is associated with stronger metformin response.
- *rs111770298*: An African ancestry-specific variant linked to weaker metformin response.
- *CPA6 rs2162145*: Associated with better metformin response, with variable prevalence across populations.[16,17]

Sulfonylureas

Key genes:

- *CYP2C9*: Encodes a major metabolizing enzyme; *CYP2C92* and *2C93** variants can elevate drug levels, raising hypoglycemia risk.
- *ABCC8 (SUR1) and KCNJ11 (Kir6.2)*: Encode KATP channel subunits. Variants such as *ABCC8 Ser1369Ala* or *KCNJ11 E23K* alter drug sensitivity and efficacy.

TABLE 1: Genetic variants influencing antidiabetic drug response.[5,15]

Drug class	*Key genes/Variants*	*Clinical impact*
Metformin	SLC22A1 rs622342, SLC47A1 rs2289669	Alters efficacy, GI side effects, population-dependent
Sulfonylureas	CYP2C9*2, *3, ABCC8 Ser1369Ala, KCNJ11 E23K	Modifies efficacy, risk of hypoglycemia, dose requirements
TZDs	CYP2C8*3, PPARG Pro12Ala, SLCO1B1, ADIPOQ	Affects exposure, glycemic effect, adverse events
DPP-4/GLP-1	GLP1R rs6923761, KCNQ1, TCF7L2	Modulates response, weight change, glycemic control
SGLT-2 inhibitors	SLC5A2, WFS1, PNPLA3, UGT1A9, UGT2B4	Influences efficacy, metabolism, side effect risk

DPP-4: dipeptidyl peptidase-4; GLP-1: glucagon-like peptide-1; (SGLT-2: sodium-glucose cotransporter-2; TZDs: thiazolidinediones)

- *TCF7L2*: Associated with reduced sulfonylurea response and higher risk of treatment failure.

Clinical effects: Genetic differences can determine dose requirements and risk of adverse reactions, with *CYP2C9* loss-of-function carriers responding to lower doses

Thiazolidinediones

Key genes:

- *CYP2C8*: Affects drug metabolism (e.g., *CYP2C8*3 alters rosiglitazone exposure)
- *PPARG (Pro12Ala)*: Associated with both reduced T2DM risk and improved glycemic response
- *SLCO1B1*: Modulates hepatic drug uptake
- *ADIPOQ*: Influences treatment effects on metabolic markers

Clinical effects: Variants can affect both efficacy and adverse events such as risk for edema

DPP-4 Inhibitors and GLP-1 Receptor Agonists

Key genes:

- *GLP-1R*: Variants like *rs6923761* (Gly168Ser) influence treatment efficacy.
- *KCNQ1*: Modulates responses to incretin-based therapies.
- *TCF7L2*: Associated with variation in incretin response.

Clinical effects: Genetic polymorphisms may affect glycemic responses and weight changes, although clinical implementation is still emerging.

SGLT-2 Inhibitors

Key genes:

- *SLC5A2*: Modulates the response to drugs like empagliflozin
- *WFS1* and *PNPLA3*: Associated with weight loss and changes in hepatic fat content on SGLT-2 inhibitor therapy.
- *UGT1A9, UGT2B4*: Crucial for drug metabolism and modulate exposure to canagliflozin.

Clinical effects: Variants influence efficacy (e.g., glucose lowering, blood pressure) and are linked to differences in side effect profiles such as weight loss or hepatic outcomes.[5,15,18]

CONCLUSION

Epigenetic mechanisms contribute to the transgenerational inheritance of T2DM. Moreover, epigenetics clarifies the interplay between an individual's genome and adverse environmental factors, such as dietary habits, physical inactivity, dysregulated circadian rhythms, and maternal nutritional status (malnutrition or obesity), which collectively contribute to the development of complex disease phenotypes, including T2DM. Emerging pharmacological interventions for T2DM are targeting the reversal of epigenetic dysregulation. However, the development of novel therapies that address T2DM pathogenesis and its complications necessitates further research to precisely identify the specific epigenetic regulators involved.

The future of diabetes management is contingent upon the integration of pharmacogenetics into standard clinical practice, enabling the synergistic application of genetic data and clinical judgment to inform individualized therapeutic strategies. Despite the complex polygenic architecture of T2DM, characterized by numerous genetic variants with modest individual effects, the clinical significance of pharmacogenetic interactions warrants significant consideration.

REFERENCES

1. Ali O. Genetics of type 2 diabetes. World J Diabetes. 2013;4(4):114-23.
2. Riggs AD, Porter TN. Overview of epigenetic mechanisms. In: Russo VEA, Martienssen R, Riggs AD (Eds). Epigenetic Mechanisms of Gene Regulation. Cold Spring Harbor, NY: Cold Spring Harbor Laboratory Press; 1996. pp. 29-45.
3. Ling C, Bacos K, Rönn T. Epigenetics of type 2 diabetes mellitus and weight change – A tool for precision medicine? Nat Rev Endocrinol. 2022;18:433-48.
4. Gujral UP, Pradeepa R, Weber MB, Narayan KMV, Mohan V. Type 2 diabetes in South Asians: similarities and differences with white Caucasian and other populations. Ann NY Acad Sc. 2013;1281(1):51-63.
5. Venkatachalapathy P, Padhilahouse S, Sellappan M, Subramanian T, Kurian SJ, Miraj SS, et al. Pharmacogenomics and Personalized Medicine in Type 2 Diabetes Mellitus: Potential Implications for Clinical Practice. Pharmacogenomics Pers Med. 2021;14:1441-55.
6. Dhawan S, Natarajan R. Epigenetics and type 2 diabetes risk. Curr Diab Rep. 2019;19:47.
7. Smith CJ, Ryckman KK. Epigenetic and developmental influences on the risk of obesity, diabetes, and metabolic syndrome. Diabetes Metab Syndr Obes. 2015;8:295-302.
8. Yajnik CS, Deshpande SS, Jackson AA, Refsum H, Rao S, Fisher DJ, et al. Vitamin B12 and folate concentrations during pregnancy and insulin resistance in the offspring: The Pune Maternal Nutrition Study. Diabetologia. 2008;51:29-38.
9. Mannar V, Boro H, Patel D, Agstam S, Dalvi M, Bundela V. Epigenetics of the Pathogenesis and Complications of Type 2 Diabetes Mellitus. touchREV Endocrinol. 2023;19(1):46-53.
10. Nakae J, Biggs WH 3rd, Kitamura T, Cavenee WK, Wright CV, Arden KC, et al. Regulation of insulin action and pancreatic beta-cell function by mutated alleles of the gene encoding forkhead transcription factor Foxo1. Nat Genet. 2002;32(2):245-53.
11. Ofori JK, Karagiannopoulos A, Nagao M, Westholm E, Ramadan S, Wendt A, et al. Human Islet MicroRNA-200c Is Elevated in Type 2 Diabetes and Targets the Transcription Factor ETV5 to Reduce Insulin Secretion. Diabetes. 2022;71(2):275-84.
12. Zhong FY, Li J, Wang YM, Chen Y, Song J, Yang Z, et al. MicroRNA-506 modulates insulin resistance in human adipocytes by targeting S6K1 and altering the IRS1/PI3K/AKT insulin signaling pathway. J Bioenerg Biomembr. 2021;53(6):679-92.
13. Roden DM, Van Driest SL. Pharmacogenetics and Pharmacogenomics. In: Brunton LL, Knollmann BC (Eds). Goodman & Gilman's: The Pharmacological Basis of Therapeutics, 14th edition. New York: McGraw-Hill Education; 2023.
14. Pearson ER. Diabetes: Is There a Future for Pharmacogenomics Guided Treatment? Clin Pharmacol Ther. 2019;106(2):329-37.
15. Samajdar SS, Maheshwari A, Tiwari A, Mukherjee S, Biswas K, Saboo B, et al., Decoding the Genetic Blueprint: Advancing Personalized Medicine in Type 2 Diabetes through Pharmacogenomics. Clin Diabetol. 2024;13(6):386-96.
16. Baye AM, Fanta TG, Siddiqui MK, Dawed AY. The Genetics of Adverse Drug Outcomes in Type 2 Diabetes: A Systematic Review. Front Genet. 2021;12:675053.
17. Srinivasan S, Yee SW, Giacomini KM. Pharmacogenetics of Antidiabetic Drugs. Adv Pharmacol. 2018;83:361-89.
18. Becker ML, Pearson ER, Tkáč I. Pharmacogenetics of Oral Antidiabetic Drugs. Int J Endocrinol. 2013;2013:686315.

3

Immunotherapy in Type 1 Diabetes: Toward Disease Modification

Banshi Saboo, Rutul Gokalani

ABSTRACT

Type 1 diabetes (T1D) is caused by the body's immune system attacking its own insulin producing cells. For years, treatment has focused only on managing blood sugar with insulin but now, a new approach is emerging with various studies and interventions. This chapter explores how immunotherapy is changing the way we think about T1D. Instead of just treating symptoms, these therapies aim to slow or even stop the disease before it fully develops. With the recent approval of teplizumab, doctors can now delay the onset of T1D in people at high risk. The chapter also looks at new and upcoming treatments, the importance of early detection, and how future care might be personalized based on a person's unique immune profile. Together, these developments offer real hope for changing the course of T1D.

Keywords: Type 1 diabetes, Immunotherapy, Disease modifiying therapy, β-cell preservation, Preclinical T1D staging, Stem cell therapy in T1D, Clinical trials in T1D.

INTRODUCTION

Type 1 diabetes (T1D) is an autoimmune disorder characterized by the selective destruction of insulin-producing pancreatic β-cells by autoreactive immune cells, predominantly T lymphocytes. Insulin deficiency results in chronic hyperglycemia, necessitating lifelong reliance on exogenous insulin and increasing the risk of complications. Although insulin therapy and glucose monitoring have progressed, these interventions fail to target the fundamental issue of autoimmunity. Disease modification in T1D involves therapeutic interventions aimed at altering the disease trajectory by preserving endogenous β-cell function or preventing or delaying disease onset, rather than merely managing glycemia. Immunotherapies have significantly improved outcomes in various autoimmune diseases, such as rheumatoid arthritis and multiple sclerosis, by specifically targeting pathogenic immune pathways. A comparable paradigm shift is occurring in T1D: Following extensive research, the initial immunotherapy teplizumab has recently received approval to postpone the onset of clinical T1D.[1] This chapter examines the rationale and evidence supporting immunotherapy in T1D, outlines current and emerging strategies for modifying disease progression, and discusses practical considerations for clinicians.

The early identification of at-risk individuals is now achievable via autoantibody screening and staging of T1D. TrialNet and similar initiatives have screened numerous relatives of individuals with T1D, facilitating the identification of presymptomatic T1D (*Stage 1*: Normoglycemia with ≥ 2 autoantibodies) and dysglycemic Stage 2 T1D prior to the manifestation of symptomatic disease. The significance of this is considerable: by the time of clinical diagnosis (Stage 3), patients typically have already lost approximately 70–90% of their β-cell mass.[2,3] Early intervention in the autoimmune process provides an opportunity to maintain residual β-cells. Postdiagnosis, the maintenance of endogenous insulin production, indicated by C-peptide levels, correlates with improved glycemic control, reduced insulin requirements, and a decrease in complications. Immunotherapeutic strategies in T1D aim to induce immune tolerance or modulate the immune response to prevent β-cell destruction, thereby prolonging the "honeymoon" phase or potentially preventing the disease in individuals at high risk. This chapter examines the mechanistic basis of these therapies, highlights key clinical trials and their outcomes, addresses current challenges, and explores future directions, including considerations beyond immunotherapy in the pursuit of a potential cure.

PATHOGENESIS OF TYPE 1 DIABETES AND RATIONALE FOR IMMUNOTHERAPY

T1D arises from a complex interplay between genetic predisposition, particularly involving human leukocyte antigen (HLA)-DR and DQ alleles, and environmental factors. The disease advances in stages: Autoimmunity without symptoms (Stage 1), dysglycemia with maintained β-cell function (Stage 2), and overt hyperglycemia (Stage 3). The autoimmune response comprises autoreactive T cells, B cells, and proinflammatory cytokines that target β-cell autoantigens such as insulin, GAD665, and IA-2 **(Fig. 1)**[4].

Maintaining residual β-cell function, even to a limited extent, can enhance glycemic control, decrease insulin needs, and mitigate the risk of complications. Immunotherapy aims to impede disease progression, extend the honeymoon phase, or potentially avert T1D in individuals at high risk.

TIMING AND TARGET POPULATION FOR IMMUNOTHERAPY IN TYPE 1 DIABETES

The timing of immunotherapy in T1D is crucial; earlier intervention, when adequate β-cell mass is preserved, has a higher likelihood of success. Two primary target populations have been identified:

1. *Individuals in the presymptomatic phase (Stages 1 and 2)*: These individuals possess two or more islet autoantibodies, regardless of the presence of dysglycemia. Their risk of progressing to clinical diabetes approaches 100%. Teplizumab has received the Food and Drug Administration (FDA) approval for delaying disease progression in individuals with Stage 2, showing efficacy in this population.[1] Current prevention trials encompass oral insulin, abatacept, hydroxychloroquine, and intranasal insulin.[5] Current strategies primarily target relatives of T1D patients; however, future methodologies may encompass wider screening in childhood or infancy to identify potential candidates at an earlier stage.
2. *New-onset T1D (within 100 days to 6 months)*: Most immunotherapy trials focus on this cohort, which generally maintains partial β-cell function. Agents such as teplizumab, rituximab, abatacept, and alefacept[6] demonstrate preservation of C-peptide levels when administered at an early stage. Immunotherapy during this period may extend the honeymoon phase and enhance glycemic control.

Age and immune profile are significant factors: Children frequently exhibit higher levels of aggressive autoimmunity compared to adolescents or adults. Responses differ according to age, HLA genotype, and immune markers. This endorses a tailored strategy—e.g., anti-CD3

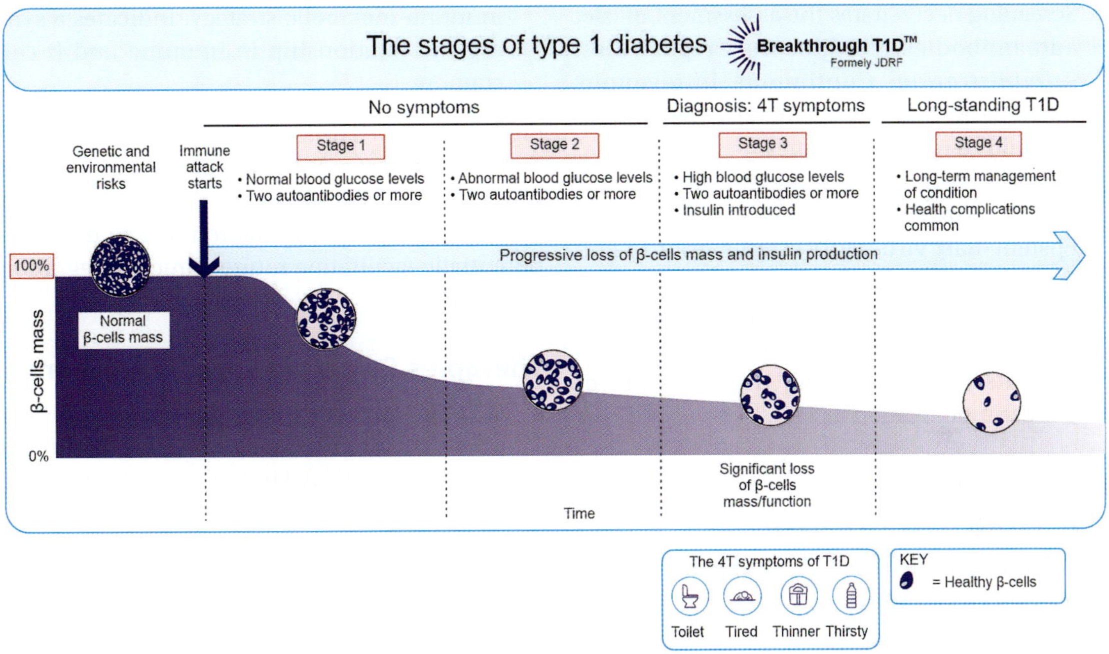

Fig. 1: Stages of type 1 diabetes (T1D) development: Timeline showing stages of development T1D. It shows how β-cells in normal level and how the triggering events such as genetic and environmental factors triggers the body's own immune system to attack the β-cells. The progression involves immune-mediated β-cell destruction, starting with normal glucose levels (Stage 1), evolving through dysglycemia without symptoms (Stage 2), to symptomatic diabetes (Stage 3, characterized by the "4Ts": Toilet, Tired, Thinner, Thirsty, and finally long-term management with increased risk of complications (Stage 4).

Source: Breakthrough T1D. The stages of type 1 diabetes. [Online] Available from https://www.breakthrought1d.org [Last accessed October, 2025].

for elevated CD8 activation, rituximab for B-cell predominance, and GAD vaccine for specific HLA types.[4]

Retreatment potential: While the majority of studies focus on single courses, continuous or repeated dosing (such as annual teplizumab) may provide enduring advantages. In established T1D with complete loss of β-cell function, the efficacy of immunotherapy is restricted unless it is integrated with regenerative approaches.

APPROVED IMMUNOTHERAPY: TEPLIZUMAB

Teplizumab, an anti-CD3 monoclonal antibody, represents the first and only FDA-approved immunotherapy for T1D as of 2024. Delaying the onset of Stage 3 diabetes is recommended for at-risk individuals in Stage 2, specifically those exhibiting two or more islet autoantibodies and abnormal glucose tolerance.[1]

The TrialNet study demonstrated that a 14-day regimen of teplizumab extended the median duration to clinical T1D by roughly 2 years.[1,2] The mechanism entails the modulation of autoreactive T cells and the enhancement of regulatory T-cell function. Adverse effects encompass rash, transient lymphopenia, and mild symptoms associated with cytokine release.

Clinical Implications

- *Patient selection*: Suitable candidates include individuals aged 8 years and older with a confirmed diagnosis of Stage 2 T1D.

- Screening necessitates the assessment of islet autoantibodies and glucose irregularities. *Administration*: Continuous intravenous infusion over 14 days; generally provided in specialized medical facilities.
- Monitoring includes complete blood count (CBC), liver function tests (LFTs), and Epstein–Barr virus (EBV) status prior to and throughout the treatment process.
- Teplizumab signifies a notable advancement by offering a preventive alternative for specific patients and confirming the principle of disease modification in T1D.[1,2]

ADDITIONAL IMMUNOTHERAPEUTIC AGENTS CURRENTLY UNDER INVESTIGATION

Monoclonal Antibodies

- Rituximab (anti-CD20), a β-cell depleting therapy, demonstrated a temporary preservation of C-peptide levels in individuals with new-onset T1D; however, it has not received approval due to its limited long-term efficacy.[7]
- Abatacept (CTLA-4-Ig) inhibits T-cell costimulation. In new-onset T1D, treatment initially delayed β-cell decline; however, the effect diminished after therapy concluded.[8]
- Golimumab (anti-TNF-α) demonstrated preservation of C-peptide levels and enhancement of remission rates in pediatric patients with newly diagnosed T1D, as evidenced by the T1GER study (Additional research may facilitate its approval).
- Ustekinumab, an anti-IL-12/23 agent, demonstrated potential for β-cell preservation in adolescents by targeting Th1/Th17 pathways. Prospective candidate for future application.[9]
- Anti-IL-21 in conjunction with liraglutide demonstrated enhanced preservation of C-peptide through a combined immune-metabolic strategy. Indicates a synergistic relationship in immune and β-cell support.

Significance in clinical practice: Although not currently approved, these agents demonstrate potential in recent-onset T1D. Several are already utilized in other autoimmune diseases, potentially facilitating future clinical integration upon approval.

Therapies Targeting Specific Antigens

- *GAD65 vaccine*: Demonstrated modest preservation of C-peptide in individuals positive for HLA-DR3. The DIAGNODE-3 trial is currently in progress, utilizing intralymphatic administration.[4]
- Oral and nasal insulin administration is intended to induce tolerance, yielding mixed outcomes. Several benefits of the subgroup have been identified.
- *Clinical relevance*: Demonstrates safety, though efficacy is limited. May play a role in the early or presymptomatic stages of T1D in the future.

Cellular Therapies

Infusion of autologous regulatory T cells Tregs in new-onset T1D has demonstrated safety and potential therapeutic benefits. The combination with rituximab demonstrated enhanced preservation of C-peptide levels.[10]

Mesenchymal stem cells (MSCs) have the potential to offer immunomodulatory effects and support for β-cells. Clinical outcomes exhibit variability.

Clinical relevance is both promising and complex. Currently, most appropriate for research environments.

Combination Therapies and Innovative Methodologies

The multifactorial nature of T1D suggests that the combination of agents may improve outcomes.

- Rituximab combined with abatacept (RELAY trial)
- Anti-IL-21 in conjunction with GLP-1 agonists[7,8,11]
- ATG combined with G-CSF[12]

BCG vaccination and low-dose IL-2 therapy[13] seek to modulate the immune system through innate or regulatory pathways, respectively. These innovative strategies are currently undergoing trials and may ultimately enhance conventional methods.

TYPE 1 DIABETES STAGES AND IMMUNOTHERAPY: KEY SUMMARY (TABLE 1)

This summary table provides a structured, stage-wise view of immunotherapy options in T1D, categorized by drug class and approval status. It is intended for clinical reference.

Key points:

- *Teplizumab* is currently the only FDA-approved immunotherapy in T1D, approved to delay progression from Stage 2 to 3.[1]
- Most therapies remain investigational and target early disease stages to preserve β-cell function.
- Antigen-specific and cell-based therapies are promising but need more efficacy data.
- Combination strategies (e.g., immune + metabolic) may offer future benefits.

This concise table should support clinicians and researchers in understanding how and when each immunotherapy might be applied in the T1D disease course.

CURRENT REGULATORY LANDSCAPE

- *Teplizumab*: FDA-approved in 2022 for delaying T1D in at-risk individuals. Not yet approved in Europe.[1]
- *Other agents*: Currently investigational. Golimumab, ustekinumab, and abatacept are among those closest to approval,[7,11,9] and other novel agents such as the tyrosine kinase inhibitor imatinib have shown beta-cell preservation in phase 2 trials.[14]

TABLE 1: Stage-wise view of immunotherapy options in type 1 diabetes (T1D), categorized by drug class and approval status.

Stage of T1D	***Clinical description***	***Approved therapy***	***Investigational therapies (with phase)***
Stage 1	Autoantibodies present, normal glucose, asymptomatic	None	Oral insulin (phase 3—no benefit shown)
Stage 2	Autoantibodies + dysglycemia, still asymptomatic	Teplizumab (anti-CD3)—FDA-approved	Low-dose ATG (phase 2) treg therapy (Phase 1–2)
Stage 3	Symptomatic hyperglycemia, insulin required	Teplizumab—being evaluated	• Rituximab (anti-CD20, phase 2) • Abatacept (CTLA4-Ig, phase 2) • Golimumab (anti-TNF, phase 2) • Baricitinib (JAK inhibitor, phase 2)[15]
Antigen-specific	Targeted tolerance to islet antigens	None approved	GAD vaccine/DIAMYD (phase 3 in HLA DR3-DQ2) proinsulin peptide (IMCY-0098, phase 2)
Cell-based therapies	Tolerance restoration or immune reset	None approved	Treg therapy (polyclonal/antigen-specific, phase 1–2) HSCT (experimental—limited use)

(ATG: anti-thymocyte globulin; FDA: Food and Drug Administration; GAD: glutamic acid decarboxylase; HSCT: hematopoietic stem cell transplantation; JAK: janus kinase; TNF: tumor necrosis factor) to restoring endogenous insulin production, moving closer to a true biological cure for diabetes.[4]

Islet Cell Transplantation

Islet cell transplantation involves isolating pancreatic islets, which contain insulin-producing beta cells, from a deceased human donor and infusing them into the portal vein of a recipient with T1D. The goal of this procedure is to restore the body's ability to produce insulin and achieve better glycemic control, often leading to a reduction in or even independence from exogenous insulin injections. The isolation process involves using special enzymes to separate the islets from the exocrine tissue of the donor pancreas, followed by purification and counting of the viable islets. Typically, multiple infusions of islets from one or more donors are required to achieve adequate beta-cell mass and sustained insulin production in the recipient. Once infused into the liver, these transplanted islets are expected to engraft and begin secreting insulin, with new blood vessels forming around them over several weeks.[5]

Despite its potential, islet cell transplantation faces several significant challenges that limit its widespread application. A primary hurdle is the severe shortage of donor pancreases, as each transplant often requires islets from multiple donors, making it an unsustainable solution for the vast number of people with diabetes. Furthermore, the procedure carries risks such as bleeding, blood clots, and portal hypertension.[6] Some recipients must undergo lifelong immunosuppressive therapy to prevent immune rejection of the transplanted islets. These powerful antirejection drugs come with considerable side effects, including increased susceptibility to infections, renal failure, and an elevated risk of certain cancers. Furthermore, a significant percentage of transplanted islets can be lost immediately post transplantation due to acute immune-mediated inflammatory reaction and lack of immediate revascularization, impacting long-term graft function and insulin independence rates.[7]

Beta Cells Derived from Stem Cells

The development of insulin-producing beta cells from pluripotent stem cells (PSCs), including embryonic stem cells (ESCs) and induced pluripotent stem cells (iPSCs), represents a groundbreaking advance in diabetes research.[8] This approach offers a potentially limitless and renewable source of beta cells, overcoming the critical scarcity of cadaveric donor pancreases that limits traditional islet transplantation. The process involves guiding PSCs through multiple stages, mimicking embryonic pancreatic development in vitro. Through certain growth factors, signaling molecules, and extracellular matrix components, scientists can direct these pluripotent cells to differentiate into definitive endoderm, primitive gut tube, posterior foregut, pancreatic progenitors, and finally, functional pancreatic beta-like cells. These laboratory-grown cells have demonstrated the ability to secrete insulin in response to glucose stimulation and reverse diabetes in preclinical animal models.[9]

One major hurdle is achieving full functional maturation of these in vitro-derived cells as they often exhibit an immature phenotype compared to native human beta cells, leading to suboptimal glucose-stimulated insulin secretion. Another critical concern is the potential for teratoma formation if undifferentiated stem cells are inadvertently transplanted. For allogeneic stem cell-derived beta cells, immune rejection remains a challenge, which requires strategies such as immune-evasive cell lines or advanced encapsulation technologies to protect the cells from the host's immune system, similar to issues encountered in traditional islet transplantation.[10]

Beta Cells Encapsulated in Semipermeable Membranes

A promising strategy to overcome the challenges of immune rejection and the need for lifelong immunosuppression in islet or stem cell-derived beta-cell transplantation is the encapsulation of these cells within semipermeable membranes. These encapsulation devices, often made from biocompatible polymers such as alginate, create a physical barrier that allows for the free diffusion of essential nutrients (such as glucose and oxygen), waste products, and secreted insulin while preventing the entry of larger immune cells, antibodies, and inflammatory molecules that would otherwise attack and destroy the transplanted cells. This process is known as immunoisolation which preserves function and minimizes the role of an immunosupressant.[11]

Various encapsulation approaches exist, categorized by their size and configuration, including microcapsules and macroencapsulation devices. Microcapsules, typically made of alginate-based hydrogels, enclose individual islets or small cell clusters in tiny spheres. It has a high surface-area-to-volume ratio for efficient diffusion. Macroencapsulation devices, on the other hand, are larger, often flat or cylindrical chambers designed to contain a larger mass of cells, with the advantage of being easily retrievable if complications arise.[12] A notable example of macroencapsulation technology is ViaCyte's PEC-Encap (also known as VC-01), which involves the encapsulation of hPSC-derived pancreatic progenitor cells (PEC-01) cells within a semipermeable membrane called the Encaptra® drug delivery system. This system is designed to allow the progenitor cells to mature into functional insulin-producing cells post implantation while shielding them from the host's immune system.[13]

Despite significant advancements, challenges remain in achieving long-term success with encapsulated beta cells. Issues include ensuring optimal oxygen and nutrient supply to the encapsulated cells, preventing pericapsular fibrotic overgrowth (a foreign body response that can encapsulate the device and impair diffusion), and maintaining the long-term integrity and permeability of the membranes.[12]

Replication of Beta Cells

The inherent capacity of pancreatic beta cells to replicate is a crucial aspect of maintaining adequate beta-cell mass throughout life. The goal is to stimulate the proliferation of existing beta cells in diabetic individuals, thereby increasing their functional beta-cell mass and improving endogenous insulin production. This approach would bypass the complexities of transplantation, such as the need for immunosuppression or donor cell sourcing. Research in this area focuses on identifying and utilizing specific growth factors and small molecules that can safely and effectively promote beta-cell division.

One prominent example of a growth factor with beta-cell proliferative effects is glucagon-like peptide-1 (GLP-1) and its analogs, which are already approved drugs for T2D. GLP-1 receptor agonists not only enhance glucose-dependent insulin secretion but have also been shown to promote beta-cell proliferation and reduce apoptosis in preclinical models. Their ability to improve beta-cell function makes them attractive candidates for regenerative strategies.[14] Another exciting discovery is harmine, a natural product that has been identified as a potent inducer of human beta-cell proliferation.[15] Harmine acts by inhibiting the dual-specificity tyrosine-phosphorylation-regulated kinase 1A (DYRK1A), a negative regulator of beta-cell proliferation.[16]

Challenges in beta-cell replication strategies include achieving sustained proliferation without adverse effects, ensuring that newly generated beta cells are fully functional and mature, and preventing uncontrolled cell growth. The precise mechanisms governing beta-cell proliferation in adults are still being studied, and identifying compounds that can selectively target beta cells for replication without affecting other cell types is critical for safety. Ongoing research aims to develop more potent and specific proliferative agents, understand the long-term effects of stimulating beta-cell growth, and translate these discoveries into safe and effective therapies that can restore normal beta-cell mass in people with diabetes. Plant-based phytochemicals have shown promising potential in promoting pancreatic beta-cell regeneration, a key therapeutic goal in diabetes management. These naturally occurring compounds—such as flavonoids, polyphenols, and alkaloids—exert antioxidant, anti-inflammatory, and antiapoptotic effects, which protect beta cells from damage and may stimulate their proliferation.[17]

Use of Reprogramming Pancreatic Cells

Beyond stimulating existing beta cells, another regenerative strategy involves the in vivo reprogramming of other pancreatic cell types into insulin-producing beta cells. The pancreas contains a variety of cell types, such as glucagon-secreting alpha cells and ductal cells, which share a common developmental lineage with beta cells. Scientists have demonstrated that by introducing specific transcription factors, these non-beta cells can be coaxed to transdifferentiate into functional beta cells. A key transcription factor in this process is Pancreatic and Duodenal Homeobox 1 (PDX1), which is crucial for pancreatic development and beta-cell maturation. PDX1 can be delivered through a viral vector, often in combination with other factors such as MafA and Ngn3.[18] Researchers have successfully converted alpha and ductal cells into insulin-producing cells in rodent models, offering an internal source for beta-cell replenishment directly within the patient's own pancreas.

The search of natural compounds, or phytochemicals, for their beta-cell proliferative properties is also gaining attraction. These compounds, derived from plants, offer a potentially safer and more accessible way for therapeutic development. Various phytochemicals have been investigated for their ability to enhance beta-cell mass and function, often through anti-inflammatory, antioxidant, or direct proliferative mechanisms. For instance, some flavonoids and polyphenols found in fruits, vegetables, and traditional medicines have shown promising effects on beta-cell survival and replication in preclinical studies.

Gene Therapy and CRISPR-based Beta-cell Replacement

Gene therapy offers a revolutionary approach to beta-cell replacement and regeneration by directly modifying genetic material to restore or enhance beta-cell function. This involves introducing new genes into cells, altering existing genes, or correcting genetic mutations that contribute to diabetes. For example, gene therapy can be used to deliver genes encoding for insulin or key transcription factors (such as PDX1, MafA, or Pax6) into pancreatic cells or other cell types, aiming to reprogram them into functional insulin-producing beta cells. Viral vectors, such as adeno-associated viruses (AAVs) or lentiviruses, are commonly used as delivery vehicles to efficiently transport these therapeutic genes into target cells. The potential benefit lies in achieving long-term, sustained insulin production without the need for repeated cell infusions or systemic immunosuppression.[18]

The advent of CRISPR-Cas9 and other gene-editing technologies has significantly advanced the precision and efficiency of genetic modifications in beta cells. CRISPR-Cas9 acts as a molecular scissor, which helps make targeted edits to the DNA sequence. This technology holds the promise of correcting specific genetic defects that cause monogenic forms of diabetes, such as maturity-onset diabetes of the young (MODY). Beyond correction, CRISPR can also be employed to enhance beta-cell survival by introducing genes that confer resistance to autoimmune attack or oxidative stress or by knocking out genes that inhibit beta-cell proliferation. For instance, researchers have successfully used CRISPR to correct a diabetes-causing genetic defect in patient-derived stem cells, which were then differentiated into functional beta cells and shown to reverse diabetes in mouse models.[19]

Despite the exciting potential, gene therapy and CRISPR-based approaches face several challenges. A key challenge is the safe and efficient delivery of genetic material to the desired target cells in vivo. Ensuring precise gene editing without unintended consequences (off-target edits) is paramount for safety. Furthermore, achieving long-term gene expression without adverse effects, such as uncontrolled cell growth or tumorigenesis, remains an area of research. Overcoming these technical and safety challenges through continued research and rigorous clinical trials will be essential for translating the promise of gene therapy and CRISPR into widely available and effective treatments for diabetes.

Autoimmunity Development/ Immunotherapies

The autoimmune destruction of beta cells is the primary cause of T1D, making the prevention or reversal of this autoimmune response a crucial aspect of developing a cure. Understanding the complex interplay of genetic predisposition and environmental triggers that lead to autoimmunity is fundamental to designing effective immunotherapies. In T1D, the immune system mistakenly identifies beta cells as foreign and launches an attack, leading to their progressive destruction. This process involves various immune cells, including T lymphocytes and B lymphocytes, and the production of autoantibodies. Therefore, immunotherapeutic strategies aim to modulate the immune system to protect existing beta cells or ensure the long-term survival of transplanted or regenerated beta cells.[20]

Immunotherapies for T1D can be broadly categorized into antigen-specific and antigen-nonspecific approaches. Antigen-nonspecific immunotherapies involve general suppression of the immune system, such as the lifelong immunosuppression required for conventional islet transplantation. While effective in preventing graft rejection, the associated side effects, including increased risk of infections, malignancies, and nephrotoxicity, significantly limit their clinical utility and the quality of life for patients. This high cost in terms of patient burden and financial expense underscores the need for more targeted and safer alternatives. Antigen-specific immunotherapies, on the other hand, aim to selectively target the immune cells or pathways involved in beta-cell destruction, leaving the rest of the immune system intact. Examples include therapies that block specific costimulation pathways essential for T-cell activation or induce regulatory T cells that can suppress autoimmune responses.[21]

Despite promising results in preclinical and early-stage clinical trials, immunotherapies face challenges in achieving long-term efficacy and ensuring safety.

CONCLUSION

The pursuit of a cure for diabetes through beta-cell replacement and regeneration is a dynamic and rapidly evolving field. From directly transplanting donor islets, with the inherent challenges of donor scarcity and lifelong immunosuppression, to the burgeoning potential of stem cell-derived beta cells offering an expandable and patient-specific source, significant strides are being made. Concurrently, efforts in stimulating endogenous beta-cell replication using growth factors such as GLP-1 and harmine, and the exciting prospect of in vivo cell reprogramming, aim to harness the body's own regenerative capacities. The precision offered by gene therapy and CRISPR-based approaches opens avenues for correcting genetic defects and enhancing beta-cell resilience. However, common threads of challenge persist across these strategies, particularly in ensuring long-term safety and sustained efficacy, overcoming immune rejection, and addressing the significant cost implications of these advanced therapies. The future likely involves a multipronged approach, potentially combining different strategies to tailor treatments to individual patient needs, ultimately striving for a durable, safe, and widely accessible cure that liberates individuals from the burden of diabetes.

TAKE HOME MESSAGE

- *Beta-cell restoration is key to diabetes cure*: Addressing the loss or dysfunction of pancreatic beta cells is fundamental to treating diabetes effectively, especially type 1.
- *Diverse strategies are evolving*: Approaches range from direct islet transplantation and stem cell-derived beta-cell therapy to stimulating the body's own beta-cell regeneration, cellular reprogramming, and gene-editing technologies such as CRISPR.
- *Immunosuppression challenges persist*: Overcoming immune rejection, whether from allogeneic transplants or autoimmune attacks, remains a critical hurdle, driving innovation in encapsulation and targeted immunotherapies.
- *Scalability and functional maturity are crucial*: Developing methods to produce sufficient quantities of fully functional beta cells and ensuring their long-term survival in vivo are ongoing areas of intensive research.
- *A combinatorial approach is the likely future*: A lasting, accessible cure will probably involve integrating multiple strategies, tailoring treatments to individual patient needs, and optimizing for safety, efficacy, and practicality.

REFERENCES

1. Ashcroft FM, Rorsman, P. Diabetes mellitus and the beta cell: the last ten years. Cell. 2012;148(6):1160-71.
2. Kahn SE, Cooper ME, Del Prato S. Pathophysiology and treatment of type 2 diabetes: perspectives on the past, present, and future. Lancet. 2014;383(9933):1068-83.
3. Grattoni A, Korbutt G, Tomei AA, García AJ, Pepper AR, Stabler C, et al. Harnessing Cellular Therapeutics for Type 1 Diabetes Mellitus: Progress, Challenges, and the Road Ahead. Nat Rev Endocrinol. 2025;21(1):14-30.
4. Hassanein A, Akhtar S. Recent advances in stem cell-based therapies for type 1 diabetes: A glimpse into the future. Biomol Biomed. 2024. https://www.bjbms.org/ojs/index.php/bjbms/article/view/12222
5. Ricordi C, Camillo, A. Islet transplantation: Immunological challenges and current perspectives. World J Transplant. 2021;11(3):57-67.
6. National Institute of Diabetes and Digestive and Kidney Diseases. (2024). Pancreatic islet transplantation. [online] Available from https://www.niddk.nih.gov/health-information/diabetes/overview/insulin-medicines-treatments/pancreatic-islet-transplantation [Last accessed September, 2025].
7. Chellappa K, Parekh V. Islet Transplantation: Current Limitations and Challenges for Successful Outcomes. J Pancreat Cancer. 2023;9(1):4-11.
8. Rezania A, Bruin JE, Arora P, Rubin A, Batushansky I, Asadi A, et al. Reversal of diabetes with insulin-producing cells derived from human embryonic stem cells. Nat Biotechnol. 2014;32(11):1121-33.
9. Pagliuca FW, Millman JR, Gürtler M, Segel M, Van Dervort A, Ryu JH, et al. Generation of functional human pancreatic β cells in vitro. Cell. 2014;159(2):428-39.
10. Millman JR, Melton DA. Recent advances in β cell differentiation from human pluripotent stem cells. Curr Opin Cell Biol. 2016;43:111-8.
11. Pepper AR, Gala-Lopez B. Islet Encapsulation: New Developments for the Treatment of Type 1 Diabetes. Front Immunol. 2022;13:869984.
12. Tomei AA, Stabler CL. Advances in islet encapsulation technologies. Nat Rev Mater. 2019;4(12):773-89.
13. ViaCyte. PEC Encap Diabetes Therapy. [online] Available from https://ontosight.ai/glossary/term/pec-encap-diabetes-therapy--67a0da106c3593987a502d17 [Last accessed September, 2025].
14. Zhou Q, Brown J, Kanarek A, Rajagopal J, Melton DA. In vivo reprogramming of adult pancreatic exocrine cells to beta-cells. Nature. 2008;455(7217):627-32.
15. Wang P, Stewart AF. (2022). Beta cell proliferation research to investigate harmine in phase 1 trial. Mount Sinai Reports. [online] Available from https://reports.mountsinai.org/article/endo2022-_3_beta-cell-harmine [Last accessed September, 2025].
16. Rosselot C, Alvarsson A, Wang P, Li Y, Kumar K, De Vita RJ, et al. (2020). The Harmine and Exendin-4 Combination Markedly Expands Human Beta Cell Mass In Vivo: Quantification and Visualization By iDISCO+ 3D Imaging. bioRxiv. [online] Available from https://www.biorxiv.org/content/10.1101/2020.07.24.220244v1 [Last accessed September, 2025].

17. Ansari P, Khan JT, Chowdhury S, Reberio AD, Kumar S, Seidel V, et al. Plant-Based Diets and Phytochemicals in the Management of Diabetes Mellitus and Prevention of Its Complications: A Review. Nutrients. 2024;16(21):3709.
18. So WY, Han W. Gene therapy targeting key beta cell regulators as a potential intervention for diabetes. EMBO Mol Med. 2024;16(7):1490-4.
19. Maxwell KG, Augsornworawat P, Velazco-Cruz L, Kim MH, Asada R, Hogrebe NJ, et al. Gene-edited human stem cell-derived β cells from a patient with monogenic diabetes reverse pre-existing diabetes in mice. Sci Transl Med. 2020;12(540): eaax9106.
20. Gitelman SE, Greenbaum CJ. Immunotherapies for prevention and treatment of type 1 diabetes. Immunotherapy. 2024;15(8):643-59.
21. Diabetes UK. Research hot topics – what are type 1 diabetes immunotherapies? [online] Available from https://www.diabetes.org.uk/our-research/about-our-research/hot-topics/immunotherapy/what-are-immunotherapies [Last accessed September, 2025].

6

Innovative Pharmacotherapy

Part A: Sodium-glucose Cotransporter-2 Inhibitors

Manoj Chawla, Purvi Chawla

ABSTRACT

Type 2 diabetes mellitus (T2DM) is a growing public health challenge, necessitating the development of newer therapeutic agents. The Sodium-glucose cotransporter-2 (SGLT-2) inhibitors are a robust class of antidiabetic agents that have been demonstrated to show pleiotropic benefits beyond glycemic control. Improvement in long-term cardiovascular and renal outcomes was seen with this class of drugs that inhibit the SGLT-2 transporters, selectively and reversibly in the proximal renal tubule causing decreased reabsorption of the filtered glucose and enhanced urinary glucose excretion (glucosuria) leading to reduced plasma glucose concentrations, independent of insulin pathways. This is a comprehensive review of the SGLT-2 inhibitors in diabetes describing the beneficial glucose lowering and cardiorenal protective actions. The recent evidence with SGLT-2 inhibitors demonstrating cardiorenal benefits in the nondiabetic population has also been included here. This analysis emphasizes on the central role of SGLT-2 inhibitors in expanding horizons beyond the glucose lowering effects, improving the overall prognosis of those with diabetes and comorbidities and complications.

Keywords: Antidiabetic, Glucose-lowering, Cardioprotection, Cardiorenal protection, SGLT-2 inhibition, Weight reduction, Mycotic infections.

INTRODUCTION

Sodium-glucose cotransporter-2 (SGLT-2) inhibitors are indeed a novel group of antidiabetic agents and have evolved into drugs offering cardiorenal protection with accruing evidence. This class of drugs represents a breakthrough in the pharmacological management of type 2 diabetes mellitus (T2DM) and has become an important pillar in modern treatment algorithms. Unlike older agents with primary efficacy restricted to glucose lowering, SGLT-2 inhibitors were found to have diverse systemic effects including improvements in weight and blood pressure, reduction in cardiovascular risk, and kidney function preservation.[1,2]

The prevalence of T2DM is increasing globally, driven by lifestyle changes, obesity, and aging populations. Achieving and maintaining glycemic control is crucial to prevent microvascular and macrovascular complications. Traditional therapies such as metformin, sulfonylureas, and insulin address hyperglycemia but often fall short in reducing cardiovascular and renal outcomes. The discovery that SGLT-2 inhibitors simultaneously address these comorbidities significantly has transformed their role to being novel agents with a multidimensional therapeutic profile.

MECHANISM OF ACTION

Sodium-glucose cotransporter-2 is a high-capacity, low-affinity sodium-dependent glucose transporter predominantly expressed in the early proximal renal tubule (S1 segment). Under normal physiological conditions, nearly 90% of the glucose filtered by the glomeruli is reabsorbed by the SGLT-2, with the remaining 10% reclaimed by SGLT-1 in the S3 segment of the tubule. By selectively inhibiting SGLT-2, these agents prevent the reabsorption of glucose, causing enhanced glucosuria. This loss of glucose translates into a daily caloric deficit of approximately 200–300 kcal, contributing to weight reduction over time.

Mechanistically, the induced glucosuria is associated with reduced plasma glucose levels both in the fasting and postprandial states.[1] The resultant osmotic diuresis promotes mild natriuresis, contributing further to reductions in both systolic and diastolic blood pressure. The improved metabolic milieu reduces glucotoxicity and lipotoxicity, potentially improving pancreatic β-cell function and peripheral insulin sensitivity. These effects are insulin-independent, making SGLT-2 inhibitors effective across the spectrum of β-cell reserve and insulin resistance.

PHARMACODYNAMICS AND PHARMACOKINETICS

Pharmacodynamically, the glucose-lowering effect of SGLT-2 inhibitors is proportional to the plasma glucose concentration and glomerular filtration rate (GFR).[3,4] Thus, there is diminished efficacy observed in patients with advanced chronic kidney disease (CKD). Pharmacokinetic profiles across the class of SGLT-2 inhibitors share common features that include rapid gastrointestinal absorption with peak plasma concentrations attained within 1–2 hours, high plasma protein binding, and extensive hepatic metabolism primarily via uridine diphosphate glucuronosyltransferase (UGT) enzymes. The elimination of half-life ranges from 10 to 17 hours, supporting once-daily dosing regimens.

Drug-drug interaction potential is low, as most SGLT-2 inhibitors do not significantly impact cytochrome P450 enzymes. Nevertheless, renal clearance of the parent drug is minimal, and the majority is excreted as inactive metabolites in urine and feces.[3-5]

CLINICAL EFFICACY IN TYPE 2 DIABETES MELLITUS

Multiple large-scale randomized controlled trials (RCTs) have demonstrated significant reductions in glycated hemoglobin (HbA1c) with SGLT-2 inhibitor therapy, typically in the range of 0.5–1.0% from the baseline levels.[6,7] These effects are evident both as monotherapy and in combination with other glucose-lowering agents, including metformin, dipeptidyl peptidase-4 inhibitors (DPP-4) inhibitors, glucagon-like peptide-1 (GLP-1) receptor agonists, thiazolidinediones, and insulin.

Weight loss of 2–3 kg is consistent across the class, primarily from the fat mass reduction, as confirmed by body composition analyses in studies. This is an important advantage over insulin secretagogues and insulin, which are associated with weight gain.

Blood pressure lowering is another consistent finding with reductions of approximately 3–5 mm Hg systolic and 1–2 mm Hg diastolic, an effect additive to standard antihypertensive therapies.

The SGLT-2 inhibitors, as a class, brought a paradigm change not only in the development of newer classes of antidiabetic agents but also in the wide-ranging clinical applications beyond glycemic control, as their multiorgan, beneficial effects were elucidated in different studies.[8]

CARDIOVASCULAR OUTCOMES

Upon release of the results of the cardiovascular outcome trials (CVOTs) with SGLT-2 inhibitors, namely the EMPA-REG OUTCOME trial, it has been determined for the first time that empagliflozin has cardioprotective effects.[4] CVOTs mandated by regulatory agencies have revealed striking benefits beyond glycemic control.[9,10] The EMPA-REG OUTCOME trial showed that empagliflozin reduced cardiovascular (CV) death by 38% and heart failure (HF) hospitalization by 35% in T2DM patients with established cardiovascular disease. The CANVAS Program with canagliflozin demonstrated a 14% reduction in major adverse cardiovascular events (MACE) and a 33% reduction in HF hospitalizations, albeit with an increased risk of lower-limb amputations. The DECLARE-TIMI study, involving dapagliflozin, enrolled a broader population including patients without established atherosclerotic cardiovascular disease (ASCVD). While there was no significant reduction in MACE, dapagliflozin reduced HF hospitalizations by 27%. These findings were reinforced by important meta-analyses, which confirmed that reductions in HF hospitalization and CV death were a class-effect of SGLT-2 inhibitors.[4,9-11]

RENAL OUTCOMES

Sodium-glucose cotransporter-2 inhibitors also confer renal benefits through multiple mechanisms: decreasing the intraglomerular hypertension via restoration of the tubuloglomerular feedback loop, lowering albuminuria, mitigating renal inflammation and fibrosis, and improving systemic hemodynamics.[12] In the CREDENCE trial with canagliflozin, it has been observed that the risk of end-stage kidney disease (ESKD) was reduced with associated decrease in doubling of serum creatinine, and renal/CV death by 30% in patients with diabetic nephropathy. In the DAPA-CKD study with dapagliflozin, these benefits seemed to be extended to both diabetic and nondiabetic CKD populations, with a 39% relative risk reduction in the composite renal endpoint.

The EMPA-KIDNEY trial with empagliflozin further confirmed renal protection even in patients without albuminuria, suggesting potential utility of empagliflozin across a wider CKD spectrum.

ROLE IN HEART FAILURE

Recent evidence now supports the use of SGLT-2 inhibitors in heart failure with reduced ejection fraction (HFrEF) and heart failure with preserved ejection fraction (HFpEF), irrespective of the diabetes status of the patients. Trials such as DAPA-HF and EMPEROR-Reduced have demonstrated significant reductions in CV death and HF hospitalizations with dapagliflozin and empagliflozin respectively, while in EMPEROR-Preserved with empagliflozin, the benefits were expanded to those with HFpEF. Improvement in biomarkers such as N-terminal pro-B-type natriuretic peptide (NT-proBNP) and left ventricular remodeling indices have been observed with improved quality-of-life scores.[11,13]

SAFETY PROFILE

Sodium-glucose cotransporter-2 inhibitors are reasonably well-tolerated. The most common adverse events associated with SGLT-2 inhibitor use are genital mycotic infections, particularly in women, due to the increased glucose content in the urinary tract. The urinary tract infections occur less frequently and are usually mild.

Volume depletion caused by SGLT-2 inhibitors leading to hypotension is more likely in the elderly patients, in those on diuretics, or with baseline low blood pressure. Modifications in the antihypertensive regimen may be required to address the same. A rare but serious adverse event includes euglycemic diabetic ketoacidosis (DKA), most often in the setting of reduced carbohydrate intake, illness, or perioperative states with indiscriminate SGLT-2 inhibitor use. Canagliflozin has been linked to increased fracture risk and amputations, warranting careful patient's selection and monitoring.

A rare yet serious genital infection called Fournier's gangrene (necrotizing fasciitis of the perineum) was added by the FDA as a warning in 2018 to all the SGLT-2 inhibitor labels. Since it is a medical emergency and life threatening, a high index of suspicion is warranted in those with diabetes and on SGLT-2 inhibitors and immediate medical attention to be sought for aggressive medical and surgical treatment.

SPECIAL CONSIDERATIONS

It is important for the renal function to be assessed prior to initiation of SGLT-2 inhibitor use and periodically thereafter. Based on the threshold of the estimated glomerular filtration rate (eGFR), SGLT-2 inhibitors may be initiated or the drug may require dose adjustments, especially when eGFR is below 45 mL/min/1.73 m^2. Recently, trials have shown that there is cardiorenal protection observed at lower eGFR levels also with SGLT-2 inhibitors.[12,13]

In addition, the vulnerable subjects like the elderly population should also be closely monitored for signs of dehydration, electrolyte imbalances, and orthostatic hypotension while being on SGLT-2 inhibitors. Since they may be used in combination with a wide range of glucose-lowering agents and antihypertensive drugs, there is caution warranted with loop diuretics due to the additive diuretic effects.

GUIDELINE RECOMMENDATIONS

The current Research Society for the Study of Diabetes in India (RSSDI), the American Diabetes Association (ADA), and the European Association for the Study of Diabetes (EASD) consensus recommend the preferential use of SGLT-2 inhibitors after metformin in patients with established ASCVD, HF, or CKD with albuminuria. They may also be considered first-line in certain high-risk individuals irrespective of the HbA1c levels. This represents a shift toward complication-centric therapy rather than a focused glucose-centric approach.

FUTURE PERSPECTIVES

Ongoing research is exploring the use of SGLT-2 inhibitors in a range of conditions including nonalcoholic fatty liver disease (NAFLD), obesity without diabetes, and acute HF. Their pleiotropic effects—ranging from improved endothelial function to reduced inflammation—suggest broader clinical application. Combination therapy with other agents, such as GLP-1 receptor agonists, may offer synergistic benefits for both metabolic and cardiovascular outcomes.

CONCLUSION

Sodium-glucose cotransporter-2 inhibitors have, thus, redefined the management of T2DM, providing a rare combination of glycemic, cardiovascular, and renal benefits. As evidence accumulates, their role is expanding into non-diabetic populations and across a spectrum of chronic diseases. Their safety, ease of administration, and multiorgan benefits support their inclusion as cornerstone therapy in modern clinical practice.

REFERENCES

1. Ferrannini E, Muscelli E, Frascerra S, Baldi S, Mari A, Heise T, et al. Metabolic response to sodium-glucose cotransporter 2 inhibition in type 2 diabetic patients. J Clin Invest. 2014;124:499-508.
2. An Y, Zhang H. SGLT-2 inhibitors: a deeper dive into their renal protective properties beyond glycemic control and proteinuria reduction. Am J Nephrol. 2025:1-13.
3. Scheen AJ. Pharmacodynamics, efficacy and safety of sodium-glucose co-transporter type 2 (SGLT2) inhibitors for the treatment of type 2 diabetes mellitus. Drugs. 2015;75(1):33-59.
4. Darwish D, Kumar P, Urs K, Dave S. Impact of SGLT-2 inhibitors on biomarkers of heart failure. Cells. 2025;14(12):919.
5. Dardi I, Kouvatsos T, Jabbour SA. SGLT2 inhibitors. Biochem Pharmacol. 2016;101:27-39.
6. Lupsa BC, Inzucchi SE. Use of SGLT2 inhibitors in type 2 diabetes: weighing the risks and benefits. Diabetologia. 2018;61(10):2118-25.
7. Scheen AJ. Sodium-glucose cotransporter type 2 inhibitors for the treatment of type 2 diabetes mellitus. Nat Rev Endocrinol. 2020;16(10):556-77.
8. Xu B, Li S, Kang B, Zhou J. The current role of sodium-glucose cotransporter 2 inhibitors in type 2 diabetes mellitus management. Cardiovasc Diabetol. 2022;21(1):83.
9. Singh AK, Singh R. Effect of background insulin therapy on cardiovascular outcomes with SGLT-2 inhibitors in type 2 diabetes: A meta-analysis of cardiovascular outcome trials. Diabetes Res Clin Pract. 2021;172:108648.
10. Yao X, Zhang H, Lu X. Meta-analysis of the efficacy and safety of SGLT-2 inhibitors in patients with heart failure and type 2 diabetes mellitus. Medicine (Baltimore). 2025;104(18):e42196.
11. Singh AK, Singh R. Do SGLT-2 inhibitors exhibit similar cardiovascular benefit in patients having reduced ejection fraction heart failure with type 2 diabetes, prediabetes and normoglycemia? Diabetes Metab Syndr. 2021;15(6):102282.
12. Zhang B, Deng L. Application of SGLT-2 inhibitors in non-diabetic CKD: mechanisms, efficacy, and safety. Front Med (Lausanne). 2025;12:1574693.
13. Singh AK, Singh A, Singh R. Have SGLT-2 inhibitors DELIVERed an EMPhatic win in heart failure and chronic kidney disease? Expert Opin Pharmacother. 2025;26(4):457-72.

Part B: GLP-1 Receptor Mono-agonists and GLP-1/GIP Dual Agonist

Awadhesh Kumar Singh, Akriti Singh

ABSTRACT

Glucagon-like peptide-1 receptor agonists (GLP-1 RAs) have emerged as a crucial therapeutic class for type 2 diabetes mellitus (T2DM) management, showcasing significant efficacy in glycemic control and weight reduction. This chapter provides an overview of the pharmacodynamics, safety profiles, and clinical outcomes associated with GLP-1 RAs over the past few years. With innovations such as once-weekly formulations and studies assessing cardiovascular (CV) benefits, this class of drugs has transformed diabetes management paradigms. Currently, GLP-1 RAs are the first-line drug in people with T2DM with high CV risk or with established CV and renal diseases. The higher strength of a few GLP-1 RAs, such as liraglutide and semaglutide, has been additionally licensed for the treatment of obesity, owing to significant weight loss. The dual agonist of GLP-1 and glucose-dependent insulinotropic polypeptide (GIP) receptors, such as tirzepatide, has shown additional weight loss compared to GLP-1 receptor mono-agonists in people with obesity. Importantly, both mono-agonists and dual agonists have nonresponders and intolerance issues as well. Thus, varied patient responses and adaptability to individual treatment plans underscore the importance of personalized medicine in diabetes and obesity care.

Keywords: GLP-1 receptor agonists, GLP-1/GIP dual agonists, Type 2 diabetes mellitus, Obesity, Cardiovascular benefits.

INTRODUCTION

Glucagon-like peptide-1 (GLP-1) is an incretin hormone secreted by the intestinal L cells in response to nutrient ingestion. It plays a critical role in glucose homeostasis through multiple mechanisms: It stimulates insulin secretion in a glucose-dependent manner, inhibits glucagon release, decreases gastric emptying, and promotes satiety. These physiological benefits have led to the development of GLP-1 receptor agonists (RAs)—synthetic analogs that enhance the action of GLP-1.[1,2]

Since the first GLP-1 RA, exenatide, was approved in 2005, this class has grown to include several agents with varied pharmacokinetic properties and dosing regimens. GLP-1 RAs have transformed the treatment landscape for type 2 diabetes mellitus (T2DM), providing not only effective glycemic control but also cardiovascular (CV) protection and weight management benefits.

The expanding body of literature examining GLP-1 RAs underscores their clinical significance. As the prevalence of T2DM rises globally, understanding GLP-1 RAs' mechanisms, benefits, and safety profiles is crucial for optimizing patient outcomes **(Fig. 1)**.

PHARMACODYNAMICS OF GLUCAGON-LIKE PEPTIDE-1 RECEPTOR AGONISTS

Glucagon-like peptide-1 receptor agonists primarily function by mimicking the effects of the endogenous incretin hormone GLP-1, thereby playing a significant role in glucose metabolism. Upon glucose ingestion, GLP-1 is released from the intestinal L cells and acts on GLP-1 receptors

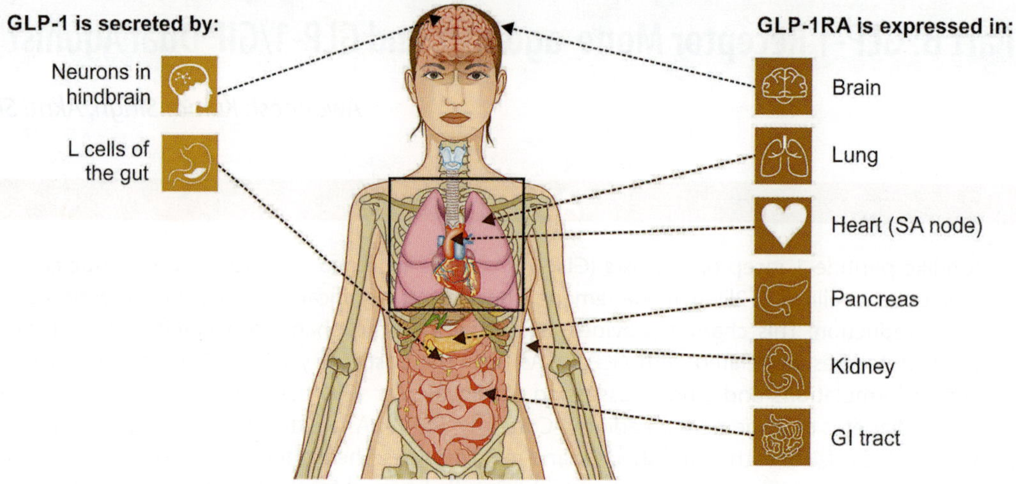

Fig. 1: Glucagon-like peptide-1 (GLP-1) secretion and receptor expression.
(GI: gastrointestinal; GLP-1 RA: GLP-1 receptor agonist; SA: sinoatrial)

found in pancreatic β cells, the central nervous system, and various peripheral tissues. The activation of GLP-1 receptors leads to several key responses.[1,2]

- *Insulin secretion*: GLP-1 RAs stimulate glucose-dependent insulin secretion. They enhance insulin release when blood glucose levels are elevated while having a minimal effect on basal insulin secretion, thereby reducing the risk of hypoglycemia.
- *Glucagon inhibition*: GLP-1 RAs suppress the secretion of glucagon—a hormone that increases blood glucose levels by promoting hepatic gluconeogenesis and glycogenolysis. This suppression helps decrease glucose output from the liver.
- *Gastric emptying*: GLP-1 RAs slow gastric emptying, leading to a more gradual absorption of glucose, thereby reducing postprandial hyperglycemia. This effect also contributes to the satiety signaling pathway.
- *Central nervous system effects*: GLP-1 receptors in the brain are implicated in appetite regulation. GLP-1 RAs signal to increase satiety and decrease food intake, facilitating weight management, which is an essential component in treating T2DM **(Fig. 2)**.

PHARMACOKINETICS

Glucagon-like peptide-1 receptor agonists display varied pharmacokinetic profiles.

- Some agents, such as exenatide (short-acting) and lixisenatide, require twice-daily administration due to their shorter half-life.
- Others, such as liraglutide, need once-daily dosing, while exenatide long-acting, dulaglutide, and semaglutide require once-weekly dosing, allowing improved patient compliance and convenience.

Research on the pharmacokinetics of these agents continues to evolve with the development of various formulations, including oral options, which aim at providing more versatile treatment strategies for patients.

OVERVIEW OF GLUCAGON-LIKE PEPTIDE-1 RECEPTOR AGONISTS

Glucagon-like peptide-1 receptor agonists are a class of medications used primarily in the treatment of T2DM and obesity. They mimic the incretin hormone GLP-1, leading to increased insulin secretion, inhibited glucagon release, delayed gastric emptying, and enhanced satiety. The primary GLP-1 RAs currently available and

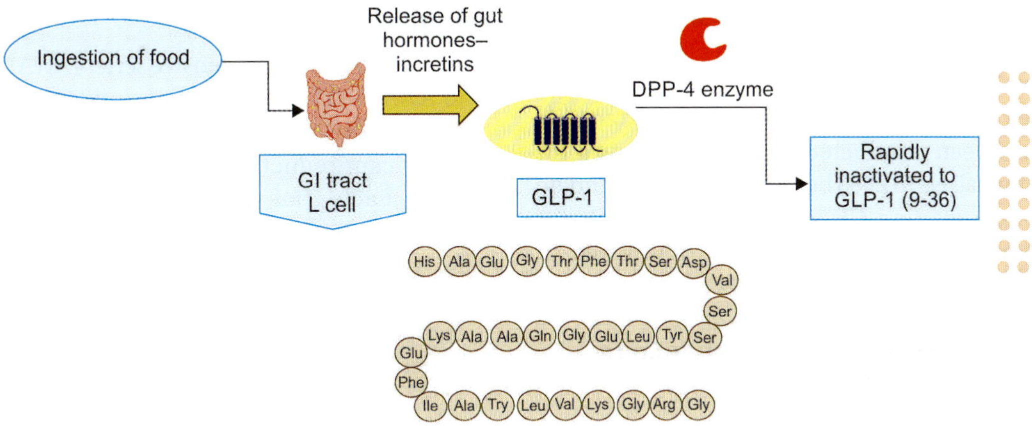

Fig. 2: Glucagon-like peptide-1 (GLP-1): Synthesis, release, metabolism, and effects.

(DPP-4: dipeptidyl peptidase 4; GI: gastrointestinal)

approved by the United States Food and Drug Administration (USFDA) are:

- Exenatide (Byetta®, Bydureon™)
- Liraglutide (Victoza®, Saxenda®)
- Dulaglutide (Trulicity®)
- Semaglutide (Ozempic®, Wegovy®, Rybelsus®)
- Lixisenatide (Lyxumia, Adlyxin™)

Albiglutide was another once-weekly GLP-1 RA that underwent an extensive phase 3 program, including a cardiovascular outcome trial (CVOT) named HARMONY Outcomes, which showed a significant reduction in the CV composite. Still, it was withdrawn due to commercial reasons. Efpeglenatide is another GLP-1 RA currently under phase 3 development, and its CVOT (AMPLITUDE-O) has yielded positive results.

OVERVIEW OF GLP-1 AND GLUCOSE-DEPENDENT INSULINOTROPIC POLYPEPTIDE RECEPTOR DUAL AGONISTS

While glucose-dependent insulinotropic polypeptide (GIP) is the primary incretin hormone in healthy individuals, causing most of the incretin effects, the insulin response to GIP is significantly reduced in T2DM. Based on these findings, the GIP was considered an appealing therapeutic target for T2DM. However, this did not click as many studies of GIP mono-agonism failed to show therapeutic benefits in people with T2DM. This concept has been evolving over recent years as it has been reported that resistance to GIP can be reversed and its effectiveness restored by improving glycemic control in association with GLP-1 RA. Since GLP-1 stimulates insulin secretion, inhibits glucagon secretion (unlike GIP, which increases glucagon), slows gastric emptying, and increases the feeling of satiety, these facts paved the way for the development of a combined GLP-1/GIP receptor agonist.

The first dual GLP-1/GIP agonist approved for the treatment of T2DM and obesity is tirzepatide, based on an extensive phase 3 development program named SURPASS (in T2DM) and SURMOUNT (in obesity) trials.

KEY CLINICAL TRIALS FOR GLUCAGON-LIKE PEPTIDE-1 RECEPTOR AGONISTS

Exenatide

Short-acting Exenatide

- *AMIGO trials*: Phase 3 AMIGO-1 to AMIGO-3 trials evaluated short-acting exenatide in various populations of T2DM and showed glycated hemoglobin (HbA1c) reduction of –0.7 to –1.0% with modest 1-3 kg weight loss.[3]

- No dedicated CVOT for short-acting exenatide has been conducted as it was approved for clinical use in 2005 before the USFDA mandate of conducting CV safety outcome trials for newer antidiabetic agents promulgated in 2007–2008.

Long-acting Exenatide (Exenatide Long-acting Release)

- *DURATION trials*: A series of phase 3 trials, DURATION-1 to DURATION-6, evaluated exenatide long-acting release (LAR) in various populations, demonstrating significant reductions in HbA1c levels ranging from 1 to 2% and notable weight loss when used as an adjunct to metformin and other treatments.[4]
- *EXSCEL trial*: CVOT showed noninferiority of exenatide LAR compared to placebo on CV end points.[5]

Liraglutide

Liraglutide in Type 2 Diabetes Mellitus (1.8 mg)

- *LEAD trials*: The LEAD program consists of six studies (LEAD-1 to LEAD-6) validating liraglutide's efficacy in glycemic control and highlighting its safety profile across diverse patient populations.[6]
- *LEADER trial*: It is the first landmark CVOT of GLP-1 RA affirming that liraglutide reduces the risk of major adverse cardiovascular events (MACE) in patients with T2DM at high CV risk.[7]

Liraglutide for Obesity (3 mg)

SCALE trials: These are series of studies validating the use of liraglutide for chronic weight management in the nondiabetic population, reporting significant weight loss and improvements in obesity-related comorbidities.[8]

Dulaglutide

- *AWARD trials*: This extensive series (AWARD-1 to AWARD-11) assessed dulaglutide's efficacy and safety, consistently demonstrating significant reductions in HbA1c and weight gain. Each trial explored various patient demographics and treatment backgrounds.[9]
- *REWIND trial*: It established dulaglutide's CV safety and confirmed reductions in MACE composite among high-risk (primarily) T2DM patients.[10]

Semaglutide

Injectable Semaglutide in Type 2 Diabetes Mellitus (0.5–1.0 mg)

- *SUSTAIN trials*: This comprehensive set of trials (SUSTAIN-1 to SUSTAIN-8) evaluated semaglutide, yielding substantial reductions in HbA1c and weight across diverse populations and comparing its effectiveness favorably against other diabetes therapies, including insulin and liraglutide.[11]
- *SUSTAIN-6 trial*: Its key findings corroborated semaglutide's CV safety and its utility in reducing CV events in high-risk populations of T2DM with a significant reduction in stroke outcome.[12]
- *FLOW trial*: This is the first GLP-1 RA trial where semaglutide showed a significant reduction in composite renal end points in people with diabetic kidney diseases.[13]
- *STRIDE trial*: It showed that semaglutide significantly improved walking in people with symptomatic peripheral arterial disease.[14]

Injectable Semaglutide in Obesity (2.4 mg)

- *STEP trials*: This series (STEP-1 to STEP-11) focused on semaglutide for weight management in obese nondiabetic populations including STEP-2 (in T2DM), confirming significant long-term weight loss (≈15–17%) and improvements in associated metabolic parameters.[15]

- *SELECT trial*: Semaglutide is the first antiobesity medication to show 20% MACE reduction in people with obesity and established cardiovascular disease (CVD). This trial paved the way to get an additional label update for semaglutide 2.4 mg to reduce CV risk in obesity with established CVD.[16]
- *STEP-HFpEF and STEP-HFpEF DM trials*: Semaglutide improves the 6-minute walk test in people with heart failure with preserved ejection fraction (HFpEF) with obesity and/or T2DM.[17]
- *ESSENCE trial*: Semaglutide showed a significant reduction in liver fibrosis in people with metabolic dysfunction-associated steatotic liver disease (MASLD).[18] This trial paved the way to get an additional label update for semaglutide 2.4 mg in people with obesity and MASLD.

Oral Semaglutide in Type 2 Diabetes Mellitus (14 mg)

- *PIONEER trials*: They are a collection of pivotal studies (PIONEER 1–10) exploring the efficacy of oral semaglutide in T2DM patients. Notably, these trials demonstrated significant reductions in HbA1c and body weight compared to placebo, empagliflozin, liraglutide 1.8 mg and sitagliptin.[19]
- *PIONEER-6 trial*: It is an essential trial focused on the CV safety of oral semaglutide, revealing it to be safe for use in high CV risk T2DM patients.[20]
- *SOUL trial*: The SOUL trial established the CV superiority outcomes with oral semaglutide, with 14% MACE reduction, contributed majorly by nonfatal myocardial infarction (MI) (26% risk) reduction.[21]

Lixisenatide

- *GetGoal trials*: This series evaluated lixisenatide in various populations, demonstrating improvements in HbA1c levels and associated weight loss compared to placebo and other conventional therapies.[22]
- *ELIXA trial*: It showed noninferiority of lixisenatide against placebo in people with established CVD.[23]

KEY OUTCOME TRIALS WITH DUAL GLP-1/GIP AGONIST TIRZEPATIDE

- *SURPASS and SURMOUNT trials*: Tirzepatide has undergone several phase 3 trials in people with T2DM (SURPASS-1 to SURPASS-6) and obesity (SURMOUNT-1 to SURMOUNT-4). Across all six SURPASS trials, tirzepatide showed a significant reduction in HbA1c ranging from –1.9 to –2.6% depending upon the dosage of tirzepatide (5–15 mg) and baseline HbA1c. Similarly, weight loss ranged from –7 to –12 kg, depending on the dosage of tirzepatide (5–15 mg) and baseline body weight across the six SURPASS trials in T2DM.[24] Across the four SURMOUNT trials, tirzepatide reduced body weight by approximately 20–21% depending on the dosage (5–15 mg) and baseline body weight, along with improvements in other metabolic parameters.[25]
- *SURMOUNT-5 trial*: This open-label head-to-head trial compared tirzepatide (10–15 mg) to semaglutide 2.4 mg and showed superior weight loss (an additional ≈6%) with the former compared to the latter.[26] Indirect analysis from STEP-1 versus SURMOUNT-1 in obesity and STEP-2 versus SURMPONT-2 in T2DM also suggests larger weight loss and HbA1c drop, respectively, with tirzepatide compared with semaglutide.[27]
- *SURPASS-CVOT trial*: The top-line results of this CVOT in T2DM with established CVD showed that tirzepatide was noninferior to dulaglutide, suggesting superiority of tirzepatide compared to a putative placebo.
- *SUMMIT-HFpEF trial*: This trial showed that tirzepatide significantly reduced (38% relative

risk reduction) the primary composite of CV death and worsening heart failure compared to placebo in obese people with HFpEF.[28]

SAFETY PROFILES AND ADVERSE EFFECTS

Overall, GLP-1 receptor mono- and dual agonists are considered safe, but they are associated with a range of adverse effects that require monitoring:

- *Gastrointestinal symptoms*: Nausea, vomiting, and diarrhea are common, particularly during the initial weeks of therapy or with dose escalation. These symptoms are believed to stem from slowed gastric emptying and can improve over time as the patient adapts.
- *Pancreatitis*: There have been reports of acute pancreatitis in patients treated with GLP-1 RAs. While this association is not conclusively established, healthcare providers are advised to monitor patients for symptoms of pancreatitis. If pancreatitis occurs, the GLP-1 RA should be discontinued immediately. In patients with a history of pancreatitis, it is prudent not to initiate GLP-1 RAs.
- *Thyroid C-cell tumors*: Long-term studies in rodents revealed an increased incidence of thyroid C-cell tumors with certain GLP-1 RAs, notably liraglutide. Although this has not been conclusively replicated in humans, caution is warranted, particularly in patients with a personal or family history of medullary thyroid carcinoma or multiple endocrine neoplasia syndrome type 2.

Monitoring these potential adverse effects is essential during both pretreatment evaluations and ongoing management. This active surveillance can help differentiate between medication-related symptoms and those stemming from other comorbidities.

CLINICAL IMPLICATIONS

The integration of GLP-1 RAs into clinical practice has far-reaching implications for the management of T2DM and obesity as highlighted by recent evidence. The key clinical implications of GLP-1 receptor mono- and dual agonist therapy are given in the following text.

Improved Glycemic Control

Glucagon-like peptide-1 receptor agonists have demonstrated significant efficacy in reducing glycemic levels among patients with T2DM. Clinical trials consistently reveal reductions in HbA1c levels, with many agents achieving reductions of 1–2% or more compared to the placebo. Meanwhile, dual GLP-1/GIP agonists appear to have even larger HbA1c reductions, ranging from 1.5 to 2.5%. Clinicians should consider early initiation of GLP-1 RAs or dual agonists for patients presenting with T2DM, particularly when glycemic targets are not met with metformin alone. Their glucose-dependent mechanism of action minimizes the risk of hypoglycemia, making them a suitable option for a wide range of patients.

Weight Management

Weight loss is a notable benefit of GLP-1 RA therapy, with many clinical trials reporting average reductions of 5–15% of the initial body weight. Because obesity is a significant contributor to insulin resistance and worsening glycemic control, the weight loss effects of GLP-1 RAs offer dual benefits. Both GLP-1 RAs and dual GLP-1/GIP agonists can be prescribed to patients with obesity or who are overweight, even in the absence of diabetes, establishing them as valuable agents in comprehensive weight management programs.

Cardiovascular Benefits

Recent trials demonstrate that GLP-1 RAs, specifically liraglutide, dulaglutide, and semaglutide, can significantly reduce the risk of major adverse CV events. (**Table 1** summarizes the results.) For patients with established CVD or at high risk for adverse outcomes due to diabetes, GLP-1 RAs can

TABLE 1: Cardiovascular outcomes with glucagon-like peptide-1 receptor agonists (GLP-1 RAs) in randomized controlled trials (RCTs).

Trial (year)	*GLP-1 RAs studied*	*Population*	*Primary end point*	*CV outcome*	*Key findings*
ELIXA (2015)	Lixisenatide (daily)	T2DM with recent ACS (<180 days)	3-point MACE (CV death, nonfatal MI, nonfatal stroke)	Neutral	Demonstrated CV safety, no added benefits versus placebo
LEADER (2016)	Liraglutide (daily)	T2DM with high CV risk	3-point MACE	Superior	13% RRR in MACE; decreased CV death by 22%, decreased all-cause mortality
SUSTAIN-6 (2016)	Semaglutide SC (weekly)	T2DM with high CV risk	3-point MACE	Superior	26% RRR in MACE; notable reduced risk of stroke (39%)
EXSCEL (2017)	Exenatide ER (weekly)	T2DM population with almost 73% with prior CVD	3-point MACE	Neutral	Did not meet the superiority
HARMONY Outcomes (2018)	Albiglutide (weekly)	T2DM with established CVD	3-point MACE	Superior	22% RRR in MACE; mainly driven by reduced MI (drug later withdrawn)
REWIND (2019)	Dulaglutide (weekly)	T2DM, broad spectrum (only 31% prior CVD)	3-point MACE	Superior	12% RRR in MACE; benefit extended to the primary prevention group
PIONEER-6 (2019)	Semaglutide oral (daily)	T2DM with high CV risk	3-point MACE	Neutral	Met noninferiority; underpowered for superiority
AMPLITUDE-O (2021)	Efpeglenatide (weekly)	T2DM with ASCVD or CKD	3-point MACE	Superior	27% RRR in MACE; reduced CV death; renal protective effects observed
SELECT (2023)	Semaglutide SC 2.4 mg (weekly)	Adults who are overweight/ with obesity without diabetes, established CVD	3-point MACE	Superior	20% RRR in MACE (HR 0.80; 95% CI 0.72–0.90); reduced all-cause mortality by 19%; reduced CV death by 15%; benefits consistent across BMI, sex, and subgroups. Landmark trial showing protection in obesity without diabetes
SOUL (2025)	Semaglutide oral (daily)	T2DM + ASCVD and/or CKD; age >50 years	3-point MACE	Superior	14% RRR in MACE (HR 0.86; 95% CI 0.770.96; $p = 0.006$); 26% reduction in nonfatal MI, 12% reduction in nonfatal stroke; 7% reduction in CV death

(ACS: acute coronary syndrome; ASCVD: atherosclerotic cardiovascular disease; BMI: body mass index; CI: confidence interval; CKD: chronic kidney disease; CV: cardiovascular; CVD: cardiovascular disease; HR: hazard ratio; MACE: major adverse cardiovascular events; MI: myocardial infarction; RRR: relative risk reduction; SC: subcutaneous; T2DM: type 2 diabetes mellitus) be integrated into first-line therapy. Their ability to address glycemic control, weight, and CV risk represents a significant advancement in the management of T2DM.

Renal Protection

The renal protective effects of GLP-1 RAs have gained attention, particularly within trials investigating their impacts on renal safety and outcomes. Emerging evidence suggests that these agents may slow the progression of diabetic kidney disease by lowering albuminuria and stabilizing renal function. Clinicians should assess the renal status of patients with diabetes and consider GLP-1 RAs as part of a multifaceted approach to managing diabetes while protecting renal health.

Safety and Monitoring

Despite their benefits, GLP-1 RAs do have potential side effects, primarily gastrointestinal symptoms such as nausea and vomiting. Serious risks, including pancreatitis and considerations around thyroid C-cell tumors, warrant vigilance. Comprehensive patient education regarding the side effects and signs of complications is essential. Ongoing monitoring for adverse events and assessment of treatment response should be a routine practice in clinical settings.

Personalized Medicine Approach

The diversity within the GLP-1 RA class allows healthcare providers to tailor therapy based on individual patient needs, preferences, and concomitant medications. Factors such as patient weight, CV risk profiles, renal function, and lifestyle should inform the selection of a particular GLP-1 RA. Engaging patients in shared decision-making facilitates discussions around therapy choices, balancing efficacy, tolerability, route of administration, and ease of use, ultimately leading to improved adherence and outcomes.

CONCLUSION

- Glucagon-like peptide-1 receptor agonists have fundamentally transformed the landscape of treatment for T2DM and obesity. Through extensive clinical trials and ongoing research, this class of medications has demonstrated substantial efficacy in improving glycemic control, promoting weight loss, and conferring CV benefits. Pivotal studies, including LEADER, REWIND, SUSTAIN-6, FLOW, SOUL, and SELECT, have established not only the effectiveness of GLP-1 RAs in achieving significant reductions in HbA1c and body weight but also their role in mitigating CV risks and preserving renal function. The CV outcomes with dual GLP-1/GIP are still to be proven in T2DM and/or obesity, but studies are ongoing. SURPASS-CVOT has demonstrated similar CV risk reduction to dulaglutide, as observed in REWIND, in individuals with T2DM, but with additional benefits in HbA1c lowering and weight loss.
- The clinical implications of these findings are profound. GLP-1 RAs and dual GLP-1/GIP agonists offer healthcare practitioners essential tools to enhance patient outcomes through personalized therapy that considers individual comorbidities, such as obesity and CVD. Their safety profiles, characterized by a low risk of hypoglycemia and additional weight loss benefits, position them favorably for use in various patient populations.
- Innovations in drug delivery systems and next-generation GLP-1 RAs may further enhance patient adherence and outcomes.
- As we advance in our understanding of metabolic diseases and the therapeutic role of GLP-1 RAs, it is vital for clinicians to stay abreast of emerging evidence and guidelines to optimize treatment strategies. The potential for integrated care models that combine GLP-1 RA therapy with lifestyle interventions and other medications offers exciting

opportunities to combat the growing global burden of diabetes and obesity.

- In conclusion, GLP-1 RAs and GLP-/GIP dual agonists symbolize a significant leap forward in diabetes and obesity management, heralding a new era of personalized, effective, and holistic patient care. Continued investment in research and commitment to clinical excellence will ensure that the transformative impact of GLP-1 receptor agonists is realized across diverse patient populations worldwide.

REFERENCES

1. Nauck MA, Quast DR, Wefers J, Meier JJ. GLP-1 receptor agonists in the treatment of type 2 diabetes—state-of-the-art. Mol Metab. 2021;46:101102.
2. Holst JJ. The incretin hormones: overview of their potential for treatment of diabetes. Diabetes Obes Metab. 2013;15(Suppl 3):35-7.
3. Htike ZZ, Khunti K, Davies M. A review of exenatide: optimizing glycemic control and associated cardiovascular risk factors in type 2 diabetes. Diabetes Ther. 2012;3(1):1-16.
4. Inaishi J, Saisho Y. Exenatide Once Weekly for Management of Type 2 Diabetes: A Review. Clin Pharmacol. 2022;14:19-26.
5. Holman RR, Bethel MA, Mentz RJ, Thompson VP, Lokhnygina Y, Buse JB, et al; EXSCEL Study Group. Effects of Once-Weekly Exenatide on Cardiovascular Outcomes in Type 2 Diabetes. N Engl J Med. 2017;377(13):1228-39.
6. Montanya E, Sesti G. A review of efficacy and safety data regarding the use of liraglutide, a once-daily human glucagon-like peptide 1 analogue, in the treatment of type 2 diabetes mellitus. Clin Ther. 2009;31(11):2472-88.
7. Marso SP, Daniels GH, Brown-Frandsen K, Kristensen P, Mann JF, Nauck MA, et al; LEADER Steering Committee; LEADER Trial Investigators. Liraglutide and Cardiovascular Outcomes in Type 2 Diabetes. N Engl J Med. 2016;375(4):311-22.
8. Mehta A, Marso SP, Neeland IJ. Liraglutide for weight management: a critical review of the evidence. Obes Sci Pract. 2017;3(1):3-14.
9. Jendle J, Grunberger G, Blevins T, Giorgino F, Hietpas RT, Botros FT. Efficacy and safety of dulaglutide in the treatment of type 2 diabetes: a comprehensive review of the dulaglutide clinical data focusing on the AWARD phase 3 clinical trial program. Diabetes Metab Res Rev. 2016;32(8):776-90.
10. Gerstein HC, Colhoun HM, Dagenais GR, Diaz R, Lakshmanan M, Pais P, et al; REWIND Investigators. Dulaglutide and cardiovascular outcomes in type 2 diabetes (REWIND): a double-blind, randomised placebo-controlled trial. Lancet. 2019;394(10193):121-30.
11. Aroda VR, Ahmann A, Cariou B, Chow F, Davies MJ, Jódar E, et al. Comparative efficacy, safety, and cardiovascular outcomes with once-weekly subcutaneous semaglutide in the treatment of type 2 diabetes: Insights from the SUSTAIN 1-7 trials. Diabetes Metab. 2019;45(5):409-18.
12. Marso SP, Bain SC, Consoli A, Eliaschewitz FG, Jódar E, Leiter LA, et al; SUSTAIN-6 Investigators. Semaglutide and Cardiovascular Outcomes in Patients with Type 2 Diabetes. N Engl J Med. 2016;375(19):1834-44.
13. Perkovic V, Tuttle KR, Rossing P, Mahaffey KW, Mann JFE, Bakris G, et al; FLOW Trial Committees and Investigators. Effects of Semaglutide on Chronic Kidney Disease in Patients with Type 2 Diabetes. N Engl J Med. 2024;391(2):109-21.
14. Bonaca MP, Catarig AM, Houlind K, Ludvik B, Nordanstig J, Ramesh CK, et al; STRIDE Trial Investigators. Semaglutide and walking capacity in people with symptomatic peripheral artery disease and type 2 diabetes (STRIDE): a phase 3b, double-blind, randomised, placebo-controlled trial. Lancet. 2025;405(10489):1580-93.
15. Bergmann NC, Davies MJ, Lingvay I, Knop FK. Semaglutide for the treatment of overweight and obesity: A review. Diabetes Obes Metab. 2023;25(1):18-35.
16. Lincoff AM, Brown-Frandsen K, Colhoun HM, Deanfield J, Emerson SS, Esbjerg S, et al; SELECT Trial Investigators. Semaglutide and Cardiovascular Outcomes in Obesity without Diabetes. N Engl J Med. 2023;389(24):2221-32.
17. Kosiborod MN, Deanfield J, Pratley R, Borlaug BA, Butler J, Davies MJ, et al; SELECT, FLOW, STEP-HFpEF, and STEP-HFpEF DM Trial Committees and Investigators. Semaglutide versus placebo in patients with heart failure and mildly reduced or preserved ejection fraction: a pooled analysis of the SELECT, FLOW, STEP-HFpEF, and STEP-HFpEF DM randomised trials. Lancet. 2024;404(10456):949-61.
18. Sanyal AJ, Newsome PN, Kliers I, Østergaard LH, Long MT, Kjær MS, et al; ESSENCE Study Group. Phase 3 Trial of Semaglutide in Metabolic Dysfunction-Associated Steatohepatitis. N Engl J Med. 2025;392(21):2089-99.

age of 35 years, exemplify the role of precision medicine—genetic identification allows targeted therapies like sulfonylureas (SUs) instead of insulin for mutations in *HNF1A* or *KCNJ11C.*[4] T2DM comprises 90–95% of cases and arises from interplay between genetic susceptibility, insulin resistance, β-cell failure, obesity, and modifiable factors like diet and exercise.[5] Genome-wide association studies (GWAS) have identified over 400 genetic loci associated with T2DM risk, clustering into pathways involving insulin secretion, lipid metabolism, and inflammation.[6] However, the lack of a meaningful application of this knowledge to improve care of patients epitomizes the challenges with precision medicine.

The American Diabetes Association (ADA) and European Association for the Study of Diabetes (EASD) Precision Medicine in Diabetes Initiative (PMDI), initiated in 2018, has issued consensus reports advocating for evidence-based subtyping and individualized therapies.[7] These include staging presymptomatic T1DM based on autoantibody presence and using clinical clusters in T2DM to forecast complications and therapeutic responses. At this time precision medicine includes multiomics integration (genomics, transcriptomics, proteomics, metabolomics, and microbiomics) and artificial intelligence (AI) for risk stratification and pharmacogenomics to reduce adverse effects.[8,9] For physicians, this entails incorporating genetic testing, biomarkers, and wearable technologies into practice to achieve patient-centered care, while navigating challenges such as data privacy, access, and equity.[10]

Although promising, precision medicine's adoption varies. Monogenic diabetes routinely benefits from genetic diagnostics, but polygenic conditions like T2DM require expansive datasets for accurate predictions.[11] In India, precision medicine initiatives are gaining traction with studies highlighting state-wise variations in diabetes incidence (e.g., higher in southern states like Tamil Nadu) and calls for integrated approaches addressing malnutrition-related diabetes, which affects underserved populations. This chapter delves into genetic subtyping, pharmacogenomics, biomarkers, personalized therapies, challenges, and future prospects, grounded in current evidence to inform clinical practice.

GENETIC FACTORS AND SUBTYPING OF DIABETES

Genetic underpinnings are central to precision diabetes medicine, facilitating subtyping that enhances risk evaluation, diagnosis, and management. GWAS and next-generation sequencing have illuminated variants clustering into key pathways: β-cell function, insulin resistance, obesity, lipodystrophy, and liver/lipid metabolism.[12]

In T1DM, genetics explain approximately 50% heritability with T1DM-GRS (>50 loci, including HLA-DR3/DR4) offering >80% diagnostic sensitivity.[13] This aids differentiation from T2DM in equivocal cases, like obese adolescents or lean seniors, cutting misdiagnosis by 5–15%.[14] T1DM staging employs GRS to pinpoint rapid progressors for trials of immunomodulators like teplizumab, delaying onset by 2–3 years.[15]

Monogenic diabetes exemplifies precision genetics with variants in *HNF1A Maturity-Onset Diabetes of the Young 3 (MODY3)*, *HNF4A (MODY1)*, and glucokinase (GCK) (MODY2) directing therapy: SUs for *HNF1A*, observation for mild GCK-MODY, and surveillance for syndromic *HNF1B* (renal cysts). In neonates <6 months, testing uncovers >80% monogenic etiology, enabling SU switch from insulin.[16] Tools like MODY probability calculators, factoring age, family history, and biomarkers, guide NGS selection, making precision medicine cost effective in the pediatric population.[17] In GDM, noninvasive fetal genotyping for GCK-MODY adjusts maternal targets to avert macrosomia.

In T2DM, over 350 loci account for 10–20% of heritability with variants like *TCF7L2 (rs7903146)* prominently linked to β-cell impairment. Ethnic differences are known; for instance, African-ancestry-specific loci such as *ZRANB3* affect β-cell mass, while South Asian cohorts exhibit heightened risk from PPARG and FTO variants.[18] The cluster approach to T2DM subtyping, pioneered by Ahlqvist et al. in 2018, is the sheet anchor of precision medicine inT2DM as it identifies distinct phenotypes with varying complication risks and treatment responses.[19] Data-driven clustering reveals subgroups like severe insulin-deficient diabetes (SIDD, elevated retinopathy risk), severe insulin-resistant diabetes (SIRD, high nephropathy risk), mild obesity-related diabetes (MOD), and mild age-related diabetes (MARD).[20] This has been subsequently extended to prediabetes, using clinical and aging/obesity-related clusters to predict progression, with high-risk groups (e.g., clusters associated with insulin resistance) benefiting from early interventions.[19]

In Middle Eastern biobanks, subtyping has implications for tailored therapies to slow complications, including sex differences and monogenic clustering.[21] Genetic partitioning complements this with polygenic risk scores (PRS) aggregated into global (gPRS) or partitioned (pPRS) forms. gPRS identifies individuals in the top 2.5% with 3.4-fold T2DM risk, while pPRS predicts pathway-specific progression, such as insulin resistance or early insulin dependence.[6] Cohorts like UK Biobank demonstrate PRS augmenting prediction beyond clinical variables, though performance wanes in non-European groups due to GWAS underrepresentation.[22] In India, cluster analyses reveal unique patterns with higher prevalence of lean T2DM necessitating adapted subtyping models.[23]

Genetic evaluation should be considered atypical cases (e.g., young nonobese onset) or with strong family histories using MODY calculators. While PRS are emerging for routine use, they excel in high-risk ethnicities such as Indians. AI integration promises refined subtyping.

PHARMACOGENOMICS AND PERSONALIZED DRUG THERAPY

Pharmacogenomics examines the genetic impact on antidiabetic drug responses, enabling tailored selection to optimize efficacy and minimize adverse reactions. In T2DM, where diverse agents are used, variants in *ADME* genes explain 30–50% of response variability.[24] *SLC22A1 (OCT1)* variants alter metformin (MF) efficacy (e.g., *rs622342* enhances response in some but not others). *ATM rs11212617* correlates with suboptimal glycemic control in Caucasians, while *TCF7L2 rs7903146* boosts response.[25] GWAS from cohorts like GoDARTS attribute 2–5% variance to these. Personalized dosing may aid 20–30% nonresponders. *CYP2C9* *2/*3 alleles reduce SU metabolism improving control but tripling hypoglycemia risk.[26] *KCNJ11 E23K* and *ABCC8 Ser1369Ala* amplify SU induced insulin secretion; *TCF7L2* reduces efficacy. Genotyping may help with dose tweaking in 8–10% of patients with risk alleles. *PPARG Pro12Ala* improves response to thiazolidinediones (20% greater HbA1c drop).[27] *NFATC2* variants have increased distal edema. *GLP1R rs6923761* predicts diminishing response to *GLP1RA*.[28] Clinically, pharmacogenetic panels can identify and enable early switching to more responsive therapies.

BIOMARKERS FOR DIAGNOSIS, PROGNOSIS, AND MONITORING

Diagnostic biomarkers including islet auto-antibodies (GAD, IA-2, and ZnT8) plus T1DM-GRS provide >90% PPV in T1DM.[29] In T2DM while C-peptide distinguishes subtypes, miRNAs (miR-200c and miR-155) can help to identify βcell dysfunction.[30] Renin-angiotensin markers for DKD guide therapy. Microbiota (butyrate-producers) and metabolites (SCFAs and TMAO) can identify dysbiosis and resistance.[31] Proteomic markers (fetuin-A, MASP) can help to predict chronic kidney disease (CKD)/cardiovascular disease (CVD) in prediabetes. Molecular sensors in wearables, such as sweat-based glucose monitors and multibiomarker trackers for lactate, pH, and electrolytes, enable noninvasive, continuous monitoring, improving early detection of hyperglycemia and heart complications.

PERSONALIZED TREATMENT APPROACHES AND TECHNOLOGIES

Subtyping and predictive responses can personalize treatment. AI approaches have been used to predict responses to *GLP1RA* and sodium-glucose cotransporter-2 inhibitors (SGLT-2i). Wearables and molecular sensors revolutionize precision with sensors tracking multiple biomarkers (e.g., glucose and cortisol) facilitating real-time adjustments; these appear to reduce hospitalizations by 20–30% in trials.[32]

RESEARCH AND EVIDENCE GAPS

Despite substantial advances, precision medicine in diabetes encounters profound research and evidence gaps that impede its full clinical translation and widespread adoption. These gaps span data quality, study design, population diversity, and integration of multifaceted factors, ultimately constraining the ability to deliver equitable, patient-centered care. A primary concern is the predominance of low-quality evidence, characterized by retrospective analyses, small sample sizes, and inconsistent reporting standards with few studies prospectively designed to test precision hypotheses.[33] For instance, while GWAS have identified numerous loci, their clinical utility remains limited due to incomplete heritability explanations (missing heritability phenomenon) and inadequate validation in real-world settings. Replication across ancestries is particularly deficient with over 90% of genetic studies focused on European populations, leading to biased polygenic risk scores that underperform in African, Asian, and Hispanic groups, exacerbating health disparities.[34]

Subtype-specific gaps are evident across diabetes forms. In monogenic diabetes, challenges include variant pathogenicity assessment, long-term genetic counseling efficacy, and understanding extrapancreatic manifestations, such as neurological or renal involvement in certain syndromes. For GDM, evidence is sparse on genetic influences, modifiable biomarkers (e.g., lifestyle-integrated omics), and head-to-head comparisons of therapeutic agents, hindering personalized prevention and interventions to prevent progression to T2DM.[35] T1DM research reveals deficiencies in prespecified subgroup analyses within immunomodulatory trials, diverse cohort representation for diagnostic algorithms, and prognostic models incorporating environmental triggers like viral exposures. In T2DM, reliance on post-hoc cluster stratifications and modest biomarker evidence (e.g., limited RCTs validating multiomics panels) necessitate larger, powered prospective trials and meta-analyses to confirm clinical benefits, such as reduced complication rates or cost savings. Cross-cutting gaps involve insufficient integration of social determinants of health (SDoH), such as socioeconomic status and access to care, alongside dynamic metabolic fluctuations (e.g., time-varying omics data) and establishing causal links between biomarkers and outcomes via Mendelian randomization or functional studies.[36] Disparities further amplify these issues with underrepresented minorities and low-income populations comprising <20% of genetic datasets, resulting in inequitable tools like PRS that may perpetuate poorer T1DM and T2DM outcomes in these groups.

Opportunities to bridge these gaps include innovative trial designs (e.g., adaptive or basket trials), machine learning for refined subphenotyping, and global collaborations for ancestry-inclusive validation, benchmarking against current standards like ADA guidelines.[37] Proposed milestones by 2030 encompass establishing diverse biobanks, regulatory frameworks for precision tools, and cost-effectiveness studies.

In resource-limited settings, such as low- and middle-income countries (LMICs) where over 80% of the global diabetes burden resides, precision medicine offers transformative potential but grapples with amplified barriers. Research output remains disproportionately low with only 0.02 studies per 1,000 disability-adjusted life years (DALYs) in sub-Saharan Africa compared to 0.95 in North America, restricting generalizability and innovation.[38] Barriers encompass financial constraints (e.g., high costs of genetic testing), data deficiencies from Eurocentric studies (leading to inapplicable PRS), sociocultural factors (e.g., stigma around genetic counseling), and infrastructural deficits for omics technologies or digital health integration. For example, in LMICs, limited access to advanced diagnostics results in underdiagnosis of monogenic forms, while heterogeneous T2DM presentations (e.g., lean phenotypes in Asia and Africa) are poorly addressed by existing models. Enablers include task-shifting to community health workers for screening, repurposing existing infrastructures from infectious disease programs (e.g., HIV biobanks for diabetes genomics), and adopting cost-effective, leapfrog technologies like mobile-based AI for risk prediction using routine clinical data. Prioritizing LMIC-led data generation, capacity building, and equity monitoring through global partnerships can mitigate disparities, ensuring precision medicine extends benefits to high-burden regions and aligns with sustainable development goals.

CONCLUSION

I have tried to explore the paradigm of precision medicine in diabetes, highlighting its role in subtyping through genetics and clusters, pharmacogenomics for drug personalization, biomarkers for diagnosis and monitoring, and technologies like wearables for treatment optimization. Challenges encompass testing access, privacy, ethnic biases. Precision medicine is poised to revolutionize diabetes through tailored, evidence-driven strategies, poised to alleviate global and India-specific burdens.

REFERENCES

1. IDF Diabetes Atlas. (2024). Diabetes Atlas. [online] Available from https://diabetesatlas.org/ [Last accessed Oct. 2025].
2. Sun H, Saeedi P, Karuranga S, Pinkepank M, Ogurtsova K, Duncan BB, et al. IDF Diabetes Atlas: Global, regional and country-level diabetes prevalence estimates for 2021 and projections for 2045. Diabetes Res Clin Pract. 2022;183:109119.
3. Tosur M, Onengut-Gumuscu S, Redondo MJ. Type 1 diabetes genetic risk scores: History, application and future directions. Curr Diab Rep. 2025;25:22.
4. Gonçalves J, Ferreira HU, Ribeiro S, Fernandes da Rocha D, Souto SB, Pedro J, et al. Challenges in diagnosis and treatment of KCNJ11-MODY. Endocrinol Diabetes Metab Case Rep. 2024;2024:e240048.
5. Elksnis A, Martinell M, Eriksson O, Espes D. Heterogeneity of metabolic defects in type 2 diabetes and its relation to reactive oxygen species and alterations in beta-cell mass. Front Physiol. 2019;10:107.
6. Suzuki K, Hatzikotoulas K, Southam L, Taylor HJ, Yin X, Lorenz KM, et al. Genetic drivers of heterogeneity in type 2 diabetes pathophysiology. Nature. 2024;627(8003):347-57.
7. Chung WK, Erion K, Florez JC, Hattersley AT, Hivert MF, Lee CG, et al. Precision Medicine in diabetes: A Consensus Report from the American Diabetes Association (ADA) and the European Association for the Study of diabetes (EASD). Diabetes Care. 2020;43:1617-35.
8. Asif HM, Nawaz A, Daniyal M. Editorial: Changing trends of precision medicine in diabetes. Front Med (Lausanne). 2025;12:1499934.
9. Franceschi R. Precision medicine in diabetes, current research and future perspectives. J Pers Med. 2022;12:1233.
10. Walter JR, Xu S, Rogers JA. From lab to life: how wearable devices can improve health equity. Nat Commun. 2024;15:123.

11. Murray Leech J, Beaumont RN, Arni AM, Chundru VK, Sharp LN, Colclough K, et al. Common genetic variants modify disease risk and clinical presentation in monogenic diabetes. Nat Metab. 2025;7:1819-29.
12. Kim H, Westerman KE, Smith K, Chiou J, Cole JB, Majarian T, et al. High-throughput genetic clustering of type 2 diabetes loci reveals heterogeneous mechanistic pathways of metabolic disease. Diabetologia. 2023;66:495-507.
13. Luckett AM, Oram RA, Deutsch AJ, Ortega HI, Fraser DP, Ashok K, et al. Utility of genetic risk scores in type 1 diabetes. Diabetologia. 2023;66:1589-600.
14. Ciężki S, Kurpiewska E, Bossowski A, Głowińska-Olszewska B. Multi-faceted influence of obesity on type 1 diabetes in children—from disease pathogenesis to complications. Front Endocrinol (Lausanne). 2022;13:890833.
15. Goldman JD, Choi H. Teplizumab: The first treatment to delay the progression of type 1 diabetes. Clin Diabetes. 2023;41:474-6.
16. Poon SWY, Chung BHY, Tsang MHY, Tung JYL. Successful transition from insulin to sulphonylurea in a child with neonatal diabetes mellitus diagnosed beyond six months of age due to C42R mutation in the KCNJ11 gene. Clin Pediatr Endocrinol. 2022;31:168-71.
17. da Silva Santos T, Fonseca L, Santos Monteiro S, Borges Duarte D, Martins Lopes A, Couto de Carvalho A, et al. MODY probability calculator utility in individuals' selection for genetic testing: Its accuracy and performance. Endocrinol Diabetes Metab. 2022;5:e00332.
18. Yaghootkar H, Whitcher B, Bell JD, Thomas EL. Ethnic differences in adiposity and diabetes risk—insights from genetic studies. J Intern Med. 2020;288:271-83.
19. Ahlqvist E, Storm P, Käräjämäki A, Martinell M, Dorkhan M, Carlsson A, et al. Novel subgroups of adult-onset diabetes and their association with outcomes: a data-driven cluster analysis of six variables. Lancet Diabetes Endocrinol. 2018;6:361-9.
20. Schrader S, Perfilyev A, Ahlqvist E, Groop L, Vaag A, Martinell M, et al. Novel subgroups of type 2 diabetes display different epigenetic patterns that associate with future diabetic complications. Diabetes Care. 2022;45:1621-30.
21. Al-Thani NM, Zaghlool SB, Toor SM, Abou-Samra AB, Suhre K, Albagha OME. Subtyping of type 2 diabetes from a large Middle Eastern biobank: Implications for precision medicine. Mol Metab. 2025;99:102195.
22. UK Biobank. (2025). From Bias to Balance: Adapting PRS Models to Non-European Populations Using Transfer Learning. [online] Available from https://www.ukbiobank.ac.uk/projects/from-bias-to-balance-adapting-prs-models-to-non-european-populations-using-transfer-learning/ [Last accessed Oct. 2025].
23. Menon R, Khan N, Charugulla S, Bassi A, Dangare P, Dedaniya A, et al. Validation of a genome-wide polygenic score for body mass index in South Asians. Front Genet. 2025;16:1603542.
24. Auwerx C, Sadler MC, Reymond A, Kutalik Z. From pharmacogenetics to pharmaco-omics: Milestones and future directions. HGG Adv. 2022;3:100100.
25. Fitipaldi H, Franks PW. Ethnic, gender and other sociodemographic biases in genome-wide association studies for the most burdensome non-communicable diseases: 2005-2022. Hum Mol Genet. 2023;32:520-32.
26. Feng Y, Mao G, Ren X, Xing H, Tang G, Li Q, et al. Ser1369Ala variant in sulfonylurea receptor gene *ABCC8* is associated with antidiabetic efficacy of gliclazide in Chinese type 2 diabetic patients. Diabetes Care. 2008;31:1939-44.
27. Della-Morte D, Palmirotta R, Rehni AK, Pastore D, Capuani B, Pacifici F, et al. Pharmacogenomics and pharmacogenetics of thiazolidinediones: role in diabetes and cardiovascular risk factors. Pharmacogenomics. 2014;15:2063-82.
28. Cui Y, Yao J, Qiu X, Guo C, Kong D, Dong J, et al. Comparative efficacy and safety of tirzepatide in Asians and non-Asians with type 2 diabetes mellitus: A systematic review and meta-analysis. Diabetes Ther. 2024;15:781-99.
29. Lampasona V, Petrone A, Tiberti C, Capizzi M, Spoletini M, di Pietro S, et al. Zinc transporter 8 antibodies complement GAD and IA-2 antibodies in the identification and characterization of adult-onset autoimmune diabetes: Non Insulin Requiring Autoimmune Diabetes (NIRAD) 4. Diabetes Care. 2010;33:104-8.
30. Ofori JK, Karagiannopoulos A, Nagao M, Westholm E, Ramadan S, Wendt A, et al. Human islet MicroRNA-200c is elevated in type 2 diabetes and targets the transcription factor ETV5 to reduce insulin secretion. Diabetes. 2022;71:275-84.
31. Cheng TY, Lee TW, Li SJ, Lee TI, Chen YC, Kao YH, et al. Short-chain fatty acid butyrate against TMAO activating endoplasmic-reticulum stress and PERK/IRE1-axis with reducing atrial arrhythmia. J Adv Res. 2025;73:549-60.
32. Liu Y, Su X, Fan P, Liu X, Pan Y, Ping J. Computationally-assisted wearable system for continuous cortisol monitoring. Sci Bull (Beijing). 2025;70:2004-13.
33. Guyatt GH, Oxman AD, Kunz R, Vist GE, Falck-Ytter Y, Schünemann HJ; GRADE Working Group. What

is 'quality of evidence' and why is it important to clinicians? BMJ. 2008;336:995-8.
34. Bogardus C. Missing heritability and GWAS utility. Obesity (Silver Spring). 2009;17:209-10.
35. Gu Y, Zheng H, Wang P, Liu Y, Guo X, Wei Y, et al. Genetic architecture and risk prediction of gestational diabetes mellitus in Chinese pregnancies. Nat Commun. 2025;16:4178.
36. Dhieb D, Anwardeen N, Velayutham D, Elrayess MA, Jithesh PV, Bastaki K. Harnessing pharmacomultiomics for precision medicine in diabetes: A comprehensive review. Biomedicines. 2025;13:447.
37. Daniells L, Mozgunov P, Barnett H, Bedding A, Jaki T. How to add baskets to an ongoing basket trial with information borrowing. Stat Methods Med Res. 2025;34:717-34.
38. Soniwala A, Kim S, Welkley J, Ho JC, Varghese JS. A large language model analysis of global inequities in precision medicine research on diabetes. Ann Epidemiol. 2025;109:25-30.

8 Achieving Type 2 Diabetes Remission—Weight Loss and Metabolic Surgery

Shashank R Joshi, Shambo Samrat Samajdar

ABSTRACT

Type 2 diabetes mellitus (T2DM) has traditionally been regarded as a progressive, lifelong condition; however, accumulating evidence now supports remission as a realistic therapeutic goal. Remission, defined by international consensus as normoglycemia without glucose-lowering medication, can be achieved through intentional weight loss, pharmacotherapy, and metabolic surgery. The pathophysiological basis for remission is anchored in improvements in insulin sensitivity, β-cell recovery, and adipose tissue remodeling. Evidence from landmark trials, such as Diabetes Remission Clinical Trial (DiRECT) and Systemic Therapy in Advancing or Metastatic Prostate Cancer: Evaluation of Drug Efficacy (STAMPEDE), underscores the role of weight reduction and bariatric procedures in both inducing and sustaining remission, with a 10–15% weight loss threshold consistently linked to robust outcomes. Comparative surgical data further highlight the superiority of Roux-en-Y gastric bypass over other procedures in achieving durable remission, especially in patients with early disease and preserved β-cell function. Predictive tools such as the Diabetes Remission Index (DRI) provide personalized estimates of remission likelihood, while emerging therapies—particularly glucagon-like peptide-1 (GLP-1) receptor agonists, dual gastric inhibitory polypeptide (GIP)/GLP-1 agonists, and combined pharmacological–surgical approaches—expand the therapeutic armamentarium. Nevertheless, challenges persist, including restricted access to surgery, socioeconomic and racial disparities, and patient and provider hesitancy. Sustaining remission demands integrated care models that incorporate multidisciplinary follow-up, digital health innovations, structured nutritional and physical activity programs, and psychological support. Looking ahead, the field is moving toward precision metabolic surgery, real-world registries, and artificial intelligence (AI)-driven personalized algorithms to ensure durable and equitable remission outcomes. Together, these advances signal a paradigm shift in T2DM management—from glucose control to disease modification.

Keywords: Type 2 diabetes mellitus, Remission, Weight loss, Metabolic surgery, GLP-1 receptor agonists.

INTRODUCTION

Conceptualizing Type 2 Diabetes Remission

The traditional view of type 2 diabetes mellitus (T2DM) as an inevitably progressive and lifelong disease has shifted significantly in recent years. Emerging evidence has established that remission of T2DM is not only possible but increasingly attainable through targeted interventions such as substantial weight loss and metabolic surgery. As a result, the therapeutic framework for T2DM is expanding to include remission as a realistic and measurable clinical goal.

The contemporary clinical definition of remission, supported by international consensus, refers to the maintenance of glycemic levels below the diagnostic thresholds for diabetes without the use of glucose-lowering medications. Specifically, complete remission is typically defined as achieving a glycated hemoglobin (HbA1c) below 6.5% and a fasting plasma glucose level under 126 mg/dL, sustained for a minimum of 3 months without pharmacological support. Partial remission refers to glycemic levels below the diabetic range but not within the normoglycemic range, also maintained without medications. When such remission is sustained for 5 years or longer, it is referred to as prolonged remission.[1]

These standardized definitions have enabled clinicians and researchers to better evaluate and monitor the efficacy of interventions aimed at reversing the metabolic dysfunction underlying T2DM, and they serve as a foundation for setting therapeutic goals beyond glycemic control alone.

Clinical Imperatives for Pursuing Remission

Prevention of Long-term Complications

Persistent hyperglycemia is a key driver of the vascular and metabolic complications associated with T2DM. Achieving remission has been associated with improvements in both microvascular and macrovascular outcomes. Reduction in glycemic exposure appears to alleviate the risk of complications such as retinopathy, nephropathy, neuropathy, cardiovascular disease, and stroke. Importantly, the potential to reverse or slow these processes is greatest when remission is achieved early in the disease course, when residual β-cell function and insulin sensitivity are more amenable to intervention.

In clinical practice, remission offers an opportunity not just for symptom control, but for genuine disease modification. By restoring glycemic regulation, even temporarily, the trajectory of long-term organ damage can be altered in a clinically meaningful way.

Enhancing Patient Quality of Life and Reducing Economic Burden

In addition to its clinical benefits, remission has significant psychosocial and economic advantages. Many individuals with T2DM face substantial treatment burdens, including daily glucose monitoring, complex medication regimens, dietary restrictions, and the psychological toll of chronic disease. Achieving remission can alleviate many of these burdens, leading to improved quality of life, reduced treatment fatigue, and greater psychological well-being.

From a healthcare systems perspective, T2DM represents a major contributor to direct and indirect healthcare expenditures. Costs related to medications, complications, hospitalizations, and lost productivity continue to escalate globally. Interventions that achieve sustained remission have the potential to reduce these costs by decreasing the need for pharmacologic therapy, limiting the incidence of complications, and decreasing healthcare utilization.[2]

Remission as a Therapeutic Target in Contemporary Diabetology

For endocrinologists and diabetologists, remission introduces a new paradigm in diabetes care. Rather than focusing exclusively on glucose control, clinical strategies can now be oriented toward inducing and sustaining a medication-free, normoglycemic state. Achieving this objective requires the integration of evidence-based modalities, including structured lifestyle interventions, antiobesity pharmacotherapy, and metabolic surgery.

Remission is most achievable in the early stages of the disease, particularly when insulin resistance and β-cell dysfunction have not progressed beyond reversibility. As such, early identification of candidates and timely implementation of remission-inducing therapies is essential.

Even in cases where permanent remission is not feasible, transient remission may still yield long-term reductions in complication risk.

Remission should therefore be considered a viable and desirable endpoint in the management of selected patients, particularly those with newly diagnosed T2DM, preserved pancreatic function, and obesity-related metabolic dysfunction. It demands a patient-centered, multidisciplinary approach and necessitates long-term follow-up to monitor for relapse and sustain health improvements.[2]

Taken together, these clinical, economic, and psychosocial imperatives as depicted in **Table 1** underscore the importance of integrating remission into modern diabetes care, thereby setting the stage for an in-depth exploration of the strategies—particularly intensive weight loss and metabolic surgery—that are most effective in achieving this therapeutic milestone.

TABLE 1: Summary of the rationale for targeting remission in type 2 diabetes mellitus (T2DM).

Dimension	*Clinical relevance*
Glycemic control	Restoration of normoglycemia without medications
Complication risk	Reduced incidence of microvascular and macrovascular complications
Quality of life	Improved physical and psychological well-being; reduced treatment burden
Health economics	Decreased long-term costs related to medications, complications, and hospitalizations
Preventive strategy	Opportunity to alter disease trajectory in early-stage T2DM

Source: Adapted from consensus interpretations and clinical findings summarized in the 2021 ADA/EASD report on T2DM remission and supported by DiRECT3 and STAMPEDE trial data.[4]

PATHOPHYSIOLOGICAL BASIS FOR REMISSION

The achievement of T2DM remission following weight loss or metabolic surgery is underpinned by several interrelated physiological improvements. These involve reversal or modulation of key pathogenic processes driving insulin resistance and β-cell dysfunction. The article presents compelling mechanistic insights that support the biological plausibility of remission, especially in the context of sustained weight loss and metabolic remodeling.

Improvement in Insulin Sensitivity

A cornerstone of T2DM remission is the enhancement of insulin sensitivity, particularly in hepatic and peripheral tissues. Weight loss and bariatric surgery rapidly reduce hepatic lipid accumulation, which leads to a marked improvement in hepatic insulin sensitivity within days. As liver fat content declines, there is a decrease in inappropriate hepatic glucose production—one of the early defects in T2DM.

Peripheral insulin sensitivity, especially in skeletal muscle, improves more gradually, often over several weeks. This is primarily mediated through reductions in ectopic fat, improvements in mitochondrial efficiency, and increased insulin-stimulated glucose uptake. These changes collectively reduce hyperglycemia and insulin demand.[5]

Beta-cell Rest and Recovery

Another central mechanism in diabetes remission is the partial restoration of β-cell function. Chronic hyperglycemia and lipotoxicity impose a substantial burden on pancreatic β-cells, leading to exhaustion and dedifferentiation. Both caloric restriction and metabolic surgery reduce this glucolipotoxic stress, allowing for β-cell "rest".

This rest is associated with recovery in first-phase insulin secretion, which is essential for postprandial glycemic control. In the context of early T2DM, β-cell plasticity enables partial functional recovery once the metabolic environment is normalized. This recovery is more robust in individuals with shorter diabetes duration, underscoring the importance of early intervention.[5]

Reduction in Adipose Tissue and Inflammatory Signals

Adipose tissue—especially visceral fat—plays a critical role in the development of insulin resistance and systemic inflammation. Substantial weight loss through diet or surgery reduces adipose mass, particularly in ectopic depots such as the liver, pancreas, and visceral compartment.

As adiposity declines, there is a corresponding reduction in the secretion of proinflammatory adipokines and cytokines [e.g., tumor necrosis factor-α (TNF-α) and interleukin-6 (IL-6)], and an increase in insulin-sensitizing factors such as adiponectin. This shift in adipokine profile contributes to improved insulin signaling and reduced systemic inflammation—both essential conditions for the restoration of normoglycemia.[6]

The qualitative remodeling of adipose tissue (e.g., improved vascularization, reduced hypoxia, and enhanced mitochondrial function) contributes to this metabolic improvement, beyond mere mass reduction.

These interconnected mechanisms—enhanced insulin sensitivity, restoration of β-cell function, and favorable remodeling of adipose tissue—collectively establish the biological foundation for achieving and sustaining remission of T2DM, particularly when initiated early in the disease course and supported by sustained metabolic interventions **(Table 2)**.

WEIGHT LOSS AS A THERAPEUTIC TARGET

The restoration of normoglycemia and potential remission of T2DM through intentional weight loss represents a paradigm shift in diabetes management. Unlike traditional pharmacotherapy aimed at glycemic control, therapeutic weight loss addresses the root metabolic dysfunction—namely, excess adiposity and its sequelae of insulin resistance and β-cell stress.

Evidence from Lifestyle Interventions: The DiRECT

The Diabetes Remission Clinical Trial (DiRECT) provides compelling evidence that structured weight management interventions can achieve sustained diabetes remission in primary care settings. In this landmark randomized controlled trial involving patients with <6 years' duration of T2DM, participants underwent a nonsurgical, calorie-restricted dietary intervention (825–853 kcal/day) followed by food reintroduction and long-term weight maintenance support.[3,7]

Key findings from DiRECT include:[3,7]

- At 12 months, *46%* of participants in the intervention group achieved diabetes remission (HbA1c < 6.5% without glucose-lowering medications).
- By 2 years, *36%* remained in remission. Among those who maintained a *weight loss ≥10 kg*, remission rates were over *80%*.
- In the 5-year extension study, participants who received continued low-intensity dietary support sustained a mean weight loss of *6.1 kg*

TABLE 2: Key pathophysiological mechanisms supporting remission.

Mechanism	***Pathophysiological reversal***
Insulin sensitivity	Improved hepatic and peripheral insulin action due to reduced ectopic fat and metabolic stress
Beta-cell recovery	Alleviation of glucolipotoxicity enables restoration of insulin secretion dynamics
Adipose tissue changes	Reduction in visceral and ectopic fat; decreased inflammatory cytokines; improved adipokine profile

and demonstrated higher rates of remission (34%) compared to those without continued support (12%).

- Notably, *participants maintaining ≥15 kg weight loss had remission rates exceeding 80% at years 1 and 2,* demonstrating a strong dose-response relationship between weight loss and glycemic remission.

These results confirm that dietary-induced weight loss, when supported with structured long-term follow-up, can serve as a potent and scalable intervention for T2DM remission—particularly in early disease and in patients not on insulin therapy.

Clinical Thresholds for Remission: The 10–15% Rule

A consistent theme across remission trials is the emergence of *10–15% body weight reduction* as a clinical threshold for achieving and sustaining remission:

- In DiRECT, individuals with ≥10% weight loss at 12 and 24 months had *remission rates of 73–81%,* with similar findings echoed in other large-scale lifestyle and bariatric cohorts.
- The *beneficial metabolic effects* of this weight loss are closely linked to reductions in liver and pancreatic fat, leading to improvements in hepatic insulin sensitivity and restoration of β-cell function.
- These thresholds have been increasingly adopted in *international guidelines* [e.g., American Diabetes Association (ADA), European Association for the Study of Diabetes (EASD), National Institute for Health and Care Excellence (NICE)] as *therapeutic targets* when aiming for remission, especially in patients with obesity and early-stage diabetes.

Importantly, even partial weight loss (<10%) confers metabolic benefits, but *remission is most robust and sustainable when weight loss exceeds 10–15% of baseline.* This reinforces the need for aggressive weight management strategies early in the treatment course of T2DM.[7]

Weight loss is not merely an adjunct in T2DM management but is now established as a *primary therapeutic modality* capable of reversing the disease in selected individuals.[8] As demonstrated in the DiRECT trial and corroborated by long-term data, achieving ≥10–15% weight loss through structured interventions is both effective and sustainable in primary care, positioning weight loss as a central target in the pursuit of diabetes remission.

METABOLIC SURGERY IN DIABETES REMISSION

Overview of Procedures

Metabolic surgery has emerged as a highly effective intervention for achieving T2DM remission in patients with obesity, primarily through mechanisms beyond weight loss, including hormonal modulation and improvement in insulin sensitivity. Several surgical procedures are currently employed, each varying in complexity, efficacy, and long-term outcomes:

- *Roux-en-Y gastric bypass (RYGB):* This procedure combines restrictive and malabsorptive mechanisms. It reduces stomach volume and reroutes the small intestine, which alters nutrient flow and enhances incretin hormone activity, contributing to early glycemic improvements independent of weight loss.
- *Sleeve gastrectomy (SG)*: It involves resecting the greater curvature of the stomach, significantly reducing gastric capacity. While it lacks the malabsorptive component, SG induces hormonal changes, including reduced ghrelin levels, contributing to appetite suppression and improved glucose metabolism.
- *Biliopancreatic diversion with duodenal switch (BPD-DS):* This is a more complex malabsorptive procedure that preserves pyloric function. It is associated with high rates of T2DM remission but also carries a greater risk of nutritional deficiencies.
- *Single anastomosis duodeno-ileal bypass with sleeve gastrectomy (SADI-S):* A more recent

modification, this procedure simplifies the duodenal switch (DS) by performing a single anastomosis, aiming to reduce complications while retaining metabolic efficacy.

Recent high-quality comparative studies have reinforced the superior efficacy of *RYGB* in achieving sustained *T2DM remission* relative to *SG*. A 2025 systematic review and meta-analysis by *Delgado et al.*, which included nine randomized trials with over 5 years of follow-up, demonstrated that RYGB resulted in significantly greater long-term excess weight loss and higher T2DM remission rates compared to SG. Although HbA1c reductions were similar between groups, RYGB offered additional benefits such as greater resolution of gastroesophageal reflux disease (GERD) symptoms—albeit with a higher incidence of late major complications.[9]

Complementing these findings, a multicenter retrospective cohort study by *Ghusn et al.* (2025) specifically evaluated patients with T2DM and diabetes-related vascular complications. The analysis revealed that RYGB was significantly more effective than SG in achieving remission, particularly among individuals with *microvascular complications*, where the odds of remission were nearly three times higher with RYGB [odds ratio (OR) 2.95]. These results underscore the importance of patient stratification and suggest that RYGB may offer a metabolic advantage in complex patient populations.[10]

Long-term Outcomes

Long-term data have increasingly emphasized the durability and limitations of diabetes remission following metabolic surgery. In a 10-year observational cohort study involving 95 individuals with T2DM, complete remission was observed in 30% of patients, with an additional 15% achieving partial remission. Importantly, 24% of those who had achieved initial remission experienced relapse over the decade-long follow-up period.

Patients with better preoperative glycemic control (lower HbA1c and fasting plasma glucose), shorter diabetes duration, and reduced reliance on antidiabetic medications were more likely to sustain long-term remission. Logistic regression analysis identified preoperative HbA1c and the number of antidiabetic agents as significant predictors of durable remission (OR 0.50 and 0.31, respectively; $p < 0.05$).

Despite some cases of relapse, patients who did not achieve formal remission still experienced significant and sustained improvements in glycemic control and medication burden over the 10-year period. Only 2% of the cohort required insulin therapy at 10 years, compared to 14% at baseline, reflecting substantial metabolic benefit beyond remission alone.[11]

These data reinforce the concept that metabolic surgery should not be deferred until late-stage T2DM. Early surgical intervention, ideally in patients with preserved β-cell function and minimal pharmacological burden, optimizes the potential for remission and long-term metabolic stability.

PREDICTORS OF REMISSION

Clinical and Biochemical Predictors

The likelihood of achieving remission of T2DM following weight loss or metabolic surgery is strongly influenced by patient-specific factors. Consistently reported predictors include:

- *Age:* Younger patients exhibit higher remission rates, largely due to preserved β-cell reserve and lower cumulative metabolic stress.
- *Duration of diabetes:* A shorter disease duration (<5 years) is among the most robust predictors of remission. For example, individuals with diabetes duration <4 years may achieve remission rates exceeding 90% after bariatric surgery, compared with <50% in those with longer-standing disease.
- *Baseline C-peptide:* Higher fasting and stimulated C-peptide levels, reflecting residual endogenous insulin secretion, are associated with improved remission likelihood.

- *Body mass index (BMI):* Higher baseline BMI and greater absolute weight loss correlate with higher remission rates, though remission can also occur in patients with BMI <35 kg/m^2.
- *Triglycerides and lipid profile:* Elevated baseline triglycerides and features of dyslipidemia are linked to lower remission probability, reflecting greater insulin resistance and metabolic derangement.

These predictors converge on the principle that remission is most feasible in patients with preserved β-cell function, shorter disease duration, and modifiable obesity-related metabolic dysfunction.[12]

Diabetes Remission Index

To improve individual risk stratification, *Ghusn et al. (2025)* developed and validated the *Diabetes Remission Index (DRI)*—a novel prognostic model designed to predict remission before and after metabolic procedures. The DRI incorporates key preoperative variables, including:

- Vascular disease burden
- Number of diabetes medications
- Insulin use
- Duration of diabetes
- Baseline HbA1c
- Fasting glucose

In a cohort of 503 patients undergoing RYGB or SG, the DRI demonstrated high predictive accuracy [area under the curve (AUC) 0.80], with external validation in 409 patients (AUC 0.78). The model provides individualized remission probabilities prior to surgery.

An enhanced version, the *Weight Loss-Adjusted Diabetes Remission Index (W-DRI)*, integrates postsurgical weight loss into the calculation, further improving predictive accuracy (AUC 0.82). This adjustment recognizes the dose-response relationship between weight loss and remission—patients achieving >15–25% weight loss show the greatest likelihood of durable remission.

Importantly, both models are accessible as an *online calculator* via the Mayo Clinic (https://newsnetwork.mayoclinic.org/dri-calculator/), enabling clinicians to incorporate evidence-based prognostic estimates into preoperative counseling and shared decision-making.[13]

Predicting diabetes remission requires careful assessment of both *clinical predictors* (age, diabetes duration, β-cell function, BMI, and lipid profile) and *validated prognostic tools* such as the DRI and W-DRI. These instruments provide practical, individualized estimates of remission probability and highlight the critical interplay between disease biology and treatment-induced weight loss. Their integration into clinical pathways **(Table 3)** offers a step toward *precision diabetology*, ensuring that metabolic surgery and intensive interventions are targeted to patients most likely to benefit.

CHALLENGES AND BARRIERS

Despite growing evidence that remission of T2DM is achievable through substantial weight loss, pharmacological advances, and metabolic surgery, several critical barriers prevent its broad adoption in clinical practice.

Access to Surgery

Although metabolic surgery provides the most durable remission outcomes, access remains limited. Insurance coverage and healthcare policy often restrict surgery to individuals with a BMI ≥ 40 kg/m^2 or ≥35 kg/m^2 with comorbidities, despite evidence showing remission is possible in patients with BMI as low as 30 kg/m^2. In publicly funded systems, long waiting lists delay intervention, reducing the likelihood of remission since early surgery is more effective. Additionally, lack of infrastructure, accredited surgical centers, and structured postoperative care further constrain access, particularly in low- and middle-income countries.

Socioeconomic and Racial Disparities

Socioeconomic inequality profoundly shapes who can benefit from remission-inducing therapies. Individuals from disadvantaged backgrounds are less likely to access specialized obesity and diabetes care, face financial constraints in

TABLE 3: Predictors of remission versus relapse in type 2 diabetes mellitus.

Category	*Predictors of remission*	*Predictors of relapse*
Demographics	Younger age	Older age
Disease duration	Shorter duration (<4–5 years)	Longer duration (≥5–10 years)
Beta-cell function	Higher baseline C-peptide; preserved first-phase insulin secretion	Low baseline C-peptide; poor β-cell reserve
Glycemic control	Lower preoperative HbA1c and fasting plasma glucose	Higher baseline HbA1c; long-standing hyperglycemia
Treatment intensity	Fewer medications; no insulin requirement	Preoperative insulin therapy; multiple antidiabetic agents
Anthropometry	Higher BMI with capacity for significant weight loss; ≥10–15% sustained weight reduction	Weight regain; insufficient early weight loss
Lipid/metabolic profile	Lower triglycerides; fewer features of metabolic syndrome	Hypertriglyceridemia; advanced metabolic syndrome
Complication burden	Absence of vascular complications; preserved microvascular function	Presence of micro- or macrovascular complications (especially nephropathy, neuropathy)
Surgical/intervention factors	Early surgery with robust postoperative support; durable weight loss	Late intervention; loss to follow-up; poor adherence to lifestyle changes

Key notes:

- *Weight loss magnitude* (>10–15% of body weight) is a critical threshold for remission, but *β-cell reserve* determines durability.
- *Diabetes Remission Index (DRI)* and *W-DRI* integrate many of these factors, offering personalized risk predictions.
- *Relapse risk* is strongly tied to poor *β*-cell function, insulin dependence, and weight regain, even after initial remission.

(BMI: body mass index; HbA1c: glycated hemoglobin; W-DRI: Weight Loss–Adjusted Diabetes Remission Index)

pursuing surgery, and often lack continuity of follow-up support. Racial disparities add a further layer of inequity: studies consistently report that Black and Hispanic patients are less likely than White patients to undergo bariatric/metabolic surgery, even after adjusting for eligibility and comorbidity profiles. Postoperative differences in remission rates may reflect both biological variation (e.g., β-cell reserve and adipose tissue distribution) and systemic inequities in long-term care.

Patient Reluctance and Provider Biases

Patient-level barriers also play a substantial role. Many individuals are reluctant to consider surgery due to fear of complications, concerns over permanent anatomical changes, or misconceptions that surgery is primarily cosmetic rather than therapeutic. At the same time, healthcare providers may contribute to underutilization. Some clinicians remain hesitant to refer eligible patients, influenced by outdated perceptions of surgical risk, limited training in obesity medicine, or unconscious biases regarding patient adherence and motivation. This results in a "treatment gap" where remission-capable interventions are under-discussed and under-offered.

The path toward widespread adoption of remission strategies for T2DM is hindered not only by clinical and biological variability but also by structural inequities, patient reluctance, and provider inertia. Overcoming these barriers requires *policy reform to broaden surgical eligibility and coverage, strategies to reduce socioeconomic and racial inequities, and improved provider education coupled with patient-centered*

The convergence of advanced technologies with personalized human care creates a scalable, patient-centered framework capable of addressing both biological and behavioral drivers of relapse. Such models represent the future of chronic disease management—shifting the paradigm from reactive treatment to proactive, sustained remission.

CONCLUSIONS AND FUTURE DIRECTIONS

The landscape of T2DM care is undergoing a profound transformation, shifting away from the traditional paradigm of *lifelong glucose management* toward a more ambitious goal of *disease modification through remission*. Evidence from weight loss interventions, pharmacological advances, and metabolic surgery has demonstrated that sustained remission is achievable in a significant proportion of patients—particularly when interventions are initiated early in the disease course and tailored to individual metabolic profiles. This evolving framework reframes T2DM from an inevitably progressive condition to a disease state with modifiable and, in some cases, reversible trajectories.

From Glucose Management to Disease Modification

The next era of diabetes care will emphasize interventions that *alter the natural history of the disease*, rather than simply controlling glycemia. Sustained weight loss, metabolic surgery, and incretin-based pharmacotherapies have proven capable of restoring insulin sensitivity, reducing glucolipotoxicity, and partially restoring β-cell function. The recognition of remission as a therapeutic target underscores the importance of *addressing underlying pathophysiology*, rather than managing hyperglycemia in isolation.

Precision Metabolic Surgery

As surgical techniques evolve, the field is moving toward *precision metabolic surgery*, where procedure selection is informed by patient-specific factors such as age, diabetes duration, β-cell reserve, adipose distribution, and vascular complications. Predictive tools such as the *DRI* and *W-DRI* represent the first steps toward personalized surgical algorithms, enabling clinicians to identify patients most likely to benefit from intervention while minimizing risk. In the future, integration of *genetic, metabolic, and digital health data* could refine surgical selection and long-term management, creating highly individualized care pathways.

Long-term Registries and Personalized Algorithms

A major limitation of current evidence is the relative paucity of *long-term, real-world outcome data* on remission durability, relapse predictors, and complication risk. Establishing *national and international registries* will be critical to monitoring outcomes, informing guidelines, and improving predictive algorithms. In parallel, advances in *AI* and *machine learning* will facilitate the development of personalized algorithms that integrate clinical, biochemical, genetic, and behavioral data to optimize therapy selection and maintenance strategies. Such approaches have the potential to enhance durability of remission while ensuring cost-effectiveness and equity in access.

CONCLUSION

The future of T2DM management lies in *integrated, personalized, and outcome-oriented strategies* that prioritize remission and long-term disease modification. By combining precision surgical approaches, advanced pharmacotherapies, digital health tools, and large-scale outcome registries, the next generation of diabetes care can move beyond glucose control to deliver durable metabolic health and prevent the long-term complications of diabetes. This shift has the potential to redefine the natural history of T2DM and transform patient lives on a global scale.

REFERENCES

1. Riddle MC, Cefalu WT, Evans PH, Gerstein HC, Nauck MA, Oh WK, et al. Consensus Report: Definition and Interpretation of Remission in Type 2 Diabetes. Diabetes Care. 2021;44(10):2438-44.
2. Rothberg A, Lean M, Laferrère B. Remission of type 2 diabetes: always more questions, but enough answers for action. Diabetologia. 2024;67(4):602-10.
3. Lean ME, Leslie WS, Barnes AC, Brosnahan N, Thom G, McCombie L, et al. Primary care-led weight management for remission of type 2 diabetes (DiRECT): an open-label, cluster-randomised trial. Lancet. 2018;391(10120):541-51.
4. Schauer PR, Bhatt DL, Kirwan JP, Wolski K, Aminian A, Brethauer SA, et al. Bariatric Surgery versus Intensive Medical Therapy for Diabetes - 5-Year Outcomes. N Engl J Med. 2017;376(7):641-51.
5. Yau B, Ghislain J, Kebede MA, Poitout V. The role of the beta cell in type 2 diabetes: new findings from the last 5 years. Diabetologia. 2025.
6. Marselli L, Piron A, Suleiman M, Colli ML, Yi X, Khamis A, et al. Persistent or Transient Human β Cell Dysfunction Induced by Metabolic Stress: Specific Signatures and Shared Gene Expression with Type 2 Diabetes. Cell Rep. 2020;33(9):108466.
7. Lean ME, Leslie WS, Barnes AC, Brosnahan N, Thom G, McCombie L, et al. 5-year follow-up of the randomised Diabetes Remission Clinical Trial (DiRECT) of continued support for weight loss maintenance in the UK: an extension study. Lancet Diabetes Endocrinol. 2024;12(4):233-46. Erratum in: Lancet Diabetes Endocrinol. 2024;12(6):e17.
8. Corrao S, Falcone F, Mirarchi L, Amodeo S, Calvo L. Type 2 Diabetes Mellitus Remission, Dream or Reality? A Narrative Review of Current Evidence and Integrated Care Strategies. Diabetes Ther. 2025;16(8):1557-79.
9. Monteiro Delgado L, Fabretina de Souza V, Fontel Pompeu B, de Moraes Ogawa T, Pereira Oliveira H, Sacksida Valladão VDC, et al. Long-Term Outcomes in Sleeve Gastrectomy versus Roux-en-Y Gastric Bypass: A Systematic Review and Meta-Analysis of Randomized Trials. Obes Surg. 2025;35(8):3246-57.
10. Ghusn W, Ma P, Ikemiya K, Salame M, Hage K, Mosleh KA, et al. Comparative effectiveness of Roux-en-Y gastric bypass and sleeve gastrectomy in achieving diabetes remission in patients with diabetes-related vascular diseases: A multicentred study. Clin Obes. 2025;15(3):e12732.
11. Meira I, Menino J, Ferreira P, Leite AR, Gonçalves J, Ferreira HU, et al. Diabetes Remission After Bariatric Surgery: A 10-Year Follow-Up Study. Obes Surg. 2025;35(1):161-9.
12. Akkus G, Tetiker T. Which predictors could effect on remission of type 2 diabetes mellitus after the metabolic surgery: A general perspective of current studies? World J Diabetes. 2021;12(8):1312-24.
13. Ghusn W, Ma P, Vierkant RA, Mundi M, Fehervari M, Ikemiya K, et al. The Diabetes Remission Index (DRI): A Novel Prognostic Calculator Model Predicting Diabetes Remission Before and After Metabolic Procedures. Ann Surg. 2025.
14. Ghusn W, Anazco D, Fansa S, Tama E, Cifuentes L, Gala K, et al. Weight loss outcomes with semaglutide based on diabetes severity using the individualized metabolic surgery score. EClinicalMedicine. 2024;72:102625.
15. Al Qassab M, Mneimneh M, Jradi A, Derbas B, Dabboussi D, Khoury Baini J, et al. The expanding role of GLP-1 receptor agonists: advancing clinical outcomes in metabolic and mental health. Curr Issues Mol Biol. 2025;47(4):285.
16. Alkhouri N, Charlton M, Gray M, Noureddin M. The pleiotropic effects of glucagon-like peptide-1 receptor agonists in patients with metabolic dysfunction-associated steatohepatitis: a review for gastroenterologists. Expert Opin Investig Drugs. 2025;34(3):169-95.
17. Pantalone KM, Xiao H, Bena J, Morrison S, Downie S, Boyd AM, et al. Type 2 diabetes pharmacotherapy de-escalation through AI-enabled lifestyle modifications: a randomized clinical trial. NEJM Catal Innov Care Deliv. 2025;6(9).
18. Shamanna P, Joshi S, Dharmalingam M, Vadavi A, Keshavamurthy A, Shah L, et al. Digital Twin in Managing Hypertension Among People With Type 2 Diabetes: 1-Year Randomized Controlled Trial. JACC Adv. 2024;3(9):101172.
19. Rein M, Ben-Yacov O, Godneva A, Shilo S, Zmora N, Kolobkov D, et al. Effects of personalized diets by prediction of glycemic responses on glycemic control and metabolic health in newly diagnosed T2DM: a randomized dietary intervention pilot trial. BMC Med. 2022;20(1):56.
20. Nakao M, Shirotsuki K, Sugaya N. Cognitive-behavioral therapy for management of mental health and stress-related disorders: Recent advances in techniques and technologies. Biopsychosoc Med. 2021;15(1):16.

9 Artificial Intelligence-driven Diabetes Care: Predictive Analytics and Personalized Interventions

Amit Kumar Dey, Avneesh Khare

ABSTRACT

Diabetes mellitus remains a major global health challenge, and traditional population-level, intermittently measured care models often fail to deliver truly individualized outcomes. This chapter reviews how artificial intelligence (AI) and machine learning (ML) are reshaping diabetes care by enabling predictive, proactive, and personalized management across the continuum—from risk stratification and early detection to real-time therapeutic optimization. It summarizes AI-based predictive analytics (including multimodal models that integrate clinical, lifestyle, and -omics data), and highlights the need for robust calibration, external validation, and bias mitigation to ensure safe generalization across diverse populations. The chapter discusses clinical validation and implementation in key domains such as diabetic retinopathy screening, AI-integrated continuous glucose monitoring (CGM), AI-supported insulin clinical decision support systems, and automated insulin delivery (AID), with evidence from trials and real-world datasets demonstrating improvements in time-in-range, HbA1c, hypoglycemia, and engagement. It also covers digital health and telemedicine platforms, ethical and regulatory considerations (privacy, transparency, fairness), health economics, and practical workflow integration challenges. Finally, future directions—including digital twins, noninvasive sensing, and explainable, equitable AI—are outlined as priorities for next-generation diabetes care.

Keywords: Artificial intelligence, Machine learning, Diabetes mellitus, Predictive analytics, Risk prediction, Continuous glucose monitoring, Automated insulin delivery/closed-loop systems, Clinical decision support systems, Digital health and telemedicine, Algorithmic bias and fairness, Explainable AI, Cost-effectiveness, Digital twins.

INTRODUCTION

Diabetes mellitus continues to pose significant challenges to global health, with rising prevalence leading to increased morbidity, mortality, and healthcare costs. Traditional models of diabetes care, dependent on population-level recommendations and intermittent data gathering, have struggled to optimize outcomes for individuals in increasingly diverse populations. The emergence of artificial intelligence (AI) and machine learning (ML) technologies within the field of diabetology heralds a new era, enabling clinicians to harness complex, multidimensional datasets for individualized prediction, monitoring, and intervention.

Artificial intelligence-driven approaches encompass predictive analytics capable of identifying at-risk individuals long before overt clinical disease, facilitating precise diagnosis of complications like retinopathy and deploying personalized interventions for glucose management using real-time systems. ML models and adaptive algorithms are now central to strategies such as continuous glucose monitoring (CGM), closed-loop (automated) insulin delivery, and digital remote care. As a result, diabetes management is shifting from reactive to proactive, personalized, and data-driven. This chapter provides an up-to-date, comprehensive review of the science, clinical validation, implementation, ethical considerations, and future directions of AI-powered diabetes care, drawing on peer-reviewed literature from the year 2022 to 2025.

ARTIFICIAL INTELLIGENCE -BASED PREDICTIVE ANALYTICS IN DIABETES CARE

Predictive Model Development and Performance

Artificial intelligence has revolutionized diabetes care by empowering clinicians to identify individuals at high risk for diabetes early in the disease process. ML models can synthesize complex risk factor combinations—including clinical, lifestyle, genomic, and metabolomic variables—to deliver nuanced predictions of diabetes onset and progression. Most modern AI-based type 2 diabetes (T2D) risk prediction models report excellent discriminative performance, with areas under the receiver-operating characteristic curve (AUC) in the 0.80–0.96 range.[1] Multimodal approaches that leverage diverse data sources, including genomics, metabolomics, and clinical variables, significantly outperform unimodal models. For instance, one study found that a model integrating genomic, metabolomic, and clinical data achieved an AUC of 0.96—markedly higher than the 0.586 AUC obtained when using genomics alone.[1]

A study from Nigeria demonstrated the efficacy of a model built from clinical symptoms and biochemical markers, producing an extraordinary 99% AUC (95% CI 97–100%) in the training set and a 94% AUC (95% CI 89–99%) in the test set, across 444 participants.[2] These robust performances indicate that AI can surpass traditional scoring systems in detecting undiagnosed cases or pinpointing high-risk individuals. Beyond static models, adaptive AI techniques—such as reinforcement learning algorithms such as RL-DITR—are gaining traction. These adaptive approaches dynamically interact with patient data, learning optimal intervention strategies over time to optimize insulin management and other therapies.[3]

Clinical Validation and Real-world Performance

For predictive analytics technologies to make an impact in clinical care, validation in diverse, real-world populations is essential. One standout area is diabetic retinopathy (DR) screening, where AI algorithms have been deployed across large-scale cohorts, screening over 251,000 individuals and demonstrating both high sensitivity and cost-effectiveness. In China, Japan, and Australia, AI-based retinal image analysis proved reliable for identifying referable DR, with benefits extending to reduced workload for ophthalmologists and consistent cost-effectiveness as measured against regional willingness-to-pay thresholds.[4]

Continuous glucose monitoring presents another sphere where AI excels. For example, the CGM froster system utilizes a transformer-based AI architecture to perform self-supervised learning on large, longitudinal CGM datasets, revealing highly individualized glucose dynamics that traditional statistical methods might miss.[5] Real-world impact is further evident in community settings: In rural India, an AI algorithm guided an SMS-based educational program targeting prediabetic individuals, resulting in an 18% improvement in fasting glucose (compared to controls) **(Table 1)**.[6]

TABLE 1: Artificial intelligence-driven diabetic retinopathy (DR) screening outcomes.[4]

Country	*Population screened*	*Sensitivity (%)*	*Cost-effectiveness*
China	120,000	95.2	Cost-saving
Japan	90,000	98.3	Below WTP threshold
Australia	41,000	94.7	Effective

(WTP: willingness-to-pay)

Implementation Challenges and Solutions

While predictive analytics bring promise, several implementation challenges remain. Chief among these is algorithmic bias and insufficient external validation. A systematic review found that only 5 of 40 published AI diabetes models provided calibration insights; only 5 had undergone external validation.[5] This is crucial for generalizability and safety in broad populations. Solutions such as federated learning—where models are trained collaboratively without exchanging raw patient data—are emerging as privacy-preserving ways to reduce bias and improve robustness.[6]

The economics of implementation pose another challenge. In low- and middle-income countries (LMICs), device costs can be prohibitive: CGM sensors may cost $300–1,000 each, while standard diabetes care in Nepal averages only $23 per patient per 6 months.[6] Thus, economic modeling and local optimization are necessary for AI technologies to achieve widespread adoption and equitable benefit.

CONTINUOUS GLUCOSE MONITORING WITH ARTIFICIAL INTELLIGENCE INTEGRATION

Real-time Data Analytics and Personalization

Integration of AI with CGM devices is shaping a new era of diabetes management. AI-enabled CGM platforms, such as Dexcom G7, have demonstrated real-world efficacy—patients with T2D (not on insulin) have shown significant improvements in time-in-range (TIR) and reductions in glycated hemoglobin (HbA1c) over 12-month follow-ups.[7] Deep learning algorithms can now analyze CGM data to not only identify episodes of dysglycemia but also model the specific impacts of foods and physical activity, providing truly personalized recommendations.[8]

State-of-the-art models incorporate dietary logs, activity trackers, and even contextual factors (illness, stress, and sleep quality), producing individualized behavioral guidance. Explainable AI research has allowed both clinicians and patients to interpret why specific glucose excursions occur and the predicted effect of various interventions.[9]

Clinical Outcomes and Effectiveness

Multiple randomized trials illustrate the effectiveness of AI-enhanced CGM. In Rwanda, a trial in type 1 diabetes (T1D) patients paired CGM with AI-driven personalized education; results included a clear increase in TIR and reduction in HbA1c compared to standard care.[10] Among 118 adults with T2D (not using insulin), provision of CGM with an AI digital therapeutic platform led to multiple improvements—greater TIR, lower average glucose, and remarkable weight loss over the study period.[11]

Comparative studies of real-time CGM (rtCGM) versus Intermittently scanned CGM (isCGM) (flash monitoring) reveal a distinct advantage for continuous approaches. rtCGM users experienced, on average, 5.6% higher TIR and 1.28% less hypoglycemia than those using intermittently scanned devices.[12] This superior performance is attributed to instant alerts and

TABLE 2: AI-CGM impact on glycemic outcomes.

Study population	*Device and platform*	*TIR gain (%)*	*HbA1c reduction*	*Additional benefit*
T1D (Rwanda)[10]	CGM + AI education	12.1	–0.8	–
T2D (US)[11]	CGM + digital application	8.4	–0.5	Weight loss
T2D (EU)[12]	rtCGM vs. isCGM	5.6	–0.3	–1.3% hypoglycemia

(HbA1c: glycated hemoglobin; TIR: time-in-range; T1D: type 1 diabetes; T2D: type 2 diabetes)

seamless data streaming, permitting early corrective action, and avoiding undetected lows **(Table 2)**.

Integration with Automated Systems

Artificial intelligence-driven CGM systems are the backbone of modern closed-loop and semi-automated insulin delivery (AID) platforms. Integration frameworks process rtCGM data, trend predictions, and behavioral analytics to automate therapeutic adjustments.[13] Many systems now support cloud-based remote access and monitoring, enabling patients and providers to review data, adjust parameters, and enact preventive changes from anywhere in the world.[14,15] Notably, predictive algorithms built into CGM platforms can warn patients of impending hypoglycemia/hyperglycemia up to 30 minutes in advance, enhancing safety and peace of mind.[16]

REAL-TIME INSULIN THERAPY OPTIMIZATION

Artificial Intelligence Clinical Decision Support Systems

Several pivotal trials confirm the clinical value of AI-powered **clinical decision support systems** (CDSS) for insulin dosing. For example, the insulin clinical decision support system; TIR: time-in-range (iNCDSS) platform demonstrated noninferiority to physician-led management (n = 149 T2D patients): 76.4% TIR for AI-managed therapy versus 73.6% for physicians (95% CI 2.7–8.0%).[9] Physician acceptance was high, with 98.9% of AI recommendations adopted, interface clarity, time-saving, and safety rated highly.[9] Other studies found that AI/ML-driven insulin optimization led to statistically significant HbA1c reductions ($p < 0.05$) and improved patient satisfaction.[11]

Automated Insulin Delivery Performance

Meta-analyses of closed-loop AID systems (65 trials; n = 3,623 patients) reveal that AI-enabled therapy outperforms conventional treatment, yielding 11.7% higher TIR and notable improvement in glycemia risk index (–3.7 points, $p < 0.01$).[12] Dual-hormonal systems—deploying both insulin and glucagon—demonstrate even greater efficacy compared to hybrid systems, with more pronounced TIR gains.[13]

Real-world Implementation Results

In pragmatic studies, Tandem Control-IQ (n = 9,451 users) achieved median TIR of 73.6% after 1 year, with 94.2% automation mode use.[14] MiniMed 780G users (n = 13,461) regularly surpassed global consensus targets, maintaining TIR >75% in long-term follow-up.[15] Real-world Omnipod 5 data (69,902 users) show that median TIR varies by glucose setpoint but consistently exceeds baseline values **(Table 3)**.[17]

AUTOMATED INSULIN DELIVERY SYSTEMS CLINICAL OUTCOMES

Pivotal Clinical Trials and Randomized Controlled Trial Results

Randomized controlled trials of AID platforms demonstrate robust gains in glycemic metrics.

consent.[24,31] Explainable AI improves trust in recommendations; models now incorporate uncertainty measures so providers can assess reliability.[31]

HEALTH ECONOMICS AND COST-EFFECTIVENESS

Cost-effectiveness Analysis Frameworks

Cost-effectiveness frameworks are crucial to demonstrate the value of AI-driven interventions in diabetes care. Recent studies in Japan show AI-based diabetic retinopathy screening achieved an incremental cost-effectiveness ratio (ICER) of ¥1,598,244 per quality-adjusted life year (QALY) (≈$11,375), well below standard willingness-to-pay thresholds.[36] These results confirm that when models emphasize higher sensitivity, for example, 96.3%, they maximize clinical outcomes and cost-effectiveness, by enabling early identification and reducing resource consumption for late-stage complications. Comparative modeling across populations further highlights that the most cost-effective AI design, though not the most accurate, offers a trade-off between population-level health gains and incremental cost, evidenced by an additional 839 QALYs gained at marginal increases in cost over 30 years.[4]

Studies from Belgium have also evaluated ICERs for hybrid digital care pathways in T2D, revealing limited probability of cost-effectiveness at current national thresholds, but demonstrating improved resource optimization as prevalence increases or algorithms become more sophisticated.[37]

Economic Impact Assessment

The broader economic impact of AI in diabetes is increasingly favorable, particularly in resource-constrained settings. Studies demonstrate that mobile health applications and remote monitoring platforms, when enhanced by AI, markedly lower costs while improving outcomes by targeting major drivers of expenditure—early diagnosis, reduced admissions, and avoidance of severe complications.[37] Value-based reimbursement models, which reward providers for achieving superior outcomes rather than high service volumes, further extend the economic justification for digital transformation.[4]

In LMICs, these interventions allow reallocation of resources toward prevention and patient engagement, strengthening health system resilience, and equity. AI-driven telemedicine strategies also reduce travel costs and indirect economic burdens for patients, offering sustainable benefits even in geographically dispersed populations.[38]

IMPLEMENTATION CHALLENGES AND SOLUTIONS

Healthcare Professional Acceptance

Provider engagement is central for successful deployment of AI in diabetes. Surveys consistently find that while most practitioners recognize the promise of AI, concerns remain regarding usability for older adults, data privacy, and the transparency of decision-making algorithms.[24] Overcoming skepticism requires targeted education about technical principles, ethical issues, and practical benefits—efforts shown to raise trust and adoption rates across clinical settings.

For example, in the iNCDSS clinical support trial, the vast majority of clinicians (98.9%) adopted system recommendations, citing a user-friendly interface and demonstrated improvements in workflow efficiency and patient safety.[9] This acceptance is further encouraged when providers are involved from the design phase, ensuring the system meets real-world requirements.

Technical and Workflow Integration

Technical challenges are most acute at the intersection of digital health systems and clinical workflows. Integration with electronic health records (EHRs), reliability, interoperability, and the need for continuous information flow are persistent hurdles.[28] Modular design, support for federated learning, and iterative codesign with clinical teams help address these issues, ensuring that systems remain relevant, safe, and effective.

The most impactful AI CDSS strategies combine automated recommendation protocols with mechanisms for human oversight and feedback. This model allows clinicians to maintain ultimate responsibility for patient care, mitigates risks associated with incorrect or opaque algorithm outputs, and promotes shared medical decision making. Continuous education and system support for both front-line staff and patients further increase digital literacy and facilitate widespread implementation.[38,39]

FUTURE DIRECTIONS AND EMERGING TECHNOLOGIES

Artificial intelligence's role in diabetes care is set to grow in sophistication and breadth. The next generation of applications includes digital twins—virtual patient models constructed from longitudinal data, supporting predictive scenario modeling and real-time optimization of insulin and lifestyle interventions.[40] Noninvasive wearable CGMs, paired with advanced algorithms, will revolutionize glycemic monitoring and feedback.[41]

Artificial intelligence-powered collaborative platforms will enable interdisciplinary care, allowing seamless sharing of risk profiles and management strategies between clinicians, educators, and patients.[42] Real-world evidence will more closely bridge the gap between research efficacy and actual performance.

Key research priorities include equitable algorithm development, robust explainability, and multisite long-term studies. Interdisciplinary collaboration, including clinicians, technologists, and regulators, will be essential to serve diverse populations safely and ethically.[40] Digital twin clinics offer promising environments for iterative testing and addressing health disparities. As validation processes, regulatory agility, and education evolve, AI will increasingly augment clinical judgment, empower patients, and deliver best-in-class outcomes worldwide.[42]

CONCLUSION

The application of AI and ML in diabetes care has transformed the management paradigm from standardized protocols to patient-centered, predictive, and adaptive strategies. AI models have demonstrated superior accuracy in predicting diabetes onset, optimizing glycemic control, detecting complications, and guiding therapy tailored to individual needs. Clinical trials and real-world deployments reveal tangible improvements in outcomes such as TIR, reductions in hypoglycemia and HbA1c, and enhanced patient engagement.

However, implementation is not without challenges—algorithmic bias, regulatory complexity, data privacy, and institutional readiness require ongoing attention. Cost-effectiveness analyses and pragmatic real-world studies affirm the value of digital health and remote monitoring, especially as scalable solutions for diverse populations. As AI integration deepens, future directions include expansion of digital twins, noninvasive sensors, transparent and explainable algorithms, and equitable access worldwide.

Clinicians should embrace the critical role of AI not only as an adjunct but as an essential component of modern diabetes care, adopting responsible, evidence-based practices while remaining alert to ethical concerns. With continued interdisciplinary collaboration, AI-driven diabetes care offers the promise of better outcomes, improved quality of life, and a new standard for chronic disease management in the 21st century.

REFERENCES

1. Wang SCY, Nickel G, Venkatesh KP, Raza MM, Kvedar JC. AI-based diabetes care: risk prediction models and implementation concerns. NPJ Digit Med. 2024;7(1):36.
2. Ojurongbe TA, Afolabi HA, Oyekale A, Bashiru KA, Ayelagbe O, Ojurongbe O, et al. Predictive model for early detection of type 2 diabetes using patients' clinical symptoms, demographic features, and knowledge of diabetes. Health Sci Rep. 2024;7(1):e1834.
3. Sen A, Mohanraj PS, Laxmi V, Ashique S, Vasudevan R, Aldahish A, et al. Advancement of artificial intelligence based treatment strategy in type 2 diabetes: A critical update. J Pharm Anal. 2025;15(6):101305.
4. Wang Y, Liu C, Hu W, Luo L, Shi D, Zhang J, et al. Economic evaluation for medical artificial intelligence: Accuracy vs. cost-effectiveness in a diabetic retinopathy screening case. NPJ Digit Med. 2024;7(1):43.
5. Lalani B, Herur R, Zade D, Collins G, Dishong DM, Mehta S, et al. Applications of artificial intelligence and machine learning in prediabetes: A scoping review. J Diabetes Sci Technol. 2025:19322968251351995.
6. Guan Z, Li H, Liu R, Cai C, Liu Y, Li J, et al. Artificial intelligence in diabetes management: Advancements, opportunities, and challenges. Cell Rep Med. 2023;4(10):101213.
7. Ji C, Jiang T, Liu L, Zhang J, You L. Continuous glucose monitoring combined with artificial intelligence: Redefining the pathway for prediabetes management. Front Endocrinol (Lausanne). 2025;16:1571362.
8. Zhang K, Qi Y, Wang W, Tian X, Wang J, Xu L, et al. Future horizons in diabetes: Integrating AI and personalized care. Front Endocrinol (Lausanne). 2025;16:1583227.
9. Ying Z, Fan Y, Chen C, Liu Y, Tang Q, Chen Z, et al. Real-time AI-assisted insulin titration system for glucose control in patients with type 2 diabetes: A randomized clinical trial. JAMA Netw Open. 2025;8(5):e258910.
10. Baker J, Cappon G, Habineza JC, Basch CH, Mey S, Malkin-Washeim DL, et al. Continuous glucose monitoring among patients with type 1 diabetes in Rwanda (CAPT1D) phase I: Prospective observational feasibility study. JMIR Form Res. 2025;9:e64585.
11. Reddy SD. The role of AI and machine learning in optimizing insulin therapy: A comparative study. Int J Community Med Public Health. 2025;12(4):1873-6.
12. Wang X, Si J, Li Y, Tse P, Zhang G, Wang X, et al. Effectiveness and safety of AI-driven closed-loop systems in diabetes management: A systematic review and meta-analysis. Diabetol Metab Syndr. 2025;17(1):238.
13. Fan W, Deng C, Xu R, Liu Z, Leslie RD, Zhou Z, et al. Efficacy and safety of automated insulin delivery systems in patients with type 1 diabetes mellitus: a systematic review and meta-analysis. Diabetes Metab J. 2025;49(2):235-51.
14. Breton MD, Kovatchev BP. One year real-world use of the control-IQ advanced hybrid closed-loop technology. Diabetes Technol Ther. 2021;23(9):601-8.
15. Passanisi S, Lombardo F, Mameli C, Bombaci B, Macedoni M, Zuccotti G, et al. Safety, metabolic and psychological outcomes of Medtronic MiniMed 780G in children, adolescents and young adults: a systematic review. Diabetes Ther. 2024;15(2):343-65.
16. Lim PY, Oh XY, Ong WQ, Jain N, Mayuren J, Pandey M, et al. Continuous glucose monitoring data for artificial intelligence-based predictive glycemic event: A potential aspect for diabetic care. Int J Diabetes Dev Ctries. 2025;45(2):272-87.
17. Forlenza GP, DeSalvo DJ, Aleppo G, Wilmot EG, Berget C, Huyett LM, et al. Real-world evidence of Omnipod 5 automated insulin delivery system use in 69,902 people with type 1 diabetes. Diabetes Technol Ther. 2024;26(8):514-25.
18. Insulet Corporation. Insulet's randomized controlled trial (OP5-003) demonstrates Omnipod 5 automated insulin delivery system is superior to pump therapy. Acton (MA): Insulet Corporation; 2024.
19. Cetin F, Sukru Goncuoglu E, Abali S, Arslanoglu I, Deyneli O, Caklili OT, et al. Early stage effectiveness of the automated insulin delivery system—is artificial intelligence really effective? Endocrinol Res Pract. 2025.
20. van Bon AC, Blauw H, Jansen TJP, Laverman GD, Urgert T, Geessink-Mennink J, et al. Bihormonal fully closed-loop system for the treatment of type 1 diabetes: a real-world multicentre, prospective, single-arm trial in the Netherlands. Lancet Digit Health. 2024;6(4):e272-80.
21. Pujante P, García AV, Villa-Fernández E, García-Villarino M, González-Vidal T, Díaz-Naya L, et al. One-year evaluation of automated insulin delivery systems in adults with type 1 diabetes. Front Digit Health. 2025;7:1596188.
22. Medtronic plc. New real-world data shows MiniMed 780G system sustains strong global performance, exceeding international targets for diabetes management. Dublin and Florence (Italy): Medtronic plc; 2024.
23. Veluvali A, Dehghani Zahedani A, Hosseinian A, Aghaeepour N, McLaughlin T, Woodward M, et al. Impact of digital health interventions on glycemic control and weight management. NPJ Digit Med. 2025;8:20.

24. Lim PC, Chong YW, Chie QT, Zainal H, Yau KA, Teoh SH. Healthcare professionals' perspectives on artificial intelligence-based mobile applications for diabetes education and behavioural management. Digit Health. 2025;11:20552076251329991.
25. Mullur RS, Hsiao JS, Mueller K. Telemedicine in diabetes care. Am Fam Physician. 2022;105(3):281-8.
26. Andrès E, Meyer L, Zulfiqar AA, Hajjam M, Talha S, Bahougne T, et al. Telemonitoring in diabetes: Evolution of concepts and technologies, with a focus on results of the more recent studies. J Med Life. 2019;12(3):203-14.
27. Lee SWH, Chan CKY, Chua SS, Chaiyakunapruk N.. Comparative effectiveness of telemedicine strategies on type 2 diabetes management: A systematic review and network meta-analysis. Sci Rep. 2017;7(1):12680.
28. Grechuta K, Shokouh P, Alhussein A, Müller-Wieland D, Meyerhoff J, Gilbert J, et al. Benefits of clinical decision support systems for the management of noncommunicable chronic diseases: Targeted literature review. Interact J Med Res. 2024;13:e58036.
29. Tandon N. (2023). Digital solutions for improving NCD care. [online] Available from https://nams-india.in/downloads/aiims-nams/2023-09-01-Dr%20Nikhil%20Tondon.pdf [Last accessed October, 2025].
30. Abràmoff MD, Tarver ME, Loyo-Berrios N, Trujillo S, Char D, Obermeyer Z, et al. Considerations for addressing bias in artificial intelligence for health equity. NPJ Digit Med. 2023;6(1):170.
31. Weiner EB, Dankwa-Mullan I, Nelson WA, Hassanpour S. Ethical challenges and evolving strategies in the integration of artificial intelligence into clinical practice. PLOS Digit Health. 2025;4(4):e0000810.
32. Joseph J. Algorithmic bias in public health AI: A silent threat to equity in low-resource settings. Front Public Health. 2025;13:1643180.
33. Benjamens S, Dhunnoo P, Meskó B. The state of artificial intelligence-based FDA-approved medical devices and algorithms: An online database. NPJ Digit Med. 2020;3:118.
34. US Food and Drug Administration. Artificial intelligence-enabled medical devices . Silver Spring (MD): FDA; 2025.
35. Palaniappan K, Lin EYT, Vogel S. Global regulatory frameworks for the use of artificial intelligence in the healthcare services sector. Healthcare (Basel). 2024;12(5):562.
36. Akune Y, Kawasaki R, Goto R, Tamura H, Hiratsuka Y, Yamada M. Cost-effectiveness of AI-based diabetic retinopathy screening in nationwide health checkups and diabetes management in Japan: A modeling study. Diabetes Res Clin Pract. 2025;221:112015.
37. Van Wilder L, De Smedt D, Sandra L, Vandormael D, Kaes J, Willems R, et al. Cost-effectiveness of a digital supportive healthcare pathway for type 2 diabetes compared to usual care in Belgium. Digit Health. 2025;11:20552076251319169.
38. Ahmed MI, Spooner B, Isherwood J, Lane M, Orrock E, Dennison A, et al. A systematic review of the barriers to the implementation of artificial intelligence in healthcare. Cureus. 2023;15(10):e46454.
39. Hassan M, Kushniruk A, Borycki E. Barriers to and facilitators of artificial intelligence adoption in health care: scoping review. JMIR Hum Factors. 2024;11:e48633.
40. Tata Elxsi. (2024). Emerging trends in diabetes care: Top technology and business insights for 2024. [online] Available from https://www.tataelxsi.com/insights/whitepaper/emerging-trends-in-diabetes-care-top-technology-and-business-insights-for-2024 [Last accessed October, 2025].
41. Murpy M. Artificial intelligence in diabetes management: Transforming care through technology. J Dia Med Care. 2024;7(5):266-8.
42. Gardner DSL, Saboo B, Kesavadev J, Mustafa N, Villa M, Mahoney E, et al. Digital health technology in diabetes management in the Asia-Pacific region: A narrative review of the current scenario and future outlook. Diabetes Ther. 2025;16(3):349-69.

10 Continuous Glucose Monitoring and Wearable Tech for Diabetes

Purvi Chawla, Supratik Bhattacharya

ABSTRACT

The integration of continuous glucose monitoring (CGM) and wearable technology has transformed the landscape of diabetes care, offering patients and clinicians real-time data with an opportunity for immediate decision making. Their use is associated with improved glycemic control, mitigating the risks of hypoglycemia and hyperglycemia, and insights into lifestyle interactions. Thus, there is enhanced and precise facilitation of insulin dosing, and in-depth patient engagement through mobile integration and automated alerts. This chapter explores the development, classifications, and functioning of CGM systems, the role of wearable tech in diabetes management, and the impact of digital health in clinical practice. Recent innovations, including closed-loop systems (artificial pancreas), smart pens, multianalyte sensors, and artificial intelligence (AI)-powered decision support tools. Clinical implications are discussed for both type 1 and type 2 diabetes, including special populations such as pregnant women and the elderly and the pandemic. Additionally, the chapter evaluates current limitations, such as device accuracy, data overload, accessibility, and cost, along with emerging solutions. This synthesis concludes with a forward-looking view of how personalized, technology-enabled diabetes management is evolving toward an integrated, patient-centric model of care.

Keywords: Continuous glucose monitoring, Wearable devices, Artificial pancreas, Diabetes technology, Glycemic variability, Digital health, Insulin delivery, Clinical outcomes.

INTRODUCTION

Diabetes mellitus, a chronic metabolic disorder, continues to be one of the pressing public health challenges globally. Despite advances in pharmacotherapy, achieving optimal glycemic control remains elusive for a large proportion of patients. Traditional self-monitoring of blood glucose (SMBG) using finger-stick methods provide limited insights into glucose trends and variability, resulting in suboptimal therapeutic decisions. In this context, the advent of continuous glucose monitoring (CGM) and wearable technologies offers a paradigm shift, allowing for real-time, dynamic, and personalized glucose data capture.[1,2] With real-time feedback to people with diabetes, they provide a decision support tool to healthcare providers and have shown superior outcomes as compared to SMBG alone.

There is increasing reliance on CGM as an important monitoring tool in terms of improving glycated hemoglobin (HbA1c), reducing hypoglycemia and improving the time in glucose range metric.[3] Initially being used as adjunctive tools requiring further fingerstick glucose tests for calibration, they are now increasingly improved in accuracy and approved for stand-alone use, since 2016. Studies have also shown that time-in-range (TIR), the glycemic metric obtained from CGM use correlates well with risk factors and complications and thus is an important marker of glycemic control in randomized trials and real-world studies.[4]

The CGM system, when integrated with insulin delivery systems or mobile health (mHealth) platforms, can facilitate timely interventions and is a step toward a fully functional artificial pancreas (AP), improves patient adherence, and reduces the risk of both short- and long-term complications. This chapter delves into the evolution, current applications, and future potential of CGM and wearable technology in diabetes care.

CONTINUOUS GLUCOSE MONITORING SYSTEMS

The CGM involves measuring interstitial glucose levels on a continuous basis and updating the glucose level display every 5–10 minutes with the information on a real-time basis. Three main components of a CGM system consist of a sensor inserted in the subcutaneous tissue, a transmitter that transfers the sensor data to the monitor and the monitor/display on a reader or person's mobile device itself, showing the glycemic information.

Importantly, CGMs aid physicians in making adjustments to the medication regimen based on the generated reports and personally for the patient in making behavioral changes to achieve the target glycemic levels. Advantages of CGMs are to detect hypoglycemic and hyperglycemic excursions, impending hypoglycemia, and wide fluctuations in glycemic levels or glycemic variability.[3] Efforts to link CGM systems with an automatically controlled insulin delivery device or insulin pump are underway to make a fully functioning AP.

TYPES AND PRINCIPLES OF CONTINUOUS GLUCOSE MONITORING

The CGM systems may be divided based on the intended use.

Professional versus Personal CGM

- Professional CGMs are clinic-owned devices providing either retrospective or real-time glucose data.
- Often they are blinded systems used for diagnostic purposes or treatment assessment, typically worn for 7–14 days.
- Personal CGMs are user-owned and provide real-time feedback and can be integrated with smartphones or insulin pumps.

Real-time versus Intermittently Scanned CGM

- Real-time CGM (rtCGM) continuously transmits data and alerts users to glucose excursions. Examples include Dexcom G7 and Medtronic Guardian CGMs.
- Intermittently scanned CGM (isCGM) (e.g., FreeStyle Libre) requires manual scanning, with a reader or mobile device in order to view the data and stores the same for up to 8 hours. It may be considered more affordable.[5]

Factory-calibrated versus User-calibrated

Modern CGMs such as Dexcom G6 and G7, FreeStyle Libre 2 and 3, and Medtronic Guardian systems 4 are factory-calibrated, eliminating the need for finger-stick calibration.

Older generation CGMs used to require fingerstick calibrations for accuracy maintenance and are outdated with limited practical applicability. **Table 1** is the summary of comparison of subcutaneous CGM devices commonly available.

- *Integration into broader health ecosystems*: Diabetes management may become part of integrated cardiometabolic health systems, tracking BP, lipid levels, and renal function.

CLINICAL IMPLICATIONS[13,14]

- *Type 1 diabetes mellitus (T1DM)*: CGM is recommended for adults and children with T1DM on insulin therapy on a continuous basis, if affording.[15] It is recommended to measure the TIR and to minimize the time-below-range (TBR) and reduce hospitalization. Intermittent use of CGMs is also found to be useful on insulin therapy.

  With the use of wearables, it is also possible to track ketones and patterns of sleep, exercise and other behavioral aspects. Features like the alarms in the wearable devices may help and reassure care providers in tracking potential hypoglycemia and preventing it.
- *Type 2 diabetes mellitus (T2DM)*: CGM is recommended for people with T2DM on oral antidiabetic drugs and basal insulin. The TIR metric guides lifestyle changes and medication regimens and helps achieve glycemic targets, reduce glycemic variability, minimize hypoglycemia, and improve quality of life. In newly diagnosed persons with diabetes, CGM use aids in identification of glycemic patterns and achievement of targets with lifestyle modifications alone.

  Wearable devices help track meals, activity levels, heart rate, blood pressure, and patterns of sleep and may offer additional support with behavioral modifications.
- *Hyperglycemia in pregnancy (T1DM/T2DM or GDM)*: CGM is recommended for all persons with T1DM in pregnancy along with HCL systems. It is also recommended to maintain a TIR ≥ 70% within 70–140 mg/dL for those with T1DM in pregnancy. CGM is also recommended for those with T2DM in pregnancy and also for those with GDM. A TIR of ≥90% within 70–140 mg/dL range should be considered as a target range for these populations.[3] Pregnancy and fetal outcomes are found to improve with the integration of technology in glycemic control.
- *In hospitalized patients*: CGM in hospitalized patients should be used with caution as certain medications and conditions such as inflammation, cancer may affect the interstitial glucose levels and may make it difficult to interpret the TIR values, thus requiring SMBG in tandem with CGM. It can assist healthcare providers in effective clinical management of diabetes for dose modifications or titration of insulin by showing the real-time glycemic information and also for detection of potential hypoglycemia. In people with diabetes posthospitalization also, insulin titration may be well managed using the CGM data generated.
- *Elderly population with T1DM or T2DM*: CGMs are effective tools for monitoring glycemia in the elderly population with T1DM or T2DM due to the high risk of hypoglycemia, hypoglycemia unawareness, and/or established cardiovascular disease and helping improve TIR [target approximately ≥50% ≤1% for TBR (54 mg/dL)]. Adherence may improve with the wearable devices and help track fall-risks.
- *Pandemic situations*: CGMs are also recommended for partial self-care in hospitals during the pandemic,[16] especially in the nonintensive care unit (non-ICU) settings and with careful validation in the ICU setting or even in quarantine, home isolation, or posthospitalization.

The clinical benefits of various CGM devices in the different patient groups is described in **Table 2**.

TABLE 2: Clinical benefits of CGM in various patient groups.

Population	*Benefits*
Type 1 DM	Reduced HbA1c, fewer hypoglycemic events
Type 2 DM	Improved TIR, behavioral awareness
Pregnant women	Better postprandial control, fetal outcomes
Children	Safety alarms, better adherence
Elderly	Support for caregivers, trend recognition

(DM: diabetes mellitus; HbA1c: glycated hemoglobin; TIR: time in range)

BARRIERS AND LIMITATIONS

- *Cost and insurance coverage*: One of the biggest barriers to successful uptake of technology, especially in the low-resource settings, is the high cost associated with sensors, transmitters, and AID systems with minimal or no coverage from insurance
- *Skin reactions and device fatigue*: Skin irritation, rashes and allergies from sensor adhesives, device dependence, and alarm fatigue may affect adherence to continuous use and also compromise on safety and effectiveness.
- *Accuracy concerns*: While improving, CGMs still lag behind blood glucose meters in certain conditions such as rapid glucose level changes.[17]
- *Data overload*: Continuous streams of data can overwhelm both patients and clinicians without appropriate interpretation tools and require regular and structured training.[18]
- *Interoperability*: The lack of harmonization in the ecosystems of all CGMs and pumps and control algorithms may be a barrier and is paving the way for integrated CGMs (iCGMs).[19]

CONCLUSION

Continuous glucose monitoring and wearable technologies have significantly enhanced the toolkit available for diabetes management. As devices become more affordable, accurate, and user-friendly, their adoption is expected to grow across all diabetes types and age groups. The synergy between data, automation, and personalized medicine heralds a new era in which diabetes care is not only more precise but also more patient-empowered. The convergence of CGM and wearable technologies have only fueled this approach further.

To fully realize this potential, stakeholders must address challenges related to cost, accessibility, training, and data literacy. With sustained innovation and cross-disciplinary collaboration, CGM and wearable tech will likely become central pillars of diabetes care in the coming decade.

REFERENCES

1. Kwon SY, Moon JS. Advances in Continuous Glucose Monitoring: Clinical Applications. Endocrinol Metab. 2025;40(2):161-73.
2. Lundgrin EL, Kelly CA, Bellini N, Lewis C, Rafi E, Hatipoglu B. Diabetes Technology Trends: A Review of the Latest Innovations. J Clin Endocrinol Metabol. 2025;110(2):S165-74.
3. Battelino T, Danne T, Bergenstal RM, Amiel SA, Beck R, Biester T, et al. Clinical targets for continuous glucose monitoring data interpretation: Recommendations from the International Consensus. Diab Care. 2019;42(8):1593-603.
4. Saboo B, Kesavadev J, Shankar A, Krishna MB, Sheth S, Patel V, Krishnan G. Time-in-range as a target in type 2 diabetes: An urgent need. Heliyon. 2021:15;7(1):e05967.
5. Heile M, Hollstegge B, Broxterman L, Cai A, Close K. Automated Insulin Delivery: Easy Enough to Use in Primary Care?. Clin Diabetes. 2020;38(5): 474-85.
6. Reddy N, Verma N, Dungan K. Monitoring Technologies- Continuous Glucose Monitoring, Mobile Technology, Biomarkers of Glycemic Control. South Dartmouth (MA): MDText.com, Inc.; 2000.

7. Heinemann L, Freckmann G. CGM versus FGM; or, continuous glucose monitoring is not flash glucose monitoring. J Diabetes Sci Technol. 2015;9(5):947-50.
8. Hartnell S, Fuchs J, Boughton CK, Hovorka R. Closed-loop technology: a practical guide. Practical Diabetes. 2021;38(4):33-9.
9. Olde Bekkink M, Koeneman M, de Galan BE, Bredie SJ. Early Detection of Hypoglycemia in Type 1 Diabetes Using Heart Rate Variability Measured by a Wearable Device. Diabetes Care. 2019;42(4):689-92.
10. Heise HM, Delbeck S, Marbach R. Non-invasive Monitoring of Glucose Using Near-Infrared Reflection Spectroscopy of Skin—Constraints and Effective Novel Strategy in Multivariate Calibration. Biosensors. 2021;11(3):64.
11. Kropff J, DeVries JH. Continuous Glucose Monitoring, Future Products, and Update on Worldwide Artificial Pancreas Projects. Diabetes Technol Ther. 2016;18,2(2):S253-63.
12. Corrao S, Janić M, Maggio V, Rizzo M. Machine learning and deep learning in diabetology: revolutionizing diabetes care. Front Clin Diabetes Healthc. 2025;6:1547689.
13. Mohan V, Joshi S, Mithal A, Kesavadev J, Unnikrishnan AG, Saboo B, Kumar P, et al. Expert Consensus Recommendations on Time in Range for Monitoring Glucose Levels in People with Diabetes: An Indian Perspective. Diabetes Ther. 2023;14(2):237-49.
14. Kong APS, Lim S, Yoo SH, Ji L, Chen L, Bao Y, et al. Asia-Pacific consensus recommendations for application of continuous glucose monitoring in diabetes management. Diabetes Res Clin Pract. 2023;201:110718.
15. Pettus J, Price DA, Edelman SV. Superiority of continuous glucose monitoring over self-monitoring of blood glucose in type 1 diabetes: A systematic review. Diabetes Technol Ther. 2015;17(3):191-7.
16. Dumitrascu AG, Perry MF, Boone RJ, Guzman MP, Chirila RM, McNally AW, et al. Continuous Glucose Monitoring for Patients with COVID-19 Pneumonia: Initial Experience at a Tertiary Care Center. Endocr Pract. 2023;29(3):155-61.
17. Marak MC, Calhoun P, Damiano ER, Russell SJ, Ruedy KJ, Beck RW. Testing the Real-World Accuracy of the Dexcom G6 Pro CGM During the Insulin-Only Bionic Pancreas Pivotal Trial. Diabetes Technol Ther. 2023;25(11):817-21.
18. Diabetes Research in Children Network (DirecNet) Study Group. Psychological aspects of continuous glucose monitoring in pediatric type 1 diabetes. Pediatr Diabetes. 2006;7(1):32-8.
19. Klonoff DC, Aaron RE, Tian T, Espinoza JC. Principles of Interoperability of Diabetes Devices. J Diabetes Sci Technol. 2024:19322968241268235.

11 Closed-loop Insulin Delivery Systems: Toward an Artificial Pancreas

Bharat Saboo, Shubhashree Patil

ABSTRACT

Closed-loop insulin delivery systems, commonly referred to as artificial pancreas systems, represent a major advancement in the management of diabetes mellitus by integrating continuous glucose monitoring, insulin pump technology, and automated control algorithms. These systems dynamically adjust insulin delivery in response to real-time glucose values, thereby reducing glycemic variability and patient burden associated with conventional insulin therapy. This chapter reviews the historical evolution of closed-loop systems, from early inpatient prototypes to modern hybrid and adaptive systems used in real-world clinical practice. It outlines the core technological components, including proportional–integral–derivative and model predictive control algorithms, and compares currently available commercial platforms such as Medtronic 780G, Tandem Control-IQ, Omnipod 5, and CamAPS FX. Evidence from randomized trials, meta-analyses, and real-world studies demonstrates consistent improvements in time in range, reductions in HbA1c, and lower hypoglycemia risk across pediatric and adult populations with type 1 diabetes, with emerging evidence in insulin-treated type 2 diabetes. The chapter also discusses regulatory pathways, economic considerations, and barriers to adoption, particularly in low- and middle-income countries. Finally, future directions including fully closed-loop systems, dual-hormone platforms, and artificial intelligence–driven personalization are explored, highlighting the potential of these technologies to advance equitable, autonomous, and precision-based diabetes care.

Keywords: Closed-loop insulin delivery, Artificial pancreas, Hybrid closed-loop systems, Continuous glucose monitoring, Insulin pumps, Model predictive control, Diabetes technology, Time in range, automated insulin delivery, Artificial intelligence in diabetes

INTRODUCTION

Diabetes mellitus, characterized by chronic hyperglycemia due to insulin deficiency or resistance, remains a leading cause of morbidity and mortality worldwide. Type 1 diabetes (T1D) and advanced type 2 diabetes (T2D) require meticulous insulin management to prevent acute and chronic complications. Traditional management strategies—multiple daily injections (MDI) or conventional insulin pumps—demand constant vigilance and manual adjustments, often resulting in suboptimal glycemic control and significant patient burden.

The development of closed-loop insulin delivery systems, colloquially termed the "artificial pancreas", represents a revolutionary approach to diabetes care by automating insulin administration based on real-time glucose monitoring and advanced control algorithms. This chapter provides a comprehensive review of the historical evolution, current technological landscape, clinical efficacy, barriers to adoption, global perspectives, and future directions of closed-loop insulin delivery systems as of 2025.[1-6]

HISTORICAL BACKGROUND

The quest for an artificial pancreas began in the mid-20th century. Arnold Kadish introduced the first prototype in 1964—a bulky, intravenous device that monitored blood glucose and infused insulin and dextrose as needed. The Biostator, developed in the 1970s, was more practical but remained hospital-bound.

Further advances in the 1990s and 2000s produced subcutaneous continuous glucose monitors (CGMs) such as the Minimed CGMs, and later Dexcom and Abbott FreeStyle Libre sensors, enabling portable closed-loop systems.[4,5] The AP@home project (2010–2015) pioneered home-based systems, demonstrating tight glycemic control and paving the way for regulatory approvals.[3,6]

CURRENT CLOSED-LOOP INSULIN DELIVERY SYSTEMS

Modern closed-loop insulin delivery systems integrate three main components—(1) a CGM, (2) an insulin pump, and (3) a control algorithm. Hybrid closed-loop (HCL) systems automate basal and correctional insulin delivery but still require manual meal announcements.[3,4]

Medtronic 780G

Uses a modified PID algorithm with Guardian 4 CGM. Offers frequent automatic boluses and target range settings (100–120 mg/dL).[5] In children, improves time-in-range (TIR) by 11.7%, HbA1c lowered by 0.4%, with slightly higher time-below-range (TBR) around 2%.[7]

Tandem Control-IQ

Employs a model predictive control (MPC) algorithm with integrated t:slim X2 pump and Dexcom G6/G7. Achieves HbA1c reductions of 0.6% and reduces glycemic variability.[2]

Omnipod 5

Tubeless patch pump with Dexcom G6 and personalized MPC algorithm. Lowers HbA1c by 0.55%, increases TIR to 68%. Approved by Health Canada in 2024.

CamAPS FX (Mylife Loop)

Adaptive MPC algorithm paired with YpsoPump and Dexcom G6/G7. CE marked since 2021, approved in Canada 2024. Ideal for young children ≥ 1 year **(Table 1)**.[7-13]

Control Algorithms and Hardware

The MPC algorithms (Tandem, Omnipod, and CamAPS) use predictive control based on glucose trends, insulin on board, and prior data.[2,5] PID algorithms (Medtronic) adjust delivery to correct current deviation from target glucose.[5]

Modern CGMs (Dexcom, Libre) communicate wirelessly with insulin pumps via Bluetooth. Pumps vary by type (tubed or tubeless/patch) and are paired through proprietary or open-source integration protocols.[1,4]

CLINICAL EFFICACY AND META-ANALYSES

Hybrid closed-loop systems in T1D improve TIR by ~10.9%, add 2.6 hours/day in range, and reduce HbA1c by ~0.5%. TBR typically decreases by 1.5% **(Table 2)**.[9-17]

The T2D patients on intensive insulin therapy show up to +15% TIR improvement and better nocturnal control.

TABLE 1: Comparison of closed-loop systems (2025).[7-13]

Feature	*Medtronic 780G*	*Tandem control-IQ*	*Omnipod 5*	*CamAPS FX (Mylife Loop)*
Algorithm	Modified PID	Model predictive control	Model predictive control	Adaptive model predictive
CGM integration	Guardian 4	Dexcom G6/G7	Dexcom G6	Dexcom G6/G7
Pump type	Tubed	Tubed (t:slim X2)	Tubeless (patch)	Tubed (YpsoPump)
Auto correction	Yes	Yes	Yes	Yes
Meal announcement	Required	Required	Required	Required
Age approval	≥7 years	≥6 years	≥2 years	≥1 year (CE Mark)
Mobile app	Yes	Yes	Yes	Yes
Unique features	Frequent auto boluses	Sleep and exercise modes	Tubeless, waterproof	Smallest pump, adaptive
Approved regions	US, EU, India	US, EU	US, Canada, EU	UK, EU, Canada

TABLE 2: Key clinical outcomes (trials and meta-analysis).[9-17]

System/Study	*Population*	*TIR (%) increase*	*HbA1c reduction (%)*	*Hypoglycemia risk change*
Medtronic 780G	Children, adults	11.7	–0.4	TBR ~ 2%
Tandem control-IQ	Adults	12.0	–0.6	TBR ~ 1%
Omnipod 5	Adults, children	11.5	–0.55	TBR ~ 1%
CamAPS FX	Adults, children	10.8	–0.5	TBR ~ 1%
Meta-analysis (2024)	Mixed	10.9 (avg)	–0.5 (avg)	↓1.5% TBR
Indian studies (pumps)	Indian T1D, T2D	8–12	–0.4 to –0.7	Improved

Patient Narratives

Kady Helme reported reduced nocturnal glucose checks and greater stability using Medtronic 670G.

John, a 36-year-old with frequent hypoglycemia, improved from TIR 55 to 72% and HbA1c 7.8 to 6.9% using Tandem Control-IQ.

Barriers to Adoption and Regulation

Regulatory processes, interoperability issues, and costs (~$5–8K/year) limit adoption especially in low- and middle-income countries (LMICs). The FDA's iCoDE project aims to standardize device connections. Equity concerns remain pronounced in rural and underserved regions **(Table 3)**.[18-21]

GLOBAL OUTLOOK AND HEALTH ECONOMICS

Europe leads adoption with broad CE Mark approvals and reimbursement.[3] North America has expanding insurance coverage and accelerated approvals for multiple systems. Asia-Pacific shows early progress but limited overall reach, particularly outside major urban centers. Africa and Latin America have limited access; pilot programs are in progress.[19-21]

TABLE 3: Barriers and solutions.[18-21]

Barrier	*Description*	*Potential solutions*
Cost	High device and consumable costs, limited insurance coverage	Subsidies, insurance expansion, local production
Training and education	Lack of provider and patient training	Structured programs, tele-education
Regulatory approval	Lengthy, complex, varies by country	Harmonized pathways, real-world data
Interoperability	Proprietary systems limit device mixing	Open protocols, regulatory mandates
Infrastructure (India/LMICs)	Patchy access to CGM, pumps, internet	Public-private partnerships, mobile health
Cultural acceptance	Device stigma, misconceptions	Peer support, awareness campaigns

TABLE 4: Ongoing clinical trials (2024–2025).

Trial name	*Location*	*Population*	*Intervention*	*Key outcome(s)*
CREATE	Canada	Pediatric T1D	Dual-hormone CL system	TIR, hypoglycemia
AiDAPT	UK	Pregnant women w/ T1D	Fully closed-loop	Maternal/Fetal outcomes
ICD-LIFE	EU	Mixed	HCL systems (real-world)	Longevity, QoL
Indian studies	India	T1D, T2D	CSII, CGM, AID	TIR, HbA1c, safety

Economic analyses predict that despite high upfront costs, closed-loop systems reduce diabetes complications (e.g., retinopathy and nephropathy) and related hospitalizations, making them cost-effective over 10 years.

FUTURE DIRECTIONS AND CLINICAL TRIALS

- Fully closed-loop systems aim to eliminate meal announcements through AI.[8,22]
- Dual-hormone pumps delivering insulin and glucagon (e.g., Beta Bionics iLet) are in phase 3 trials.
- AI-augmented algorithms integrate biometric and behavioral data for personalized dosing **(Table 4)**.[7]

CONCLUSION

Closed-loop insulin delivery systems have transformed diabetes care, improving glycemic outcomes, reducing hypoglycemia, and enhancing quality of life across diverse populations. Continued advances promise fully autonomous artificial pancreas systems, further improving patient independence and health equity.[3,6,8]

REFERENCES

1. Templer S. Closed-Loop Insulin Delivery Systems: Past, Present, and Future Directions. Front Endocrinol. 2022;13:919942.
2. Thabit H, Hovorka R. Closed-loop insulin delivery in type 1 diabetes. Curr Diab Rep. 2012;12(6):737-44.
3. Charpentier G, Bismuth E, Joubert M, Renard E, Tubiana-Rufi N, Chaillous L, et al. Practical implementation of automated insulin delivery systems in 2025: A French position statement update. Diabetes Metab. 2025;51(1):101637.

4. Ware J, Hovorka R. Closed-loop insulin delivery: update on the state of the field and emerging technologies. Expert Rev Med Devices. 2022;19(11):859-75.
5. Ware J. Recent advances in closed-loop insulin delivery. Curr Opin Endocrinol Diabetes Obes. 2022;29(1):1-7.
6. Kadiyala N, Hovorka R, Boughton CK. Closed-loop systems: recent advancements and lived experience. Expert Rev Med Devices. 2024;21(1):1-12.
7. Passanisi S, Lombardo F, Mameli C, Bombaci B, Macedoni M, Zuccotti G, et al. Safety and Metabolic Outcomes of Medtronic 780G in in Children, Adolescents and Young Adults: A Systematic Review. Diabetes Ther. 2023;15(12):343-65.
8. Ware J, et al. Real-World HCL Outcomes: Tandem and Omnipod Lead HbA1c Reduction. J Diabetes Sci Technol. 2025;19(1):45-53.
9. Oliva Morgado Ferreira R, Trevisan T, Pasqualotto E, Schmidt P, Pedrotti Chavez M, et al. Efficacy of the hybrid closedloop insulin delivery system in children and adolescents with type 1 diabetes: a meta-analysis with trial sequential analysis. Arch Endocrinol Metab. 2024;68:e230280.
10. Akturk HK, Snell-Bergeon J, Shah VN. Efficacy and Safety of Tandem Control IQ Without User-Initiated Boluses in Adults with Uncontrolled Type 1 Diabetes. Diabetes Technol Ther. 2022;24(10):779-83.
11. Kovatchev B, Castillo A, Pryor E, Kollar LL, Barnett CL, DeBoer MD, et al. Neural-Net Artificial Pancreas: A Randomized Crossover Trial of a First-in-Class Automated Insulin Delivery Algorithm. Diabetes Technol Ther. 2024;26(6):375-82.
12. "An Incredible Burden Has Been Lifted": Kady Helme's Artificial Pancreas Journey. NIH MedlinePlus. 2017.p.17.
13. Phillip M, Nimri R, Bergenstal RM, Barnard-Kelly K, Danne T, Hovorka R, et al. Consensus Recommendations for the Use of Automated Insulin Delivery Technologies in Clinical Practice. Endocr Rev. 2023;44(2):254-80.
14. Bergenstal RM, Garg S, Weinzimer SA, Buckingham BA, Bode BW, Tamborlane WV, et al. Safety of a Hybrid Closed-Loop Insulin Delivery System in Patients with Type 1 Diabetes. JAMA. 2016;316(13):1407-8.
15. Breton MD, Kanapka LG, Beck RW, Ekhlaspour L, Forlenza GP, Cengiz E, et al. A Randomized Trial of Closed-Loop Control in Children with Type 1 Diabetes. N Engl J Med. 2020;383(9):836-45.
16. Brown SA, Kovatchev BP, Raghinaru D, Lum JW, Buckingham BA, Kudva YC, et al. Six-Month Randomized, Multicenter Trial of Closed-Loop Control in Type 1 Diabetes. N Engl J Med. 2019;381(18):1707-17.
17. Hovorka R, et al. Closed-Loop Insulin Delivery in Adults with Type 1 Diabetes. Diabetes Care. 2014;37(5):1204-11.
18. Kesavadev J, Saboo B, Krishna MB, Krishnan G. Evolution of insulin delivery devices: from syringes to smart insulin pens and insulin pumps in India. J Assoc Physicians India. 2020;68(12):51-5.
19. Kesavadev J, Das AK, Unnikrishnan R, Joshi SR, Ramachandran A, Shamsudeen J, et al. Use of Insulin Pumps in India: Suggested Guidelines Based on Experience and Cultural Differences. Diabetes Technol Ther. 2010;12(10):823-31.
20. Phillip M, et al. Barriers to Adoption of Closed-Loop Systems and Solutions. Diabetes Technol Ther. 2025.
21. Singh K, Chakma T, Ray S, Vaidh N, Shrivastava S. Exploring the viability of newer technologies in care and management of tribal diabetes in India. Int J Res Med Sci. 2024;12(4):1321-6.
22. Medscape. (2025). How close is fully closed-loop automated insulin delivery? [online] Available from https://www.medscape.com/viewarticle/how-close-fully-closed-loop-automated-insulin-delivery-2025a10008623 [Last accessed October, 2025].

SUGGESTED READINGS

1. Wang X, Si J, Li Y, Tse P, Zhang G, Wang X, et al. Effectiveness and safety of AI-driven closed-loop systems in diabetes management: a systematic review and meta-analysis. Diabetol Metab Syndr. 2025;17(1):238.
2. Fan W, Deng C, Xu R, Liu Z, Leslie RD, Zhou Z. Efficacy and Safety of Automated Insulin Delivery Systems in Patients with Type 1 Diabetes Mellitus: A Systematic Review and Meta-Analysis. Diabet Metabol J. 2025;49(2):235-51.
3. Hughes MS, Levy CJ. The Future of Automated Insulin Delivery Systems. Endocr Pract. 2025;31(9):1162-70.
4. Royston C, Hovorka R, Boughton CK. Closed-loop therapy: recent advancements and potential predictors of glycemic outcomes. Expert Opin Drug Deliv. 2025;22(6):875-92.

12

Telemedicine and Digital Health in Diabetes Management

Anil Kumar Virmani, Vinayak Hiremath

ABSTRACT

The management of diabetes has undergone significant transformation through the advent of telemedicine and digital health technologies, offering innovative, patient-focused solutions. The implementation of these solutions has enhanced access, optimized glycemic control, and tackled health disparities.

The impact of diabetes on 89.8 million individuals in India, projected to rise to 156.7 million by 2050, underscores the critical need for the development of care models that prioritize scalability and accessibility. Individuals are empowered to take charge of their health conditions by utilizing digital innovations such as mobile health applications, wearable technology, and artificial intelligence.

Telemedicine enables the execution of virtual consultations, facilitates remote monitoring, and allows for real-time adjustments to treatment plans. The application of these technologies supports patients in adhering to their prescribed treatments, facilitates patient education, and addresses the disparities in care for underserved medical populations.

Recent studies indicate a significant decrease in HbA1c levels along with enhanced patient satisfaction, even in the face of challenges such as digital literacy, data protection, and infrastructure limitations. This chapter provides a comprehensive overview, encompassing implementation techniques, patient perspectives, global case studies, and effective solutions to challenges, all aimed at ensuring that diabetes care is equitable and sustainable.

Future research should focus on long-term outcomes, economic viability, and cultural adaptability to optimize these technologies. By integrating telemedicine and digital health, healthcare systems can transform diabetes management, ensuring equitable, personalized, and sustainable care.

Keywords: Telemedicine, digital health, Mobile health, Wearable devices, Artificial intelligence, Health disparities, Patient engagement.

INTRODUCTION

Diabetes, a chronic metabolic and vascular disorder, affects millions globally, with significant implications for micro- and macrovascular complications. According to the International Diabetes Federation (IDF) Atlas, India has 89.8 million people with diabetes in 2025, projected to increase to 156.7 million by 2050.[1] Traditional diabetes management relies on in-person consultations and standardized protocols, which often fail to account for individual patient differences in metabolism, lifestyle, and disease progression. Barriers such as geographical distance, financial constraints, and time limitations hinder access, particularly in rural and underserved areas where specialized care is scarce. These challenges are compounded by a reactive care model that responds to glucose fluctuations after they occur, missing opportunities for proactive intervention.

The solution to these challenges is Telemedicine and Digital health. Telemedicine facilitates electronic health data exchange, enabling virtual consultations, remote monitoring, and real-time treatment adjustments. Digital health tools, including mobile health (mHealth) applications, wearable devices such as continuous glucose monitors (CGMs), and artificial intelligence (AI)-driven analytics, empower patients to actively manage their condition. The COVID-19 pandemic accelerated telehealth adoption, with programs like the Veterans Health Administration demonstrating improved access and outcomes for rural populations with multimorbidity, including diabetes.[2] In India, initiatives such as NanoHealth and Apollo Hospitals' telehealth services have bridged care gaps, particularly during the pandemic.

This chapter explores the role of telemedicine and digital health in diabetes management, it provides practical frameworks, actionable solutions to challenges, and a balanced focus on technology and human factors. The goal is to offer a comprehensive guide for healthcare providers, policymakers, and researchers to leverage these technologies for equitable, personalized, and sustainable diabetes care.

TELEMEDICINE IN DIABETES MANAGEMENT

Definition and Modalities

Patient outcomes can be improved by the electronic exchange of health information, known as telemedicine, which is of three types:

1. *Synchronous telemedicine*: Real-time virtual consultations via video or phone
2. *Asynchronous telemedicine*: Transmission of medical data (e.g., glucose readings) for later assessment
3. *Remote monitoring*: Continuous data collection from devices like CGMs[3]

These modalities enhance access, reduce travel burdens, and facilitate timely interventions, particularly for underserved populations.

Enhancing Access to Care

Telemedicine bridges geographical and socioeconomic barriers by enabling remote consultations with specialists. A 2024 systematic review found telemedicine as effective as in-person visits for glycemic control in rural communities, with adoption accelerated by the COVID-19 pandemic.[4] In India, NanoHealth leverages mobile connectivity and community health workers to deliver chronic disease management, improving access for 70% of participants. Globally, teleretinal screening in the United States has increased diabetic retinopathy detection by 30% in rural areas.[5] In Kenya, SMS-based reminders and mobile apps have improved medication adherence by 25% in low-resource settings.[6]

Improving Glycemic Control

Remote monitoring tools like CGMs provide real-time glucose data, enabling proactive treatment adjustments. A 2023 meta-analysis reported a weighted-mean HbA1c reduction of –0.59 (95% CI –0.84 to –0.35, p <–0.001) with telemedicine interventions, indicating high certainty of evidence.[7] CGMs reduce hypoglycemic and hyperglycemic episodes, enhancing patient safety. For instance, AI-integrated CGMs can predict glucose trends, preventing complications like hypoglycemia.[8]

Facilitating Patient Education and Self-management

Telemedicine platforms offer diverse functionalities:

- *Tele-education*: Virtual training on nutrition, exercise, and medication adherence
- *Teleconsultation*: Real-time specialist consultations

A 2023 study found a cost-benefit ratio of 1.5:1 in urban underserved areas due to reduced emergency visits.[14] In India, BeatO has minimized clinic visits, saving 20% in patient costs.[10] Further research is needed for rural settings.[15]

ADDRESSING CHALLENGES

- *Digital literacy*: Community-based training and user-friendly interfaces can bridge the digital divide.[13]
- *Data privacy*: Adopt AES-256 encryption, blockchain, and GDPR/HIPAA compliance.[13]
- *Infrastructure*: Invest in mobile connectivity and interoperable platforms.[6]

Patient perspective: Patients report high satisfaction (78%) with telemedicine but emphasize the need for hybrid models.[10,16]

Global case studies:
- *India*: Apollo Hospitals' telehealth services improved access for 70% of underserved patients.[10]
- *US*: Teleretinal screening reduced blindness risk by 30%.[5]
- *Kenya*: Mobile health initiatives increased adherence by 25%.[6]

CONCLUSION

Telemedicine and digital health have revolutionized diabetes management by offering flexible, patient-centered care. These technologies improve access, personalize treatment, and enhance glycemic control, with HbA1c reductions of up to 0.59%.[7] In India, initiatives such as NanoHealth and Apollo Hospitals demonstrate scalability, while global examples from the US and Africa highlight universal applicability.[5,6] Challenges such as digital literacy, data privacy, and infrastructure limitations require collaborative solutions, including training, encryption, and partnerships.[13] Patient perspectives underscore the importance of hybrid care models.[10,16] Future research should focus on long-term outcomes, cost-effectiveness, and cultural adaptability.[15,17] By integrating telemedicine and digital health, healthcare systems can ensure equitable, sustainable, and effective diabetes care, transforming the lives of millions.[18-20]

REFERENCES

1. Anjana RM, Unnikrishnan R, Deepa M, Pradeepa R, Tandon N, Das AK, et al. Metabolic non-communicable disease health report of India: the ICMR-INDIAB national cross-sectional study (ICMR-INDIAB-17). Lancet Diabetes Endocrinol. 2023;11(7):474-89.
2. Heyworth L, Kirsh S, Zulman D, Ferguon JM. Expanding access through virtual care: the VA's early experience with Covid-19. NEJM Catal. 2020;1(4).
3. Dhediya R, Chadha M, Bhattacharya AD, Godbole S, Godbole S. Role of telemedicine in diabetes management. J Diabetes Sci Technol. 2023;17(3):775-81.
4. Wakefield BJ, Turvey CL. Evaluating the impact of telemedicine on glycemic control in rural communities. J Rural Health. 2024;40(2):123-30.
5. Liu TYA, Wolf RM. Telemedicine in diabetes care. Am Fam Physician. 2022;105(3):281-8.
6. Canali S, Schiaffonati V, Aliverti A. Challenges and recommendations for wearable devices in digital health: data quality, interoperability, health equity, fairness. PLOS Digit Health. 2022;1(10):e0000131.
7. De Groot J, Wu D, Flynn D, Robertson D, Grant G, Sun J. Efficacy of telemedicine on glycaemic control in patients with type 2 diabetes: A meta-analysis. World J Diabetes. 2021;12(2):170-97.
8. Ayers AT, Ho CN, Kerr D, Cichosz SL, Mathioudakis N, Wang M, et al. Artificial intelligence to diagnose complications of diabetes. J Diabetes Sci Technol. 2024;19(1):246-64.
9. Rosta L, Menyhart A, Mahmeed WA, Al-Rasadi K, Al-Alawi K, Banach M, et al. Telemedicine for diabetes management during COVID-19: what we have learnt, what and how to implement. Front Endocrinol (Lausanne). 2023:14:1129793.
10. Agarwal P, Mukerji G, Desveaux L, Ivers NM, Bhattacharyya O, Hensel JM, et al. Mobile App for Improved Self-Management of Type 2 Diabetes: Multicenter Pragmatic Randomized Controlled Trial. JMIR Mhealth Uhealth. 2019;7(1):e10321.
11. Borgen I, Småstuen MC, Jacobsen AF, Garnweidner-Holme LM, Fayyad S, Noll J, et al. Effect of the Pregnant+ smartphone application in women with gestational

diabetes mellitus: a randomised controlled trial in Norway. BMJ Open. 2019;9(11):e030884.
12. Yu X, Wang Y, Liu Z, Jung E. Technological functionality and system architecture of mobile health interventions for diabetes management: a systematic review and meta-analysis. Front Public Health. 2025;13:1549568.
13. Mumtaz H, Riaz MH, Wajid H, Saqib M, Zeeshan MH, Khan SE, et al. Current challenges and potential solutions to the use of digital health technologies in evidence generation: a narrative review. Front Digit Health. 2023;5:1203945.
14. Smith J, Brown K, Patel R. Effectiveness of telemedicine in urban medically underserved areas: a retrospective study. Inform Med Unlocked. 2023;40: 101316.
15. Lee JY, Lee SWH. Telemedicine cost-effectiveness for diabetes management: a systematic review. Diabetes Res Clin Pract. 2022;188:109928.
16. Eberle C, Stichling S. Impact of telemedical care on quality of life in people with diabetes. J Clin Med. 2023;12(4):1542.
17. Gordon BA, Benson AC, Bird SR, Fraser SF. Resistance training improves metabolic health in type 2 diabetes: a systematic review. Diabetes Res Clin Pract. 2009;83(2):157-75.
18. Kerr D, Gabbay RA. Challenges and opportunities in using telehealth for diabetes care. Diabetes Spectr. 2022;35(1):33-40.
19. Correia JC, Meraj H, Teoh SH, Waqas A, Ahmad M, Lapão LV, et al. Telemedicine to deliver diabetes care in low- and middle-income countries: a systematic review and meta-analysis. Bull World Health Organ. 2021;99(3):209-219B.
20. Patel R, Huang J, Hsueh L, Gopalan A, Millman A, Franklin I, Reed M. Telemedicine's Impact on Diabetes Care During the COVID-19 Pandemic: A Cohort Study in a Large Integrated Healthcare System. J Diabetes. 2025;17(5):e70096.

13

Public Health Strategies for Diabetes Prevention

Ranjit Mohan Anjana, Akshay Subramanian A, Viswanathan Mohan

ABSTRACT

The International Diabetes Federation (IDF) estimates that there are 589 million people living with diabetes worldwide as of 2024, and this number is expected to increase to 853 million by the year 2050. As diabetes is associated with considerable morbidity and mortality as well as costs to the individual and society, it is imperative to employ effective public health strategies at population level to counter the increasing prevalence of diabetes. Individuals at risk of diabetes progress from normoglycemia through stages of intermediate hyperglycemia (prediabetes) before they develop frank diabetes, providing a window of opportunity for primary prevention. It has now been unequivocally shown that lifestyle modification, with or without medication, can delay or prevent the progression from prediabetes to diabetes. However, translating these findings into real life is challenging and requires reorientation of health policy as well as intersectoral coordination between various stakeholders. Several such initiatives have been launched at the National and State level in India, holding out promise for diabetes prevention at the population level.

Keywords: Public, Strategies, Diabetes, Prevention.

INTRODUCTION

Diabetes is a silent chronic noncommunicable disease (NCD) that occurs either when the pancreas does not produce enough insulin or when the body cannot effectively use the insulin it produces. Uncontrolled diabetes is characterized by chronic hyperglycemia that can, over time, lead to serious damage to various organs and culminate in severe morbidity or even mortality.

MAGNITUDE OF THE PROBLEM

The International Diabetes Federation (IDF) estimates that there are 589 million people living with diabetes worldwide as of 2024, and this number is expected to increase to 853 million by the year 2050. The prevalence is particularly high and is increasing rapidly in low- and middle-income countries compared to high-income countries.[1]

In India, the large, nationally representative—Indian Council of Medical Research-India Diabetes (ICMR-INDIAB) study—showed that there were 101 million individuals with diabetes, much higher than the previously reported figures.[2]

NEED FOR PREVENTING DIABETES

Diabetes and its complications are a leading cause of morbidity and mortality worldwide. The IDF Diabetes Atlas[1] estimates 3.4 million annual deaths from diabetes complications worldwide as of 2024. Individuals with diabetes have higher all-cause mortality and mortality due to cardiovascular disease (CVD), cancer, chronic lower respiratory diseases, cerebrovascular disease, and kidney disease.[3] Further morbidity occurs due to limb amputations and vision loss following proliferative diabetic retinopathy, diabetic cataract, or glaucoma.

Globally, the average annual medical expenditure for people with diabetes is around $19,736, with about $12,022 attributed to diabetes itself.[4] Costs increase with complications, with patients with greater number of complications incurring higher expenses. The costs for insulin and medications as well as inpatient care necessitated by the presence of serious complications, represents a serious financial drain on individuals in countries like India, where medical expenses need to be borne out of pocket.

NATURAL HISTORY OF DIABETES

The natural history of diabetes is characterized by gradual progression from normal glucose tolerance through a stage of intermediate hyperglycemia or prediabetes [defined as impaired glucose tolerance (IGT) or impaired fasting glucose (IFG)], then to clinical diabetes and finally to the stage of complications. Prediabetes is that stage in an individual where the blood glucose level is higher than the normal but not high enough to be diagnosed as diabetes.

Individuals with fasting glucose between 100 and 125 mg/dL are considered to have IFG while those with 2-hour post-load blood glucose (during an oral glucose tolerance test) between 140 and 199 mg/dL are considered to have IGT. IFG and IGT can occur in isolation, or together (combined IFG and IGT). With the increasing use of glycated hemoglobin (HbA1c) for diagnosis of diabetes, individuals with HbA1c between 5.7 and 6.4% are considered to be "at risk of diabetes", yet another phenotype of prediabetes.

The progression from prediabetes to type 2 diabetes (T2D) is not inevitable and does not occur at the same rate in all populations, occurring at high levels in populations such as Pima Indians and Asian Indians.[5] There is now sufficient evidence to show that pharmacological and nonpharmacological interventions can prevent or slow the progression of prediabetes to diabetes. Many of these interventions can also reduce cardiovascular risk in individuals with prediabetes. Therefore, there is an urgent need to identify individuals with prediabetes so that prompt preventive measures can be implemented in them. However, most people with prediabetes are asymptomatic and can only be identified by screening. The need for screening is particularly high in populations with high prevalence of T2D, such as Asian Indians. **Figure 1** depicts the stages of prevention of diabetes.

In general, there are four levels of prevention for any disease: Primordial prevention, primary prevention, secondary prevention, and tertiary prevention.

The prevention of emergence of the risk factors for a disease is called primordial prevention. When the risk factors are already present in an individual, the measures taken to prevent the individual from developing the disease are called primary prevention. Once the disease has developed in a person, early and prompt diagnosis with adequate treatment will help in preventing or delaying the complications. This is called secondary prevention. When the patient has ended up with complications of the disease, providing proper rehabilitation and disability limitation to ensure quality of life becomes a priority. This is tertiary prevention. Preventing individuals with prediabetes from developing T2D is an example of primary prevention. **Figure 2** shows the complexity of diabetogenic factors.

EVIDENCES FOR TYPE 2 DIABETES PREVENTION

Da Qing Study

The Da Qing study conducted in China[6] attempted to demonstrate feasibility of prevention of T2D.

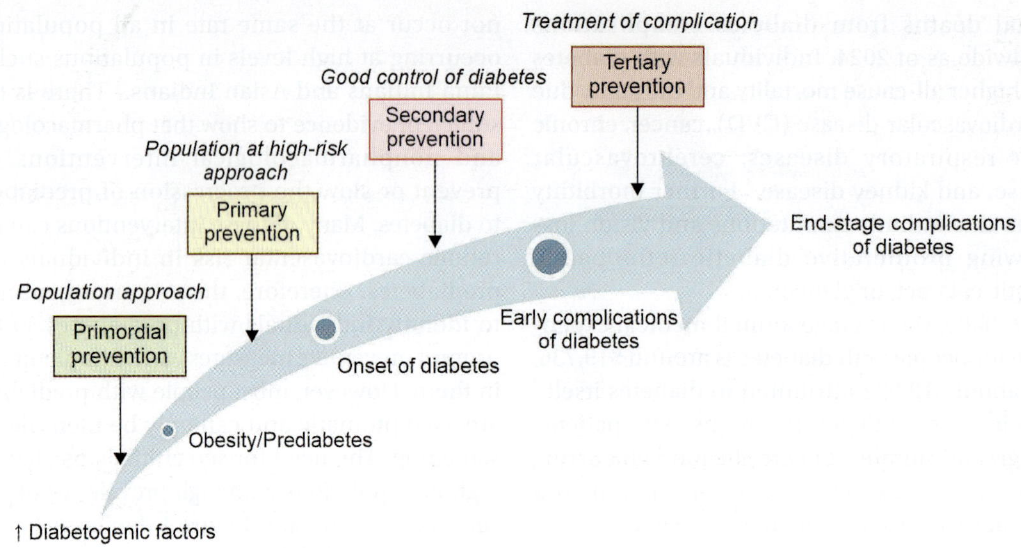

Fig. 1: Stages of diabetes prevention.

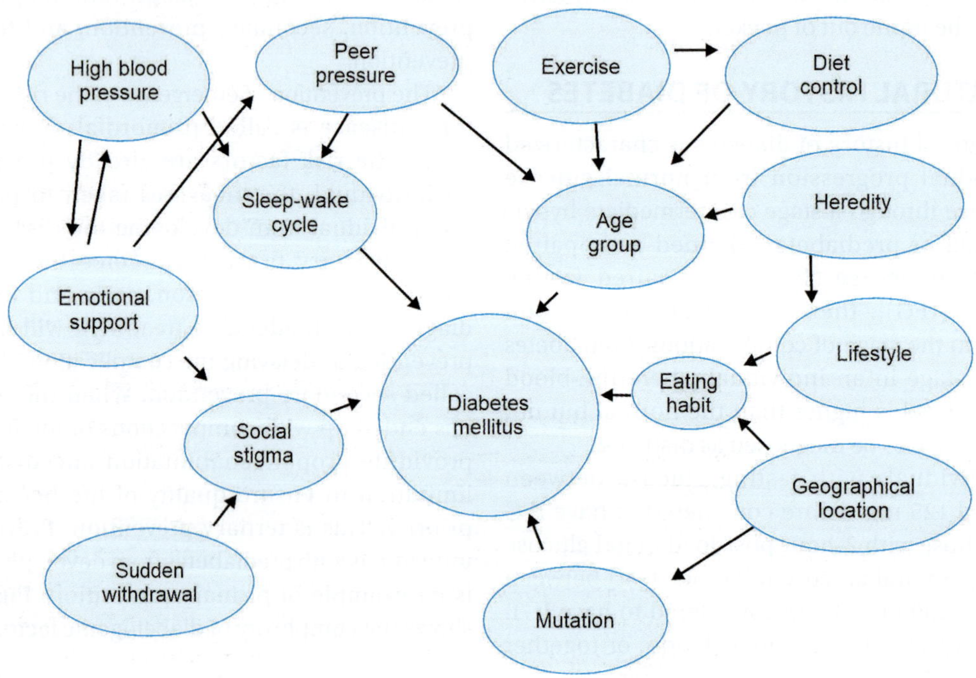

Fig. 2: Multifactorial causation of diabetes.

This was a cluster randomized trial in which 577 adults with IGT attending 33 clinics were randomly assigned to four groups: Control, diet, exercise, and diet plus exercise for 6 years. At the end of the study period, individuals randomized to diet, exercise and diet, and exercise had a lower risk of developing diabetes by 31.5, 46, and 42% compared to those assigned to control. Subsequently, participants were followed to assess the long-term effects of intervention on the incidence of diabetes, CVD events, composite microvascular complications, CVD death, all-cause mortality, and life expectancy. At the end of the 30 years of follow-up, the combined intervention group had a median delay of about 3.96 years for T2D onset, fewer cardiovascular events and deaths, and lesser incidence of microvascular complications.

Finnish Diabetes Prevention Study

In the Finnish DPS,[7] 522 individuals with IGT were randomized to intervention group (individualized counseling aimed at reducing weight, total intake of fat, and intake of saturated fat and increasing intake of fiber and physical activity) or control group and followed up for a mean duration of 3.2 years. At the end of follow-up, individuals randomized to the intervention group had a 58% lower risk of diabetes compared to the control group. These benefits were maintained at the 7-year follow-up, with 43% risk reduction in progression to T2D compared to nonintervention.

Diabetes Prevention Program

The United States (US) Diabetes Prevention Program (DPP)[8] was a large randomized controlled trial evaluating the effects of lifestyle intervention or metformin on modifying the risk of T2D in individuals at high risk. The DPP enrolled 3,234 individuals with prediabetes and assigned them to one of three groups: Placebo, lifestyle intervention, and metformin. After a mean follow-up of 2.8 years, individuals randomized to lifestyle modification had a 58% lower, and those randomized to metformin, 31% lower risk of developing T2D as compared to those assigned to placebo. The long-term follow-up of the DPP, the DPP-Outcomes Study (DPP-OS) showed that the benefits of lifestyle intervention and metformin were maintained for up to 15 years, albeit attenuated (27% risk reduction in the lifestyle group and 18% in the metformin group).

Indian Diabetes Prevention Program

This prospective community-based study analyzed if progression to diabetes can be influenced by interventions among Asian Indians with IGT. Study participants (n = 531) were randomized into four different groups—(1) control, (2) lifestyle modification, (3) metformin, and (4) lifestyle modification plus metformin. The study concluded[9] that combination of lifestyle intervention along with metformin was associated with the greatest risk reduction for T2D (relative risk reduction of 28.2%).

Diabetes-community Lifestyle Intervention Program

This study[10] tested the effectiveness, cost-effectiveness, and acceptability of a stepwise model of diabetes prevention with lifestyle modifications as a continuous intervention in the targeted group, and metformin added only when needed (stepwise addition of 500 mg metformin twice a day to those who were at highest risk of conversion to T2D after 4 months or more of follow-up). Participants with prediabetes (IGT, IFG, or both IFG and IGT) (n = 578) were randomly assigned into intervention and control groups. While those in the control group received only the standard of care, the intervention was put to rigorous lifestyle modification with 16 weekly classes and an additional 8 weeks of maintenance classes. At the end of the 3-year follow-up period, only 25.7% of those among the intervention group progressed to T2D compared with 34.9% of those in the control group. This program also provided clues for the sustainability of these lifestyle modification programs, as it utilized the services of lay "diabetes ambassadors" who helped in training and motivating participants.

ARE WE TREATING EARLY OR PREVENTING?

Several randomized trials (including some of those listed above) have made use of medications to prevent the development of T2D, in addition to lifestyle modifications, with varying results. These medications include the antidiabetic drugs metformin, acarbose, rosiglitazone, and nateglinide and the renin–angiotensin–aldosterone system blockers, ramipril and valsartan. While some of the newer antidiabetic agents (such as the glucagon-like peptide 1 receptor agonists and glucagon-like peptide–glucose-dependent insulinotropic peptide dual receptor agonists) have been shown to reduce the incidence of diabetes, these findings have emerged predominantly from weight loss trials and not from formal diabetes prevention trials. The use of antidiabetic drugs to prevent diabetes raises an important question: In the name of preventing T2D, are we merely initiating pharmacotherapy for hyperglycemia earlier? Also, none of the drugs mentioned above are approved for prevention of diabetes, although some national diabetes associations do provide guidance supporting this indication. The case is often made that popping a daily pill is easier and more convenient for the individual than undertaking the significant lifestyle modifications that have been shown to be necessary to prevent diabetes. Such an argument fails to take into consideration, issues regarding the sustainability, cost-effectiveness, and long-term safety of pharmacotherapy, with particular reference to the newer agents. Lifestyle modification, on the other hand, has benefits not only in preventing diabetes but also other metabolic conditions such as hypertension, dyslipidemia, and obesity. As will be seen below, there is now evidence that less stringent lifestyle modifications than those trialled in randomized prevention programs might suffice to prevent diabetes at the population level. Therefore, for most individuals with prediabetes, lifestyle change should be the initial intervention of choice.

TRANSLATING RESULTS OF CLINICAL TRIALS INTO PRACTICE: WHAT IS THE EVIDENCE?

As discussed earlier, bringing into practice intensive lifestyle modification interventions (such as those described in the trials above) in large populations is largely impractical. It requires logistics, trained human resources and the need for societal adjustments coupled with health system strengthening. However, some population-based interventions in advanced countries provide hope that this can indeed be achieved.

United Kingdom National Health Service Diabetes Prevention Program

The United Kingdom National Health Service Diabetes Prevention Program (UK NHS DPP) aims to integrate diabetes prevention into routine health care. It offers individuals with prediabetes and others at high risk with 9–12 months of behavioral modification intervention sessions for adopting a healthier lifestyle, aiming at weight reduction and counseling to improve physical activity and to develop habits of healthier eating. Participants who signed up to the program had significant reductions in HbA1c, body mass index (BMI), body weight, triglycerides and increased high-density lipoprotein (HDL)-cholesterol with a nonsignificant reduction in systolic blood pressure.[11] These sessions are based on the NICE guidelines and participants are referred by general practitioners. This program has been shown to be cost-effective and represents a major advance toward diabetes prevention being employed at a population level.

National Diabetes Prevention Program

The National Diabetes Prevention Program (National DPP) has been implemented since 2012 by the Centers for Disease Control (CDC) in the US. It focuses on structured lifestyle interventions targeting weight loss and increased physical activity. It has demonstrated significant success in reducing diabetes incidence among adults with prediabetes. In one study from the University of Michigan,[12] enrollees had lower odds of developing T2D (40% lower at 1 year and 20% lower at 2 years) compared to nonenrollees. Overall, the National DPP has demonstrated that a structured lifestyle intervention program can effectively lower T2D risk at the population level and can be cost-effective.

However, both these population-based programs have been conducted in developed countries. Whether similar programs can be successfully planned and implemented in resource-constrained settings is yet to be determined.

EVIDENCE FROM INDIA; SMALL CHANGES CAN LEAD TO BIG BENEFITS!

Dietary Changes

Hippocrates has rightly said "Let food be thy medicine and medicine be thy food". What he meant to emphasize was the profound correlation between what we eat and its impact on health. Diet is not just about calories (quantity of food) but also about the quality of the food. A good curated medical nutrition therapy will largely help in achieving and maintaining the required weight of the individual for age, thereby also helping in improving insulin sensitivity and reducing risk of T2D. A healthy diet is characterized by a balanced intake of both macronutrients and micronutrients. Various dietary approaches to treating and preventing diabetes employ drastic changes in the composition of the diet, such as total removal of carbohydrates or avoidance of all processed foods. Such diets, although effective, are not sustainable and their long-term safety has also been called into question.

Data from ICMR - INDIAB study suggest[13] that even minimal modification of dietary macronutrient intake can help to prevent diabetes in those with prediabetes, or even lead to remission of diabetes in those who have newly developed the disorder. For instance, it has been shown that reducing the carbohydrate content of the diet to 50–56% total daily energy intake and increasing protein intake to 18–20% can help individuals with prediabetes return to normal glucose tolerance. Similarly, a carbohydrate content of 54–57% and protein,16–20% was shown to prevent progression of prediabetes to T2D. These dietary intakes do not represent a major deviation from the typical Asian Indian diet and should therefore be easy for individuals to adopt and follow over the long term.

Physical Activity

Physical activity levels have declined worldwide on account of urbanization, automation of occupations, and availability of motorized transport. In developed countries, part of this decline has been compensated by increases in leisure-time physical activity (LTPA). However, in developing countries such as India, levels of LTPA are abysmally low[14] rendering the population at high risk of developing metabolic diseases such as obesity and T2D. Low levels of physical activity also make diabetes prevention challenging.

Many reasons have been given for the low levels of LTPA in India. In addition to lack of awareness, these include lack of time, lack of places to exercise, unfavorable weather, and safety concerns. These issues are particularly relevant among women and girls, in whom societal norms pose an additional barrier to exercising. In order to improve physical activity levels among women and girls and thereby reduce their risk of diabetes and other metabolic disorders, a novel high-intensity interval training (HIIT) dance routine called THANDAV has recently been introduced.[15] THANDAV is a 10-minute HIIT routine consisting of four loops including a 2 minutes high [80–90% of maximum heart rate (HR)] and a 30 seconds low (50–60% of maximum HR). The movements are choreographed in a simple and repetitive manner so that they can be done in a loop without much stress. THANDAV has been shown to favorably impact parameters such as step count, skeletal muscle mass, fat mass, blood pressure, sleep, and stress levels in adolescent girls and may represent an easily scalable, culturally acceptable approach to diabetes prevention in this population.

ROLE OF PUBLIC HEALTH POLICY

The current global pandemic of T2D is a direct consequence of the obesogenic environment that exists today in most parts of the world. While the ultimate responsibility for health lies on the individual, the role of other stakeholders such as local and national governments cannot be forgotten.

Global Initiatives to Improve Metabolic Health

Taking cognizance of the burgeoning epidemic of NCDs, the World Health Organization (WHO) proposed a Global Action Plan on Physical Activity (GAPA)[16] in 2018. This plan aims at reducing physical inactivity by 15% by the year 2030. The strategies under this plan include creating active societies by mass awareness campaigns, developing active environments by providing safe parts and cycling paths, promoting active people by community-based programs and building active systems via policy support and workforce training.

The WHO's Global Strategy on Diet, Physical Activity and Health,[17] unveiled in 2004, urges governments to implement policies to promote healthy diets (low in sugar, salt, and fat and high in fiber), increase physical activity in daily routines and in schools, and support public education and food labeling reforms.

Initiatives in the Indian Context

There is much that health policy can do to slow down the spread of diabetes in developing countries like India. The explosive increase in T2D in India mainly occurred following the liberalization and globalization policies adopted by the government in the early 1990s. These policies, doubtless, contributed to the prosperity of the nation, but brought other problems in their wake. Higher levels of disposable income led to increased discretionary expenditure on items such as junk foods and high-calorie, low nutritional value foods that suddenly became available consequent to opening up of the economy. Parallelly, there was a shift away from labor-intensive occupations and nonmotorized transport, reducing levels of physical activity in the occupational and transport domains. All these have led to burgeoning obesity rates and rising prevalence of T2D.

While one cannot argue in favor of a return to the conditions of 1950s or 1960s, there needs to be a clearsighted policy on improving the metabolic health of the population so that India's gains in healthcare over the last 75 years are not compromised by a tsunami of NCDs. In recent years, the Government of India has prioritized NCD prevention and management in its national health policies. The National Multi-sectoral Action Plan (NMAP)[18] for NCDs was launched in 2017 to promote lifestyle modification as a core strategy for NCD prevention. This plan encourages intersectoral collaboration between health, education, urban planning, and agriculture to tackle the growing epidemic of NCDs in India.

- *Policy on diet:* Awareness needs to be created on healthy eating. In a country where, until recently, the main issue was not having enough to eat, the new paradigm of overnutrition demands out-of-the-box solutions. Enforcing food labeling (and training consumers to read them) and instituting sugar and fat taxes (as has already been done by several states) will motivate adoption of healthier diets. Of course, healthier foods need to be made more easily available, accessible, and affordable. In this context, Government needs to rethink the easy availability of refined cereals through the public distribution system and consider providing healthier options such as pulses, legumes and vegetables through the system, so that the less well-off can also eat healthy. Awareness on healthy diets should be inculcated from childhood. In this context, the recent initiative by the Central Board of Secondary Education (CBSE) to promote healthy eating in schools, in particular by cutting down sugar intake, is timely and welcome. Healthier meals can also be provided through the "mid-day meal scheme" operational in many states of India. The "Eat Right India" movement,[19] led by the Food Safety and Standards Authority of India (FSSAI), focuses on reducing trans fat, sugar, and salt in the diet, promoting fortified foods, and nutrition labeling and public awareness.

- Encouraging physical activity from a young age is essential to prevent the development of prediabetes and T2D. With the enormous industrialization and overcrowding prevalent in a populous country like India, sometimes finding the right space for exercise becomes challenging. The government again needs to allocate more resources and infrastructure into finding large spaces for physical activity, such as public parks. Emphasis should be laid on improving the built environment[20] by promoting walkable and bicycle-friendly cities. Schools should be required to allocate sufficient time for physical activity. Initiatives such as THANDAV can be adopted to bring physical activity within the reach of individuals who would otherwise be excluded. The Fit India Movement[21] launched in 2019, is a national campaign to encourage citizens to adopt physically active lifestyles. This is being implemented in schools, workplaces, and communities.
- In spite of all the above efforts, some individuals in the population will develop prediabetes. The objective in these cases should be to identify them at the earliest possible stages such that they can adopt intensive lifestyle changes and delay or prevent T2D. As prediabetes is a silent condition, it can only be picked up by screening using a blood test. At the population level, it is impractical to screen all adults; it would be more cost-effective to identify individuals at high risk using validated tools such as the Indian Diabetes Risk Score (IDRS), and direct screening and prevention efforts to them. Screening for diabetes and prediabetes should be incorporated into primary care across India.

CONCLUSION

In conclusion, delaying/preventing the onset of T2D in India can be achieved by lifestyle intervention with or without medication in individuals found to have prediabetes. This can be integrated into primary healthcare across the country. However, arresting the diabetes epidemic in India ultimately demands correction of the obesogenic environment in the country. This can only be achieved by multisectoral coordination including the health, transport, food, and education sectors.

REFERENCES

1. International Diabetes Federation. (2025). IDF Diabetes Atlas 2025. [online] Available from https://diabetesatlas.org/resources/idf-diabetes-atlas-2025/ [Last accessed September, 2025].
2. Anjana RM, Unnikrishnan R, Deepa M, Pradeepa R, Tandon N, Das AK, et al. Metabolic non-communicable disease health report of India: the ICMR-INDIAB national cross-sectional study (ICMR-INDIAB-17). Lancet Diabetes Endocrinol. 2023;11(7):474-89.
3. Li S, Wang J, Zhang B, Li X, Liu Y. Diabetes Mellitus and Cause-Specific Mortality: A Population-Based Study. Diabetes & Metabolism Journal 2019;43(3):319.
4. Bommer C, Sagalova V, Heesemann E, Manne-Goehler J, Atun R, Bärnighausen T, et al. Global Economic Burden of Diabetes in Adults: Projections From 2015 to 2030. Diabetes Care. 2018;41(5):963-70.
5. Anjana RM, Shanthi Rani CS, Deepa M, Pradeepa R, Sudha V, Divya Nair H, et al. Incidence of Diabetes and Prediabetes and Predictors of Progression Among Asian Indians: 10-Year Follow-up of the Chennai Urban Rural Epidemiology Study (CURES). Diabetes Care. 2015;38(8):1441-8.
6. Pan XR, Li GW, Hu YH, Wang JX, Yang WY, An ZX, et al. Effects of diet and exercise in preventing NIDDM

in people with impaired glucose tolerance. The Da Qing IGT and Diabetes Study. Diabetes Care. 1997;20(4):537-44.

7. Tuomilehto J, Lindström J, Eriksson JG, Valle TT, Hämäläinen H, Ilanne-Parikka P, et al. Prevention of Type 2 Diabetes Mellitus by Changes in Lifestyle among Subjects with Impaired Glucose Tolerance. N Engl J Med. 2001;344(18):1343-50.
8. Crandall JP, Dabelea D, Knowler WC, Nathan DM, Temprosa M; DPP Research Group. The Diabetes Prevention Program and Its Outcomes Study: NIDDK's Journey Into the Prevention of Type 2 Diabetes and Its Public Health Impact. Diabetes Care. 2025;48(7):1101-11.
9. Ramachandran A, Snehalatha C, Mary S, Mukesh B, Bhaskar AD, Vijay V. The Indian Diabetes Prevention Programme shows that lifestyle modification and metformin prevent type 2 diabetes in Asian Indian subjects with impaired glucose tolerance (IDPP-1). Diabetologia. 2006;49(2):289-97.
10. Weber MB, Ranjani H, Staimez LR, Anjana RM, Ali MK, Narayan KMV, et al. The Stepwise Approach to Diabetes Prevention: Results From the D-CLIP Randomized Controlled Trial. Diabetes Care. 2016;39(10):1760-7.
11. Ravindrarajah R, Sutton M, Reeves D, Cotterill S, Mcmanus E, Meacock R, et al. Referral to the NHS Diabetes Prevention Programme and conversion from nondiabetic hyperglycaemia to type 2 diabetes mellitus in England: A matched cohort analysis. PLoS Med. 2023;20(2):e1004177.
12. Herman WH, Villatoro C, Joiner KL, McEwen LN. Retention and outcomes of National Diabetes Prevention Program enrollees and non-enrollees with prediabetes: The University of Michigan experience. J Diabetes Complications. 2023;37(8):108527.
13. Anjana RM, Srinivasan S, Sudha V, Joshi SR, Saboo B, Tandon N, et al. Macronutrient Recommendations for Remission and Prevention of Diabetes in Asian Indians Based on a Data-Driven Optimization Model: The ICMR-INDIAB National Study. Diabetes Care. 2022:dc220627.
14. Strain T, Flaxman S, Guthold R, Semenova E, Cowan M, Riley LM, et al. National, regional, and global trends in insufficient physical activity among adults from 2000 to 2022: a pooled analysis of 507 population-based surveys with 5·7 million participants. Lancet Glob Health. 2024;12(8):e1232-e1243. Erratum in: Lancet Glob Health. 2025;13(2):e202.
15. Anjana RM, Nitika S, Jagannathan N, Vinothini D, Yuvarani K, Mohan V, et al. A Novel High-Intensity Short Interval Dance Intervention (THANDAV) for Non-Communicable Disease Prevention Tailored to Asian Indian Adolescent Girls. J Diabetes Sci Technol. 2025;19(4):1035-50.
16. WHO. (2018). Let's be active, the global action plan on physical activity 2018-2030. [online] Available from www.who.int. or https://www.who.int/initiatives/gappa [Last accessed September, 2025].
17. WHO. (2004). Global Strategy on Diet, Physical Activity and Health. [online] Available from www.who.int. or https://www.who.int/publications/i/item/9241592222 [Last accessed September, 2025].
18. Ministry of Health & Family Welfare, Government of India. (2023). Operational Guidelines: National Programme for Prevention and Control of Non-Communicable Diseases (2023-2030). [online] Available from Mohfw.gov.in or https://www.mohfw.gov.in/sites/default/files/NP-NCD%20Operational%20Guidelines_0.pdf [Last accessed September, 2025].
19. Food Safety and Standards Authority of India (FSSAI). Eat Right India. [online] Available from https://eatrightindia.gov.in/ [Last accessed September, 2025].
20. Aarthi GR, Begum TSM, Moosawi SA, Kusuma D, Ranjani H, Pradeepa R, et al. Associations of the built environment with type 2 diabetes in Asia: a systematic review. BMJ Open. 2023;13(4):e065431.
21. FIT India Movement: Ministry of Education (MoE) Activities [Internet]. Education.gov.in. 2024. Available from https://dsel.education.gov.in/en/fit-india. [Last accessed September, 2025].

14

Global Initiatives and Policies in Diabetes Care

Amit Gupta, Sanjay Agarwal, Soumyaranjan Mohanty

ABSTRACT

Diabetes mellitus represents a critical global public health challenge, with its prevalence quadrupling over the past four decades. Addressing disparities in prevention, treatment accessibility, and long-term management requires coordinated policies and international collaboration. This chapter comprehensively reviews key global initiatives in diabetes care, including the WHO Global Diabetes Compact and the coverage targets adopted at the 75th World Health Assembly (WHA). It also examines updates to the WHO Essential Medicines List and regionally tailored programs. Guideline frameworks such as the International Diabetes Federation (IDF) Global Clinical Practice Recommendations and the American Diabetes Association (ADA) Standards of Care are discussed, alongside emerging digital health innovations such as artificial intelligence (AI)-based predictive tools and telemonitoring. Case studies from India, the UK, and Africa illustrate national adaptations of these strategies. Clinical implications emphasize the importance of integrating policies into primary care, ensuring affordable access to medicines, and delivering culturally relevant education. Notable advances, including the inclusion of glucagon-like peptide 1 (GLP-1) receptor agonists in the WHO Essential Medicines List and AI-enabled risk prediction models, reflect progress while highlighting persistent inequities in resource-limited settings. The chapter concludes with recommendations to strengthen implementation, promote equity, and align global diabetes goals with national health priorities.

Keywords: Diabetes care, WHO Global Diabetes Compact, Essential medicines list, IDF guidelines, ADA standards of care, Health policy, Global health.

INTRODUCTION

Diabetes mellitus has emerged as one of the most urgent public health challenges of the 21st century. Over the past four decades, the global prevalence of diabetes has surged dramatically, with the number of adults living with the condition increasing from approximately 108 million in 1980 to over 537 million in 2021, representing a fourfold rise.[1] Projections by the International Diabetes Federation (IDF) estimate that this number will reach 783 million by 2045, with the most significant increases expected in low- and middle-income countries (LMICs).[2] This alarming trend highlights the critical need for coordinated, global strategies that focus on equitable and sustainable prevention, diagnosis, and management of diabetes.

The burden of diabetes is multifaceted, encompassing both clinical and societal dimensions. It is associated with microvascular complications such as retinopathy, nephropathy, and neuropathy, and substantially elevates the risk of macrovascular complications, including ischemic heart disease and stroke. Consequently, individuals with diabetes face a twofold to threefold increased risk of cardiovascular disease (CVD) compared to those without diabetes.[3] Beyond health impacts, diabetes imposes a considerable economic burden. In 2021, global health expenditure on diabetes reached USD 966 billion, marking a 316% increase over the past 15 years.[4] While healthcare systems in high-income countries (HICs) bear the majority of these costs, the financial impact is disproportionately severe in LMICs, where constrained health budgets and high out-of-pocket expenditures exacerbate the challenge.

A critical aspect of the diabetes epidemic is the gap in diagnosis and care. According to the IDF Diabetes Atlas 2023, nearly 50% of adults with diabetes remain undiagnosed globally, and the figure rises to over 60% in LMICs.[2] Undiagnosed and untreated diabetes contributes substantially to preventable morbidity and mortality. Furthermore, inequalities in access to essential medicines such as insulin, glucose-monitoring devices, and novel pharmacotherapies exacerbate disparities in health outcomes. For example, a WHO report from 2022 highlighted that while insulin has been available for over a century, many patients in LMICs still lack affordable and reliable access to this life-saving drug.[5]

The growing burden of diabetes has prompted urgent calls for global cooperation, leading to the establishment of several international initiatives and policy frameworks. The World Health Organization (WHO) has taken a central role, particularly through the launch of the Global Diabetes Compact in 2021, which seeks to unify governments, civil society, and private sector partners toward achieving measurable global targets by 2030.[6] Similarly, the 75th WHA in 2022 adopted the first-ever global diabetes coverage targets, including goals to diagnose 80% of people with diabetes and ensure 100% of individuals with type 1 diabetes have access to affordable insulin.[7] These initiatives represent a paradigm shift in acknowledging diabetes not only as a clinical condition but also as a priority for global health security, equity, and sustainable development.

Alongside WHO's efforts, other global and regional organizations have intensified their contributions. The IDF continues to provide guidance through its Clinical Practice Recommendations, most recently updated in 2025, which emphasize adaptable, evidence-based interventions across diverse healthcare systems.[8] The American Diabetes Association (ADA) has also advanced the global dialogue by expanding the applicability of its Standards of Care to international contexts, underscoring the importance of integrating obesity management, psychosocial support, and cardiovascular risk reduction into comprehensive diabetes care.[9]

The COVID-19 pandemic further highlighted the vulnerabilities of people living with diabetes. Not only were individuals with diabetes at greater risk of severe outcomes from SARS-CoV-2 infection, but the pandemic also disrupted essential diabetes services worldwide, from screening and routine follow-up to medication supply chains.[10] These disruptions reinforced the need for resilient, integrated health systems capable of sustaining chronic disease management during global crises. They also accelerated innovations in telemedicine, digital health, and remote patient monitoring, which are now increasingly being recognized in global policy frameworks.

In parallel, the global policy landscape for diabetes has been influenced by the inclusion of newer pharmacological agents in essential medicine frameworks. The WHO's decision in 2025 to add glucagon-like peptide 1 receptor agonists (GLP-1 RAs) and rapid-acting insulin analogs to its essential medicines list marks a significant milestone in broadening the spectrum of affordable therapeutic options.[11] These developments illustrate how global policies can catalyze both innovation and access, provided that equitable distribution mechanisms are ensured.

At the national level, countries have begun adapting these global frameworks to their specific contexts. For instance, India has operationalized large-scale noncommunicable disease (NCD) clinics and partnered with the World Diabetes Foundation (WDF) and WHO to improve access to diagnostics and essential medicines in underserved regions.[12] In Africa, WHO's Regional Office has launched implementation roadmaps to integrate diabetes care into primary health systems, though challenges such as supply-chain weaknesses and workforce shortages persist.[13] Meanwhile, HICs like the United Kingdom are piloting artificial intelligence (AI)-based predictive tools within their national health systems, aimed at identifying individuals at high risk of type 2 diabetes years before onset.[14] Together, these examples demonstrate how global initiatives are translated into diverse national strategies, tailored to local epidemiology, resources, and capacities.

This chapter will explore these global initiatives and policies in detail, with a focus on their objectives, implementation, and clinical implications. It will also examine recent advances in digital health and pharmacotherapy, discuss persistent gaps in access and equity, and highlight emerging strategies for integrating diabetes care into broader health system strengthening efforts. By synthesizing recent evidence and policy developments, this chapter aims to provide a comprehensive understanding of the global response to diabetes and identify future directions for research, practice, and policymaking.

GLOBAL POLICY FRAMEWORKS AND INITIATIVES

The accelerating diabetes epidemic has garnered unprecedented global attention from policymakers, international organizations, and advocacy groups. Over the past decade, key stakeholders including the WHO, the United Nations (UN), and nongovernmental organizations such as the IDF and the WDF have led multiple initiatives aimed at harmonizing efforts in the prevention, diagnosis, and treatment of diabetes globally. These frameworks emphasize not only effective disease control but also prioritize equity, sustainability, and the integration of diabetes care into broader NCD agendas.

WHO Global Diabetes Compact (2021)

The WHO Global Diabetes Compact, launched in April 2021, represents a landmark step in positioning diabetes as a central component of global health policy.[6] The compact calls for:

- Political commitment at the highest levels to address diabetes as part of NCD prevention.
- Universal access to essential medicines and technologies, including insulin, glucose monitoring, and oral therapies.
- Primary healthcare integration, ensuring that diabetes care is not siloed but part of comprehensive health services.
- Accountability and monitoring through global targets and indicators. Importantly, the compact aligns with the sustainable development goals (SDGs), particularly goal 3, which seeks to reduce premature mortality from NCDs by one-third by 2030.

Global Coverage Targets for 2030

At the 75th WHA in May 2022, member states endorsed the first-ever global diabetes coverage targets, designed to be achieved by 2030.[7] These include:

- 80% of people with diabetes diagnosed
- 80% of people with diagnosed diabetes achieving good glycemic control
- 80% achieving blood pressure control
- 60% of adults with diabetes aged 40 years or older receiving statin therapy
- 100% of people with type 1 diabetes having access to affordable insulin and self-monitoring of blood glucose.

TABLE 1: WHO global coverage targets for diabetes by 2030.

Target no.	*Coverage indicator*	*2030 goal*
1	Proportion of people with diabetes who are diagnosed	80%
2	Proportion achieving glycemic control	80%
3	Proportion achieving blood pressure control	80%
4	Adults ≥ 40 years receiving statin therapy	60%
5	Type 1 diabetes patients with access to insulin and monitoring	100%

Source: World Health Organization. First-ever global coverage targets for diabetes adopted at the 75th World Health Assembly. Geneva: WHO; 2022.

These targets are ambitious but provide a benchmark for countries to align national policies with global commitments **(Table 1)**.

WHO Essential Medicines List (EML) Updates (2025)

A landmark advancement in global diabetes policy was the inclusion of GLP-1 RA (such as semaglutide and tirzepatide) and rapid-acting insulin analogs in the WHO Model List of Essential Medicines in 2025.[11] This decision was driven by robust evidence demonstrating these agents' efficacy in reducing cardiovascular risk and improving glycemic control.

The addition of GLP-1 RA is particularly significant due to their dual benefits of enhancing blood sugar regulation and promoting weight loss, which is crucial given the strong link between obesity and diabetes. However, challenges remain in ensuring equitable access to these medications, as their high-cost limits availability, especially in LMICs. The WHO's endorsement presents an opportunity for governments to negotiate better pricing and for global procurement mechanisms to integrate these therapies into essential medicine supply chains.

Regional WHO Adaptations

The WHO Regional Offices have tailored the Global Diabetes Compact to local contexts:

- *Africa (AFRO)*: A framework launched in 2023 prioritizes strengthening primary care systems, improving supply chains, and training health workers.[13]
- *America (PAHO)*: Focus on health equity, particularly in underserved rural and indigenous populations.
- *Europe (EURO)*: Emphasis on harmonizing digital health strategies and leveraging electronic health records.
- *South-East Asia (SEARO)*: Focused on integrating diabetes care into maternal and child health programs, given the region's rising gestational diabetes prevalence.

Role of Nongovernmental Organizations

The IDF and WDF play critical roles in complementing WHO's policy frameworks:

- The IDF continues to play a pivotal role in global advocacy, education, and the dissemination of clinical guidelines. Its 2025 global clinical practice recommendations for type 2 diabetes emphasize flexibility and advocate for low-cost, practical strategies tailored to the needs of LMICs.[8]
- Meanwhile, the WDF, in partnership with governments and the WHO, invests heavily in capacity-building initiatives. For instance, its 2024 collaboration with the Government of India aims to achieve 75% access to essential diagnostics and medicines in targeted districts.[12] These partnerships highlight how nongovernmental organizations effectively

address gaps left by international governance, especially in resource-constrained settings.

Integration into Broader NCD Frameworks

Global diabetes policy is increasingly embedded in the larger NCD prevention and control agenda. Diabetes shares common risk factors with other NCDs—such as tobacco use, unhealthy diet, physical inactivity, and alcohol misuse—making integrated policy approaches cost-effective and sustainable.[15] This has been evident in the WHO Global NCD Action Plan (2013–2030), where diabetes targets are aligned with goals for CVD and obesity prevention.

Challenges in Policy Implementation

Despite progress, several challenges hinder effective global implementation:

- *Resource inequities*: Insulin remains unavailable or unaffordable in many LMICs.
- *Health system fragmentation*: Diabetes care often lacks integration into primary health services.
- *Monitoring gaps*: Many countries lack reliable data systems to track progress toward global targets.
- *Pharmaceutical access*: While GLP-1 RA are now on the EML, their cost poses a barrier to scaling up.
- *Cultural barriers*: Policies often overlook gender, literacy, and cultural norms that influence self-care practices. Addressing these challenges requires cross-sectoral action, including innovative financing models, stronger governance, and active community participation.

CLINICAL GUIDELINES AND STANDARDIZATION

Clinical guidelines serve as the backbone of diabetes care, translating research evidence into structured, practical recommendations for clinicians, policymakers, and health systems. They define diagnostic thresholds, treatment algorithms, monitoring schedules, and preventive strategies. Yet, global diabetes care remains heterogeneous, shaped by differences in health system capacities, drug availability, cultural contexts, and economic priorities. Over the past 5 years, several organizations have revised their guidelines to emphasize patient-centered, resource-sensitive, and outcome-driven strategies.

American Diabetes Association Standards of Care (2025)

The ADA Standards of Care in Diabetes are updated annually and considered the global benchmark for evidence-based clinical practice. The 2025 edition introduced several key revisions:[9]

- *Diagnosis*: Emphasis on HbA1c ≥ 6.5% confirmed by repeat testing; fasting plasma glucose ≥ 126 mg/dL; or 2-hour oral glucose tolerance test (OGTT) ≥ 200 mg/dL.
- *Screening*: Universal screening recommended starting at age 35, with earlier testing for high-risk groups (obesity, family history, and gestational diabetes).
- *Pharmacologic therapy*: First-line treatment remains metformin, but strong preference for GLP-1 RA or SGLT-2 inhibitors in patients with CVD, chronic kidney disease (CKD), or obesity.
- *Technology*: Integration of continuous glucose monitoring (CGM) and hybrid closed-loop insulin pumps into care, particularly for type 1 diabetes.
- *Comorbidities*: Broader focus on mental health, social determinants of health, and sleep quality. While comprehensive, ADA guidelines often reflect high-resource settings, posing challenges for implementation in LMICs.

International Diabetes Federation Global Clinical Practice Recommendations (2025)

The IDF guidelines, revised in 2025, aim to provide a more resource-sensitive alternative to the ADA.[8] Distinguishing features include:

- *Tiered recommendations*: Care is stratified into basic, standard, and comprehensive levels, acknowledging variation in national health resources.
- *Essential medicines*: Emphasis on metformin, sulfonylureas, and human insulin as core therapies in resource-limited settings.
- *Nutrition and lifestyle*: Stronger focus on culturally adapted dietary advice and community-level interventions.
- *Primary care empowerment*: Encouragement of task-shifting, training nurses, and community health workers to deliver diabetes education and monitoring.
- *Technology use*: While acknowledging benefits of CGM and insulin pumps, IDF recognizes these may be inaccessible in LMICs and prioritizes cost-effective alternatives. This pragmatic framework is particularly influential in LMICs where ADA standards may be aspirational but unrealistic.

World Health Organization Package of Essential Noncommunicable Disease Interventions (PEN)

The WHO's Package of Essential Noncommunicable Disease Interventions (PEN) protocols, updated in 2023, integrate diabetes care into primary health care as part of a broader NCD framework.[16] Key features include:

- *Simplified protocols*: Clear algorithms for diagnosis and follow-up suitable for use by nonspecialist health workers.
- *Affordable essential medicines*: Ensuring uninterrupted supply of metformin, sulfonylureas, human insulin, and antihypertensive agents.
- *Risk-based management*: Prioritization of high-risk groups for intensive management (e.g., those with diabetes and hypertension).
- *Task-shifting*: Expanding roles of nonphysician health workers in screening, counseling, and follow-up.
- *Health system integration*: Linking diabetes care with maternal health, tuberculosis, and HIV programs for efficiency. PEN is crucial for countries where resources are constrained and physician density is low, offering a standardized but flexible blueprint.

National Guidelines and Regional Adaptations

While global guidelines provide overarching frameworks, national adaptations are essential to ensure feasibility and cultural fit.

- *India*: The RSSDI (Research Society for the Study of Diabetes in India) 2024 guidelines emphasize early screening (age 30+), integration with rural health missions, and use of fixed-dose combinations to enhance adherence.[17]
- *United Kingdom (NICE, 2023)*: Focus on individualized HbA1c targets (6.5–7.5%) and strong emphasis on weight management, including pharmacologic and bariatric options.[18]
- *Latin America*: Regional adaptations often integrate diabetes guidelines with obesity and hypertension programs due to overlapping risk factors. Such localized strategies bridge the gap between evidence and practice, reflecting national epidemiology, healthcare infrastructure, and cultural behaviors **(Figs. 1 and 2)**.

Toward Standardization: Common Ground Across Guidelines

Despite differences, several converging themes have emerged:

- Early detection is critical, with most guidelines recommending opportunistic screening starting at age 30–35.
- Lifestyle modification remains the cornerstone of diabetes prevention and management.

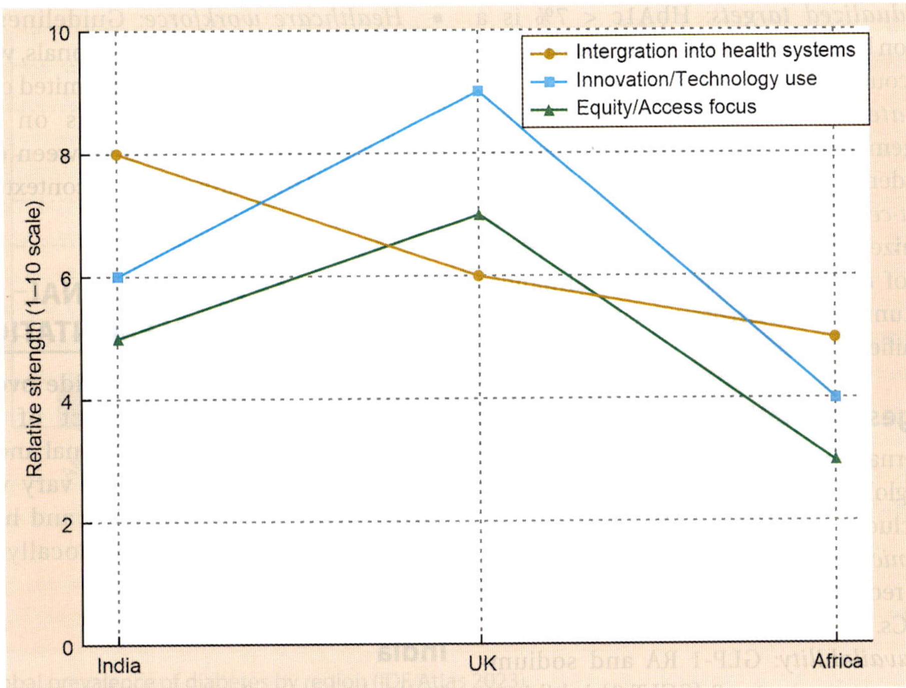

Fig. 1: Comparative policy implementation models.

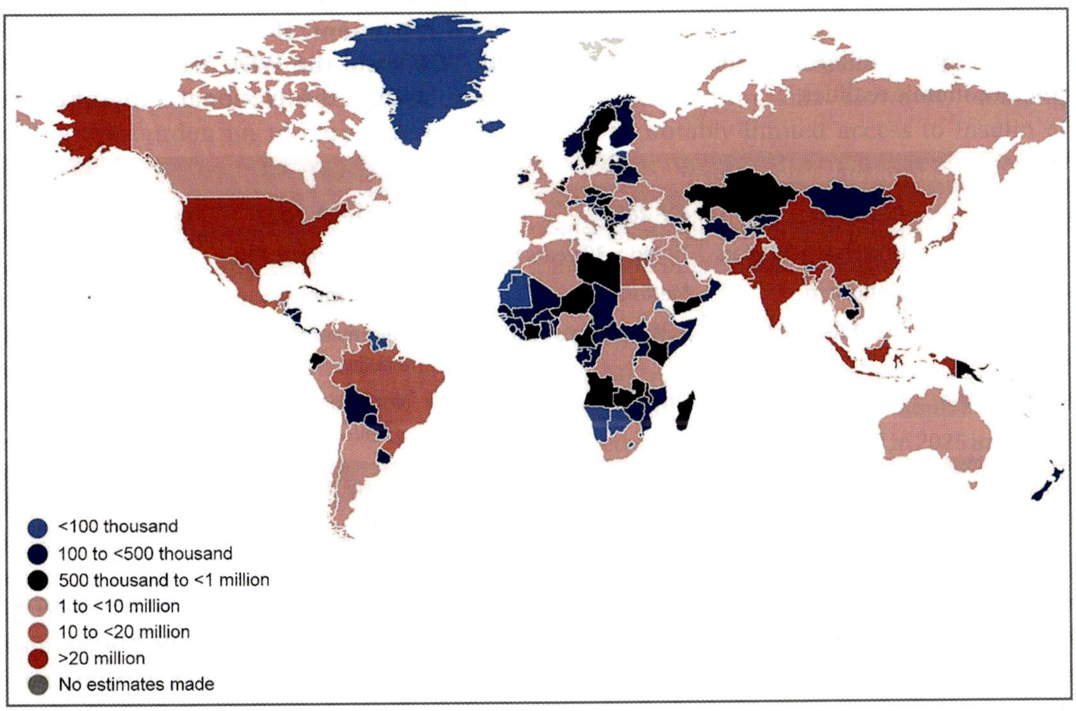

Fig. 2: Estimated total number of adults (20–79 years) with diabetes in 2024.

intervention over 7.8 years of follow-up.[1] Importantly, glycemic control alone has limited impact on macrovascular events, as evidenced by the ACCORD, ADVANCE, and VADT trials, suggesting that strategies must extend beyond glucose lowering to include other cardiovascular risk factors.[2]

Recent Advances

Newer glucose-lowering agents such as SGLT-2 inhibitors and GLP-1 receptor agonists have transformed the landscape of cardiovascular risk management in diabetes. Multiple large cardiovascular outcome trials (CVOTs), including EMPA-REG OUTCOME, CANVAS, DECLARE-TIMI 58, and REWIND, have demonstrated that these agents significantly reduce the risk of cardiovascular death, myocardial infarction, and heart failure hospitalization, independent of glucose control.[2,3] The American Diabetes Association and European Society of Cardiology now recommend the early use of these cardioprotective agents in individuals with diabetes and established ASCVD.[2,6]

Clinical Implication

Despite advances in therapy, the burden of IHD remains high in diabetes, partly due to delayed diagnosis, under-recognition of atypical presentations, and lower rates of evidence-based treatment application in real-world settings. Stress testing with myocardial perfusion imaging, coronary calcium scoring, and CT angiography are increasingly utilized for early detection of subclinical disease in high-risk diabetic individuals.[6] Future strategies aiming to integrate precision medicine, genetic risk profiling, and early aggressive intervention may further improve outcomes in this high-risk group.

HYPERTENSION IN DIABETES

Hypertension is highly prevalent among individuals with diabetes, affecting approximately 70–80% of adults with type 2 diabetes, and significantly amplifies the risk of both macrovascular and microvascular complications.[1] The coexistence of hypertension and diabetes synergistically accelerates the development of atherosclerosis, heart failure, chronic kidney disease, and retinopathy, making blood pressure management a critical component of comprehensive cardiovascular risk reduction strategies. Epidemiological studies, including data from the UKPDS and ADVANCE trials, demonstrate that even modest elevations in blood pressure are associated with substantial increases in cardiovascular events in diabetic individuals.[1,2]

The pathophysiology of hypertension in diabetes is multifactorial, involving insulin resistance, activation of the renin–angiotensin–aldosterone system (RAAS), increased sympathetic nervous system activity, endothelial dysfunction, and sodium retention.[1,3] Obesity, a common comorbidity in type 2 diabetes, further exacerbates blood pressure elevations through adipokine-mediated mechanisms and mechanical effects on vascular resistance. Notably, diabetic patients often exhibit a nondipping nocturnal blood pressure pattern and increased arterial stiffness, both of which contribute to heightened cardiovascular risk.[1,3]

Clinical guidelines recommend a blood pressure target of <130/80 mm Hg for most individuals with diabetes, based on a balance between cardiovascular benefit and the risk of treatment-related adverse events such as hypotension, syncope, and electrolyte abnormalities.[2,6] The ACCORD BP trial evaluated intensive versus standard blood pressure control in type 2 diabetes and found that targeting a systolic blood pressure of <120 mm Hg did not significantly reduce the primary composite cardiovascular outcome compared to a target of <140 mm Hg, although a significant reduction in stroke risk was observed.[2] Subsequent meta-analyses suggest that systolic blood pressure lowering to below 130 mm Hg is beneficial, particularly for reducing stroke, coronary events, and progression of nephropathy.[3,6]

Pharmacologic management typically begins with agents that block the RAAS pathway, such as angiotensin-converting enzyme inhibitors (ACE inhibitors) or angiotensin receptor blockers (ARBs), which have demonstrated cardiovascular and renal protective effects in diabetic populations beyond blood pressure lowering alone.[2,6] Thiazide-like diuretics and calcium channel blockers are often added as second-line agents when blood pressure goals are not achieved, and combination therapy is commonly required in most patients with diabetes and hypertension. Beta-blockers may be appropriate in individuals with coronary artery disease or heart failure but are generally not preferred as initial therapy for hypertension in the absence of compelling indications.[2,3]

Nonpharmacologic strategies, including dietary sodium reduction, weight loss, increased physical activity, moderation of alcohol intake, and adoption of dietary patterns such as the DASH diet, are essential adjuncts to medication in achieving optimal blood pressure control.[1] Despite clear evidence supporting aggressive hypertension management in diabetes, real-world data indicate that blood pressure control remains suboptimal in many populations, with treatment inertia, medication nonadherence, and social determinants of health contributing to gaps in care.[2,6]

Recent Advances

The BPROAD (Blood Pressure Reduction in Obese and Diabetic patients) trial evaluated the impact of intensive versus standard blood pressure control in individuals with type 2 diabetes and obesity. The study found that while intensive systolic blood pressure lowering (target <130 mm Hg) resulted in modest improvements in microvascular outcomes, it did not significantly reduce the incidence of major adverse cardiovascular events (MACE) compared to a standard target (<140 mm Hg). Moreover, the intensive arm was associated with a higher risk of treatment-related adverse effects, including hypotension and electrolyte disturbances. Given the strong relationship between blood pressure and cardiovascular outcomes in diabetes, effective hypertension control represents a cornerstone of any strategy aimed at reducing the burden of ischemic heart disease, stroke, heart failure, and kidney disease in this high-risk population. Future research directions include optimizing individualized blood pressure targets based on comorbidity profiles, integrating emerging biomarkers of vascular injury, and improving the implementation of guideline-directed care across diverse clinical settings **(Flowchart 2)**.[3,6]

HEART FAILURE IN DIABETES

Heart failure is a major and growing complication of diabetes mellitus, with individuals with diabetes experiencing a two- to fivefold increased risk of developing heart failure compared to the general population.[1] Diabetes contributes to both heart failure with reduced ejection fraction (HFrEF) and heart failure with preserved ejection fraction (HFpEF), through multiple mechanisms including chronic hyperglycemia, myocardial fibrosis, microvascular dysfunction, autonomic neuropathy, and an altered metabolic substrate utilization that impairs myocardial energetics.[1,2] Importantly, heart failure often develops in diabetic individuals independent of ischemic heart disease, reflecting the unique diabetic cardiomyopathy phenomenon.

Recent Trials

In the context of diabetes management, several CVOTs have substantially reshaped the approach to heart failure prevention and treatment. The EMPA-REG OUTCOME trial first demonstrated that empagliflozin significantly reduced hospitalization for heart failure and cardiovascular death in individuals with type 2 diabetes and established ASCVD.[2] Subsequent trials such as CANVAS, DECLARE-TIMI 58, and VERTIS-CV confirmed consistent heart failure benefits with SGLT-2 inhibitors, particularly in reducing heart

TABLE 1: Cardiovascular outcome trials (CVOTs) in diabetes.

Trial name	*Drug*	*Class*	*Main population*	*Primary outcome*	*Key results*
EMPA-reg outcome	Empagliflozin	SGLT-2 inhibitor	T2DM with ASCVD	3P-MACE	↓ MACE, ↓ CV death (38%), ↓ HF hospitalization,
CANVAS	Canagliflozin	SGLT-2 inhibitor	T2DM, high CV risk	3P-MACE	↓ MACE, ↑ amputation risk
DECLARE-tIMI 58	Dapagliflozin	SGLT-2 inhibitor	T2DM, broad risk	3P-MACE, HF	↓ HF hospitalization, neutral MACE
VERTIS-CV	Ertugliflozin	SGLT-2 inhibitor	T2DM with ASCVD	3P-MACE	Noninferior, no major MACE reduction
DAPA-HF	Dapagliflozin	SGLT-2 inhibitor	HFrEF (± T2DM)	HF outcomes	↓ HF hospitalization, ↓ CV death
EMPEROR-reduced	Empagliflozin	SGLT-2 inhibitor	HFrEF (± T2DM)	HF outcomes	↓ HF hospitalization
EMPEROR-preserved	Empagliflozin	SGLT-2 inhibitor	HFpEF (± T2DM)	HF outcomes	↓ HF hospitalization
LEADER	Liraglutide	GLP-1 receptor agonist	T2DM with high CV risk	3P-MACE	↓ MACE (13%)
SUSTAIN-6	Semaglutide	GLP-1 receptor agonist	T2DM	3P-MACE	↓ Stroke risk
REWIND	Dulaglutide	GLP-1 receptor agonist	T2DM, moderate risk	3P-MACE	↓ MACE (12%)
AMPLITUDE-O	Efpeglenatide	GLP-1 receptor agonist	T2DM with CVD/CKD	3P-MACE	↓ MACE (27%)
SOUL trial	Oral semaglutide	GLP-1 receptor agonist	T2DM, broad CV risk	3P-MACE	↓ MACE (~14%)
ORIGIN	Insulin glargine	Insulin	T2DM and prediabetes	3P-MACE	Neutral effect
DEVOTE	Insulin degludec	Insulin	T2DM with high CV risk	3P-MACE	Noninferior to glargine
FIDELIO-DKD[9]	Finerenone	MR antagonist	T2DM with CKD	Renal, CV	↓ Kidney events, ↓ MACE (18%)
FIGARO-DKD[10]	Finerenone	MR antagonist	T2DM with early CKD	CV outcomes	↓ CV events (13%)
SUMMIT-HFpEF[8]	Tirzepatide	Twincretin (GIP/GLP1)	HFpEF + obesity	HF outcomes	↓ HF worsening, ↓ CV death
FLOW Trial[11]	Semaglutide	GLP-1 receptor agonist	T2DM with CKD	Renal, CV	↓ MACE (~14%, preliminary)

(ASCVD: atherosclerotic cardiovascular disease; CKD: chronic kidney disease; CVD: cardiovascular disease; GLP-1: glucagon-like peptide-1; MACE: major adverse cardiovascular event; T2DM: type 2 diabetes mellitus) for most adults with diabetes aged 40–75 years, regardless of baseline LDL-C levels, especially if additional ASCVD risk factors are present. For individuals with multiple ASCVD risk factors or those aged 50–70 years, high-intensity statin therapy is advised to achieve greater LDL-C reductions.[7]

In cases where LDL-C targets are not met with maximally tolerated statin therapy, the addition of nonstatin agents such as ezetimibe or proprotein convertase subtilisin/kexin type 9 (PCSK9) inhibitors may be considered. The IMPROVE-IT trial demonstrated that adding ezetimibe to statin therapy provided incremental benefits in reducing cardiovascular events.

For patients with elevated triglyceride levels (≥500 mg/dL), fibrate therapy may be employed to reduce the risk of pancreatitis. However, the combination of fibrates with statins should be approached cautiously due to potential adverse effects. Omega-3 fatty acid supplementation, particularly icosapent ethyl, has shown promise in reducing cardiovascular events in high-risk patients with elevated triglycerides, as evidenced by the REDUCE-IT trial.[12]

Lifestyle modifications remain a cornerstone in managing diabetic dyslipidemia. Dietary interventions focusing on reducing saturated fat and cholesterol intake, increasing physical activity, and achieving weight loss can significantly improve lipid profiles and reduce cardiovascular risk **(Table 2)**.

PERIPHERAL ARTERIAL DISEASE IN DIABETES

Peripheral arterial disease is a frequent but often underdiagnosed complication of diabetes mellitus, characterized by the progressive narrowing and occlusion of peripheral arteries, primarily affecting the lower extremities. Diabetes is a major independent risk factor for PAD, with prevalence estimates ranging from 20 to 30% among older adults with diabetes.[13] The pathophysiology of PAD in diabetes involves a combination of atherosclerosis, endothelial

TABLE 2: ADA 2025 guidelines on management of dyslipidemia in patients with diabetes mellitus.[2]

Recommendations for statin and combination treatment in adults with diabetes:

Age	*ASCVD*	*Recommended statin intensity ând combination treatment**
<40 years	No	None[†]
	Yes	High: If LDL cholesterol ≥70 mg/dL despite maximally tolerated statin dose, consider adding additional LDL-lowering therapy (such as ezetimibe or PCSK9 inhibitor)[#]
≥40 years	No	Moderate[‡]
	Yes	High: If LDL cholesterol ≥70 mg/dL despite maximally tolerated statin dose, consider adding additional LDL-lowering therapy (such as ezetimibe or PCSK9 inhibitor)

*In addition to lifestyle therapy.

^For patients who do not tolerate the intended intensity of statin, the maximally tolerated statin dose should be used.

†Moderate-intensity statin may be considered based on risk-benefit profile and presence of ASCVD risk factors. ASCVD risk factors include LDL cholesterol ≥100 mg/dL (2.6 mmol/L), high blood pressure, smoking, chronic kidney disease, albuminuria, and family history of premature ASCVD.

#High-intensity statin may be considered based on risk-benefit profile and presence of ASCVD risk factors.

‡Adults aged <40 years with prevalent ASCVD were not well represented in clinical trials of non-statin-based LDL reduction. Before initiating combination lipid-lowering therapy, consider the potential for further ASCVD risk reduction, drug-specific adverse effects, and patient preferences.

(ASCVD: atherosclerotic cardiovascular disease; LDL: low-density lipoprotein)

embedded in international guidelines as first-line agents in individuals with high cardiovascular risk, independent of glycemic thresholds.

Despite these advances, implementation gaps persist in real-world clinical practice. Suboptimal blood pressure control, therapeutic inertia, underuse of statins and cardioprotective agents, and disparities in access to care continue to limit the full realization of cardiovascular risk reduction in diabetes. Moving forward, patient-centered care models, digital health interventions, and population-level strategies to improve adherence and equity will be essential.

In conclusion, reducing CVD in diabetes requires a shift from siloed treatment paradigms toward comprehensive, individualized, and evidence-based care. Through early recognition, aggressive multifactorial risk factor control, and the judicious use of proven pharmacotherapies, it is possible to markedly reduce cardiovascular morbidity and mortality in the diabetic population. The integration of newer therapies, lifestyle interventions, and systems-based approaches into routine practice offers a hopeful trajectory in the ongoing fight against cardiovascular complications in diabetes.

REFERENCES

1. Holt RIG, Flyvbjerg A (Eds). Textbook of Diabetes, 6th edition. Hoboken, New Jersey: Wiley; 2024. pp. 681-4.
2. American Diabetes Association Professional Practice Committee. Cardiovascular disease and risk management: Standards of Care in Diabetes—2025. Diabetes Care. 2025;48(Suppl. 1):S207-38.
3. Joseph JJ, Deedwania P, Acharya T, Aguilar D, Bhatt DL, Chyun DA, et al. Comprehensive management of cardiovascular risk factors for adults with type 2 diabetes. Circulation. 2022;145:e722-59.
4. Ozkan B, Ndumele CE. Addressing cardiovascular risk in diabetes: It's more than the sugar. Circulation. 2023;147:1887-90.
5. Low Wang CC, Hess CN, Hiatt WR, Goldfine AB. Clinical Update: Cardiovascular Disease in Diabetes Mellitus: Atherosclerotic Cardiovascular Disease and Heart Failure in Type 2 Diabetes Mellitus - Mechanisms, Management, and Clinical Considerations. Circulation. 2016;133(24):2459-502.
6. Kelsey MD, Nelson AJ, Green JB, Granger CB, Peterson ED, McGuire DK, et al. Guidelines for cardiovascular risk reduction in patients with type 2 diabetes. J Am Coll Cardiol. 2022;79:1849-57.
7. American Diabetes Association. 10. Cardiovascular Disease and Risk Management: Standards of Medical Care in Diabetes—2023. Diabetes Care. 2023;46(Suppl 1):S158-90.
8. Packer M, Zile MR, Kramer CM, Baum SJ, Litwin SE, Menon V, et al. Tirzepatide for Heart Failure with Preserved Ejection Fraction and Obesity. N Engl J Med. 2025;392(5):427-37.
9. Bakris GL, Agarwal R, Anker SD, Pitt B, Ruilope LM, Rossing P, et al. Effect of Finerenone on Chronic Kidney Disease Outcomes in Type 2 Diabetes. N Engl J Med. 2020;383(23):2219-29.
10. Pitt B, Filippatos G, Agarwal R, Anker SD, Bakris GL, Rossing P, et al. Cardiovascular Events with Finerenone in Kidney Disease and Type 2 Diabetes. N Engl J Med. 2021;385(24):2252-63.
11. McGuire DK, Marx N, Mulvagh SL, Deanfield JE, Inzucchi SE, Pop-Busui R, et al. Oral Semaglutide and Cardiovascular Outcomes in High-Risk Type 2 Diabetes. N Engl J Med. 2025;392(20):2001-12.
12. Bhatt DL, Steg PG, Miller M, Brinton EA, Jacobson TA, Ketchum SB, et al. Cardiovascular Risk Reduction with Icosapent Ethyl for Hypertriglyceridemia. N Engl J Med. 2019;380(1):11-22.
13. Jude EB, Eleftheriadou I, Tentolouris N. Peripheral arterial disease in diabetes—a review. Diabet Med. 2010;27(1):4-14.
14. Fowkes FG, Rudan D, Rudan I, Aboyans V, Denenberg JO, McDermott MM, et al. Comparison of global estimates of prevalence and risk factors for peripheral artery disease: an updated systematic review and analysis. Lancet. 2013;382(9901):1329-40.
15. Bradbury AW, Adam DJ, Bell J, Forbes JF, Fowkes FG, Gillespie I, et al. Bypass versus angioplasty in severe ischemia of the leg (BASIL) trial: survival outcomes. J Vasc Surg. 2010;51(5 Suppl):5S-17S.
16. Bonaca MP, Catarig AM, Houlind K, Ludvik B, Nordanstig J, Ramesh CK, et al. Semaglutide and walking capacity in people with symptomatic peripheral artery disease and type 2 diabetes (STRIDE): a phase 3b, double-blind, randomised, placebo-controlled trial. Lancet. 2025;405(10489):1580-93.
17. Caruso P, Maiorino MI, Longo M, Porcellini C, Matrone R, Digitale Selvaggio L, et al. Liraglutide for Lower

Limb Perfusion in People With Type 2 Diabetes and Peripheral Artery Disease: The STARDUST Randomized Clinical Trial. JAMA Netw Open. 2024;7(3):e241545.

18. Gerstein HC, Miller ME, Byington RP, Byington RP, Goff DC Jr, Bigger JT, et al. Effects of intensive glucose lowering in type 2 diabetes. N Engl J Med. 2008;358(24):2545-59.
19. Turnbull F, Neal B, Algert C, Byington RP, Goff DC Jr, Bigger JT, et al. Effects of different blood pressure-lowering regimens on major cardiovascular events in individuals with and without diabetes mellitus: results of prospectively designed overviews of randomized trials. Arch Intern Med. 2005;165(12):1410-9.
20. Zelniker TA, Wiviott SD, Raz I, Im K, Goodrich EL, Bonaca MP, et al. SGLT2 inhibitors for primary and secondary prevention of cardiovascular and renal outcomes in type 2 diabetes: a systematic review and meta-analysis of cardiovascular outcome trials. Lancet. 2019;393(10166):31-9.

17 Diabetic Kidney Disease: Advances in Prevention and Treatment

TEO Boon Wee Jimmy

ABSTRACT

The renin–angiotensin–aldosterone system (RAAS) inhibitors have long been the mainstay of pharmacological treatment in patients with diabetic kidney disease (DKD), based on their proven efficacy in slowing the progression of chronic kidney disease (CKD). Despite RAAS inhibitor treatment, DKD remains the leading cause of end-stage kidney disease (ESKD) and new therapeutic approaches are necessary. This chapter provides an overview of the pharmacological management of DKD, with a focus on newer medications such as sodium–glucose cotransporter-2 (SGLT-2) inhibitor, nonsteroidal mineralocorticoid antagonist (nsMRA), and glucagon-like peptide type 1 receptor agonists (GLP-1RAs).

These medications target different pathways involved in the pathophysiology of DKD and may have synergistic effects when used in combination. Developing evidence supports the use of several therapeutic agents to reduce the residual risk of DKD progression. Newer agents such as endothelin-1 receptor A antagonists have shown potential renoprotective effects, but remain under investigation. However, inconsistent definitions for composite kidney outcomes may limit the direct comparison of the clinical trials. Overall, this chapter aims to inform clinicians and researchers on the current therapeutic advancements, challenges, and future directions to improve renal outcomes in the management of DKD.

Keywords: Diabetic kidney disease, Combination therapy, Clinical trials, Renal outcomes, Renoprotective effect.

INTRODUCTION

Over the past two decades, the main treatment approach to diabetic kidney disease (DKD) is largely influenced by the major trials of renin–angiotensin–aldosterone system (RAAS) inhibitors. The Captopril Collaborative Study, the Irbesartan Diabetic Nephropathy Trial (IDNT), and the Reduction of Endpoints in NIDDM with the Angiotensin II Antagonist Losartan (RENAAL) have shown that angiotensin-converting enzyme (ACE) inhibitors and angiotensin receptor blockers (ARBs) significantly slow the progression of chronic kidney disease (CKD) in addition to their antihypertensive properties.[1-3] All three trials used composite primary endpoints focused on clinically relevant renal outcomes. The endpoints included doubling of serum creatinine and progression to end-stage kidney disease (ESKD). The RENAAL and IDNT trials also incorporated all-cause mortality into their composite measures. These studies exclusively enrolled DKD patients with proteinuria reinforcing the renoprotective efficacy of RAAS inhibitor. These three landmark trials formed the standard of care till 2019. A recent study further supports the continuation of RAAS inhibitor in advanced and progressive CKD conferring slower glomerular filtration rate (GFR) decline.[4] Despite RAAS inhibitor treatment, the overall reduction of risk in CKD progression, ESKD, and death was modest in this high-risk patient group. Thus, more potent and efficacious therapies are needed for DKD **(Table 1)**.

THEMATIC/TOPICAL SECTIONS

In recent years, there are substantial therapeutic advancements in managing DKD, improving patient outcomes, and disease control. In 2025, the four options for managing DKD include RAAS inhibitor, sodium–glucose cotransporter-2 (SGLT-2) inhibitor, nonsteroidal mineralocorticoid antagonist (nsMRA), and glucagon-like peptide type 1 receptor agonists (GLP-1RA). Three key phase 3 randomized, placebo-controlled trials analyzing SGLT-2 inhibitor, namely CREDENCE, DAPA-CKD, and EMPA-KIDNEY, led changes in clinical practice guidelines. The CREDENCE trial demonstrated that treatment with canagliflozin resulted in a significant 30% relative risk reduction in the primary composite outcome, which included kidney failure and major cardiovascular (CV) events.[5] The DAPA-CKD and EMPA-KIDNEY trials evaluated both diabetic and nondiabetic CKD patients, confirming the safety and cardiorenal benefits of dapagliflozin and empagliflozin compared to placebo.[6,7]

The FIDELIO-DKD and FIGARO-DKD trials analyzed the effects of the nsMRA, finerenone, on over 13,000 patients with DKD.[8,9] FIDELIO-DKD reduced the risk of ESKD and CKD progression by 20 and 23%, respectively.[8] The FIGARO-DKD trial showed 14% reduction in cardiovascular morbidity and mortality.[9] The FLOW trial showed that semaglutide compared to placebo (GLP-1RA) reduced the risk of the primary kidney outcome events by 24%.[10]

Although these trials were conducted at different times, the combined use of these medications contributed to a more comprehensive, multitarget approach to DKD management, aiming to preserve kidney function.[11] This is because all these medications act on different pathways involved in DKD influencing hemodynamic perturbation, reducing inflammation and fibrosis, and stabilizing metabolic dysregulation.[12] Several trials have explored combination strategies involving the four major medication types for DKD with proven cardiorenal benefits. For example, for both DECREASE and ROTATE trials, patients administered with dapagliflozin paired with exanetide or eplerenone showed a 40 and 50% reduction of proteinuria, respectively. In the FLOW trial, about 15% of the population were taking SGLT-2 inhibitor at baseline, and there was no adverse impact on the primary kidney outcome. The SMART-C meta-analysis, encompassing 12 SGLT-2 inhibitor trials with over 3,000 patients on baseline GLP-1RA therapy, also demonstrated a reduction in CKD progression. An analysis on the main trials of SGLT-2 inhibitor, nsMRA, and GLP-1RA estimated a reduction of 58% in CKD progression compared to using RAAS inhibitor alone and a 35% relative risk reduction in major CV events.[11] Thus, the combination of these medications generally offers a greater effect of reducing GFR decline from approximately 4–6 mL/min with RAAS inhibitor alone to around 3 mL/min today.[12] Most recently, the CONFIDENCE trial recently demonstrated that the combination of an SGLT-2 inhibitor and finerenone produced a 29% greater reduction in the urinary albumin-to-creatinine ratio (UACR) compared with finerenone alone (ratio 0.71; 95% CI 0.61–0.82; $p < 0.001$), and a 32% greater reduction compared with empagliflozin alone (ratio 0.68; 95% CI 0.59–0.79; $p < 0.001$).[13]

RECENT ADVANCES

Several medications are noted in the therapy of DKD. Among the many pharmacological approaches that are explored, endothelin-1 receptor A antagonists and bardoxolone methyl

TABLE 1: Primary renal outcomes in phase 3 trials.

Trial	*Intervention*	*N*	*Type of patients: DKD only, both DKD and non-DKD*	*Primary outcome type*	*Results*
RENAAL (2001)[1]	Losartan vs. placebo	1,513	DKD patients only (T2D + proteinuric CKD)	• Doubling of serum creatinine • ESKD • Death from any cause	• Losartan group had a 16% risk reduction in the primary composite endpoint • Risk of ESKD alone was • No significant effect on overall mortality
IDNT (2001)[2]	Irbesartan vs. amlodipine vs. placebo	1,715	DKD patients only (T2D + proteinuric CKD)	• Doubling of serum creatinine • ESKD • Death from any cause	• Irbesartan reduced the risk of the primary composite endpoint by 20% compared to placebo and 23% compared to amlodipine • Amlodipine had no significant renal benefit
Captopril collaborative study (1993)[3]	Captopril vs. placebo	409	DKD patients only (type 1 diabetes + proteinuric nephropathy)	• Doubling of serum creatinine • ESKD	• Captopril reduced the risk of doubling of serum creatinine by 48% • Fewer patients reached ESKD in the captopril group • Blood pressure reductions were similar in both groups, indicating a renoprotective effect beyond BP lowering
CREDENCE (2019)[5]	Canagliflozin vs. placebo	4,401	DKD only (T2D + proteinuric CKD)	• Doubling of serum creatinine • ESKD • Renal or CV death	• 30% relative risk reduction in the primary composite outcome • Reduced hospitalization for heart failure and CV events
DAPA-CKD (2020)[6]	Dapagliflozin vs. placebo	4,304	Both DKD and non-DKD (include proteinuric CKD)	• ≥50% decline in eGFR • ESKD • Renal or CV death	• 39% relative risk reduction in the primary outcome • Benefits seen in both DKD and non-DKD patients • Lower risk of death from any cause
EMPA-KIDNEY (2022)[7]	Empagliflozin vs. placebo	6,609	Both DKD and non-DKD (eGFR <45 mL/min/1.73 m^2 regardless of albuminuria, or eGFR 45 to <90 mL/min/1.73 m^2 with UACR ≥200 mg/g)	• ≥40% decline in eGFR • Sustained eGFR of <10 mL/min/1.73 m^2 • ESKD • Renal or CV death	• 28% relative risk reduction in the primary outcome • Benefit seen across DKD and non-DKD patients • Reduced hospitalization for heart failure

Continued

Continued

Trial	*Intervention*	*N*	*Type of patients: DKD only, both DKD and non-DKD*	*Primary outcome type*	*Results*
FIGARO-DKD (2021)[9]	Finerenone vs. placebo	7,352	DKD only (T2D + proteinuric CKD)	*CV composite*: • CV death • Nonfatal • Myocardial infarction • Stroke • Hospitalization for heart failure	Reduction of 13% risk of primary outcome
FIDELIO-DKD (2020)[8]	Finerenone vs. placebo	5,674	DKD only (T2D + proteinuric CKD)	*Renal composite*: • ESKD • Sustained ≥40% eGFR decline • Renal death	Reduction of 18% risk of primary outcome
FLOW (2024)[10]	Semaglutide vs. placebo	3,533	DKD only (T2D + proteinuric CKD)	• ≥50% eGFR decline • ESKD • Renal or CV death	24% lower primary outcome risk
SONAR (2019)[14]	Atrasentan vs. placebo	2,648	DKD only (T2D + proteinuric CKD)	• Doubling of serum creatinine (sustained for ≥30 days) • ESKD • Renal death	• Atrasentan significantly reduced the risk of the primary renal outcome compared to placebo • Increased rate of hospitalizations for heart failure observed in the atrasentan group • Short-term albuminuria reduction without marked sodium retention
AYAME (2022)[16]	Bardoxolone methyl vs. placebo	1,013	DKD only (T2D)	*Time to onset of*: • ≥30% decrease in eGFR from baseline • ESKD	• Bardoxolone methyl did not significantly reduce the primary outcome compared to placebo • No significant differences between bardoxolone methyl and placebo in secondary renal and CV outcomes

(CKD: chronic kidney disease; CV: cardiovascular; DKD: diabetic kidney disease; ESKD: end-stage kidney disease; eGFR: estimated glomerular filtration rate; T2D: type 2 diabetes)

have been studied more prominently due to potential renoprotective effects. The phase 3 SONAR trial used atrasentan which has a higher efficacy and selectivity to ET-A receptors. The trial demonstrated favorable short-term outcomes, indicating that low-dose atrasentan effectively reduced albuminuria without inducing significant sodium retention. As for long-term outcomes,

disease outcomes in type 2 diabetes. N Engl J Med. 2020;383(23):2219-29.
9. Pitt B, Filippatos G, Agarwal R, Anker SD, Bakris GL, Rossing P, et al. Cardiovascular events with finerenone in kidney disease and type 2 diabetes. N Engl J Med. 2021;385(24):2252-63.
10. Perkovic V, Tuttle KR, Rossing P, Mahaffey KW, Mann JFE, Bakris G, et al. Effects of semaglutide on chronic kidney disease in patients with type 2 diabetes. N Engl J Med. 2024;391(2):109-21.
11. Neuen BL, Yeung EK, Rangaswami J, Vaduganathan M. Combination therapy as a new standard of care in diabetic and nondiabetic chronic kidney disease. Nephrol Dial Transplant. 2025;40(Supplement_1): i59-69.
12. Naaman SC, Bakris GL. Diabetic nephropathy: Update on pillars of therapy slowing progression. Diabetes Care. 2023;46(9):1574-86.
13. Agarwal R, Green JB, Heerspink HJL, Mann JFE, McGill JB, Mottl AK, et al. Finerenone with empagliflozin in chronic kidney disease and type 2 diabetes. N Engl J Med. 2025;393(6):533-43.
14. Heerspink HJL, Parving HH, Andress DL, Bakris G, Correa-Rotter R, Hou FF, et al. Atrasentan and renal events in patients with type 2 diabetes and chronic kidney disease (SONAR): a double-blind, randomised, placebo-controlled trial. Lancet. 2019;393(10184):1937-47.
15. Maruno S, Tanaka T, Nangaku M. Exploring molecular targets in diabetic kidney disease. Kidney Res Clin Pract. 2022;41(Suppl 2):S33-S45.
16. Nangaku M, Takama H, Ichikawa T, Mukai K, Kojima M, Suzuki Y, et al. Randomized, double-blind, placebo-controlled phase 3 study of bardoxolone methyl in patients with diabetic kidney disease: design and baseline characteristics of the AYAME study. Nephrol Dial Transplant. 2023;38(5):1204-16.
17. Kyowa Kirin. (2023). Kyowa Kirin Announces Phase III Study Results of bardoxolone methyl (RTA 402) in Japan and Discontinuation of Development . [online] Available from https://www.kyowakirin.com/media_center/news_releases/2023/e20230510_01.html [Last accessed September, 2025].
18. Levin A, Agarwal R, Herrington WG, Heerspink HL, Mann JFE, Shahinfar S, et al. International consensus definitions of clinical trial outcomes for kidney failure: 2020. Kidney Int. 2020;4:849-59.
19. Cannon CP, Pratley R, Dagogo-Jack S, Mancuso J, Huyck S, Masiukiewicz U, et al. Cardiovascular outcomes with ertugliflozin in type 2 diabetes. N Engl J Med. 2020;383(15):1425-35.
20. van Raalte DH, Bjornstad P, Heerspink HJL, Persson F, Cherney DZI. Importance of standardizing renal outcomes in clinical trials: Illustration by recent sodium glucose cotransporter 2 inhibitor studies. Kidney Int. 2021;99(3):768-70.

18 Diabetic Retinopathy and Neuropathy: Protecting Vision and Nerve Health

Vijay Viswanathan, Reshma Mirshad

ABSTRACT

Diabetes, a systemic disease, is associated with several serious secondary complications. It is one of the rapidly growing health challenges faced by people globally, 589 million people were affected by diabetes 2024, an alarming figure projected to reach 853 million by 2050. Diabetic retinopathy and diabetic neuropathy, significant microvascular complications, are prevalent in patients with diabetes due to prolonged hyperglycemia. Diabetic retinopathy affects over 100 million individuals globally and is the most common cause of blindness in working-age individuals. While diabetic peripheral neuropathy (DPN) is present in up to two-thirds of people with diabetes, it often leads to foot ulcers, infections, and amputations. Both conditions are driven by poor glycemic control, uncontrolled hypertension, dyslipidemia, nephropathy, male sex, and obesity. Recent advancements, including anti-vascular endothelial growth factor (VEGF) agents, corticosteroid implants, gene therapy, artificial intelligence-driven screening tools, wearable devices, and neuromodulation, are reshaping management strategies. Despite these innovations, optimal outcomes rely heavily on prevention through lifestyle modifications, regular screenings, glycemic control, and a multidisciplinary care approach. This review highlights the current understanding, emerging technologies, and future directions for managing DR and DPN to reduce disease burden and enhance patient outcomes.

Keywords: Diabetes, Diabetic retinopathy, Diabetic neuropathy, Diabetic peripheral neuropathy, Nonproliferative diabetic retinopathy, Proliferative diabetic retinopathy, Diabetic macular edema.

INTRODUCTION

Diabetes is one of the most formidable noncommunicable diseases, with an estimated 589 million people affected by diabetes in 2024, an alarming figure projected to reach 853 million by 2050.[1] It is a multifactorial complex disease with many secondary complications, including diabetic retinopathy (DR), diabetic neuropathy, diabetic nephropathy, and diabetic foot. In 2020, an estimated 103.12 million adults worldwide were reported to have had DR, while 28.54 million had vision-threatening diabetic retinopathy (VTDR), and these numbers are projected to rise to 160.50 million and 44.82 million by 2045.[2] DR causes extensive damage to the retina. Thus, DR remains the leading cause of severe vision loss in working-age adults. DR progresses from nonproliferative to proliferative stages, with increasing risk of irreversible retinal damage and visual impairment if left untreated.[3]

plexiform layer. They form a circinate ring around a microaneurysm.

- Soft exudates (cotton wool spots) are located in the retinal nerve fiber layer (axoplasmic debris) and represent focal infarcts of the precapillary arterioles.
- Intraretinal microvascular abnormalities are direct connections between retinal arterioles and venules, bypassing the capillary network and appear near regions of capillary closure. IRMAs remain within the retina without crossing major vessels and do not show leakage on fluorescein angiography.
- Neovascularization at the disk (NVD) is the formation of new blood vessels at or extending up to one disk diameter from the optic disk. Neovascularization elsewhere (NVE) is the formation of new blood vessels beyond one disk diameter from the optic disk.[17]

As peripheral neuropathy is prevalent among patients with diabetes, the American Diabetes Association (ADA) recommends that clinicians evaluate type 2 diabetic patients at the time of diagnosis. For type 1 diabetic patients, assessment should be done 5 years after diagnosis and then annually.[12]

A complete medical history should be obtained, including systemic diseases such as diabetes, obesity, dyslipidemia, and hypertension. Clinicians should also assess a systematic review and the medications taken by patients, as these could be underlying causes of DPN. Other common risk factors for DPN should also be considered. Peripheral neuropathy has characteristic features, such as burning, numbness, or tingling in the feet, which worsen at night.[18] Approximately 80% of DPN patients present with symptoms such as numbness, tingling, pain, and/or weakness that begin in the feet, spread proximally in a length-dependent manner, reaching the knees, and eventually involve the upper limb digits (characterized by stocking and glove distribution).[19]

A lower extremity examination is also conducted. It includes evaluation of muscle strength, reflexes, and sensation, including light touch with a monofilament, vibratory sensation, and proprioception. Checking for dry or cracked skin may also be done, as it may represent autonomic neuropathy. Pedal deformities such as hammertoes suggest motor neuropathy.[20]

Temperature changes or pinprick testing are used to assess small fiber sensation. A patient's risk for developing ulcers is determined by their ability to feel pressure. Although protective sensation is lost after sensory impairment, the standard Semmes–Weinstein 5.07 monofilament test, which measures 10 g of pressure, may still be sensed even after developing a neurotrophic ulcer. Large fibers are assessed through vibratory sensation.[19] Autonomic neuropathy also occurs in diabetes and can affect various systems, such as the gastrointestinal, cardiovascular, and genitourinary systems.

MANAGEMENT

The foremost step in managing a case of NPDR is maintaining proper glycemic control and regular intake of antidiabetic medications. Regular eye examinations are crucial for detecting ocular abnormalities. Any other associated systemic disorders should be addressed. A detailed systemic investigation should be done to look for other systemic side effects of diabetes mellitus. For a case of very mild nonproliferative diabetic retinopathy (NPDR), follow-up is recommended every year. For mild-to-moderate NPDR, follow-up is needed every 6 months. For severe-to-very severe NPDR, follow-up is required within 2–4 months. Data reveal that 16% of cases of mild NPDR and 23% of cases of moderate NPDR progress to proliferative stages within 4 years, while 50% of severe NPDR and 75% of cases of very severe NPDR progress to proliferative diabetic retinopathy (PDR) within 1 year.[18]

Previously, panretinal photocoagulation (PRP) was considered the best treatment option for PDR cases. Recent studies have evaluated the role of intravitreal anti-VEGF injections in cases of PDR. For low-risk PDR without DME, careful 2–4 monthly follow-ups are needed. For high-risk PDR without DME, panretinal photocoagulation should be initiated. For PDR with DME, a combination of intravitreal anti-VEGF injections and PRP sessions should be considered. In high-risk PDR where complete photocoagulation is not possible, cryopexy or vitrectomy should be considered.[21] Pars plana vitrectomy should be considered for advanced eye diseases where other treatment modalities have not been effective in resolving the symptoms.

Diabetic peripheral neuropathy management is initiated with preventive measures, followed by conservative, pharmacologic, and interventional therapies. The first line of conservative therapy includes physical therapy, weight-bearing exercises and Tai Chi massage therapy. The second-line therapy involves health management through strict glycemic control, a healthy diet and weight loss if needed. The third-line therapy consists of minimally invasive treatments, such as acupuncture and transcutaneous electrical nerve stimulation (TENS).

In pharmacological therapy, the first-line agents are gabapentinoids (e.g., pregabalin, gabapentin) and duloxetine. The second-line agents include serotonin and norepinephrine reuptake inhibitors (e.g., venlafaxine), tricyclic antidepressants (e.g., amitriptyline), tapentadol, an 8% capsaicin patch, and a 5% lidocaine patch. The third- and fourth-line agents are tramadol, opioid and intravenous agents (e.g., lidocaine, ketamine). In interventional therapy, the first-line treatment includes dorsal column spinal cord stimulation. Other neuromodulation therapies, such as burst spinal cord stimulation, dorsal root ganglion spinal cord stimulation, and peripheral nerve stimulation, fall under the second line of treatment. The third-line therapy constitutes the use of intrathecal drug delivery systems such as intrathecal morphine, fentanyl, or hydromorphone and intrathecal ziconotide.[12]

RECENT ADVANCES IN EVALUATION AND FUTURE DRUG PROSPECTS

Recent studies implicate the role of personalized health management applications in managing diabetes, such as blood glucose monitoring apps and telemedicine platforms. Data reveals that these applications have significantly improved glycemic control in people with diabetes.[22] Wearable devices, such as smart bracelets and smartwatches, also play a crucial role in managing diabetes. They deliver data, thereby encouraging patients to make adjustments that eventually help prevent the progression of DR.[23] In recent years, AI technology has demonstrated the ability to detect early lesions of DR with high accuracy, which significantly aids in diagnosis.[24]

Several innovative approaches have been discovered recently in the management of DR. Receptor-interacting protein kinase 1 (RIP1 kinase) inhibitors have been shown to prevent retinal damage. Thus, evidence reveals that RIP1 kinase inhibitors will play a crucial role in managing DR.[25] Gene therapies have emerged as a revolutionary field, particularly in the areas of gene editing technology and gene transfer therapy, which hold promise as future treatment modalities for DR, as evidenced by numerous research studies.[26] Stem cell therapy can also provide significant treatment options by repairing retinal tissue damage and restoring its normal function. Sodium-glucose cotransporter-2 (SGLT-2) inhibitors may be beneficial in the early stages of DR by preventing vascular congestion and reducing capillary blood flow.[27]

Skin biopsies are used to understand the underlying neurodegenerative mechanisms behind DPN. Therefore, it emphasizes the importance of diagnosing DPN. In vivo corneal confocal microscopy (IVCCM) has demonstrated good diagnostic utility in both subclinical and clinical DPN.[28] Nerve conduction studies (NCS) and nerve excitability testing (NET) have been developed for assessing large-fiber DPN. Perception threshold tracking (PTT) has been designed to assess nerve excitability testing of small sensory nerve fibers.[29] Microneurography can be used to investigate painful DPN.[30] Electrically evoked cortical responses can be helpful in the early detection of DPN as they provide a direct measure of both peripheral and central conduction.[31]

Novel targeted drugs are emerging drugs for the management of DPN that restore normal neurological function and at least slow down disease progression by targeting specific pathogenic mechanisms including SGLT-2 inhibitors (empagliflozin, canagliflozin), GLP-1 receptor agonists (liraglutide, exenatide, dulaglutide), aldose reductase inhibitor (ranirestat), Anti-AGEs (benfotiamine), PKC inhibitor (ruboxistaurin), PARP inhibitor (actovegin), voltage-gated sodium and calcium channel blockers (vixotrigine, mirogabalin), angiotensin II type 2 receptor antagonists, erythropoietin analogs, μ-opioid receptor agonists, dual enkephalinase inhibitor, β-adrenoceptor antagonist (Nebivolol), α2-adrenoceptor agonists (clonidine gel), monoclonal antibody against NGF (fulranumab), anti-inflammatory agents (salsalate), and combination nutraceuticals (Metanx). Recently, stem cell therapy and gene therapy have been shown to repair nerve damage.[32] **Table 2** presents recent advancements and clinical significance in DR and neuropathy.

TABLE 2: Recent advancements and clinical significance in diabetic retinopathy and neuropathy.

Category	*Advancement*	*Clinical significance*
Pharmacological therapy	• Antivascular endothelial growth factor (anti-VEGF) agents • SGLT-2 inhibitors for neuroprotection	Improves retinal edema and prevents progression; supports vascular integrity in DR and DPN
Steroid implants	Sustained-release dexamethasone and fluocinolone implants	Reduces retinal inflammation; long-acting, lowers injection frequency
Gene therapy	Adeno-associated viruses (AAV)-mediated gene transfer targeting angiogenesis and nerve regeneration	A promising long-term solution for DR and DPN, currently in the trial phase
Stem cell therapy	Regenerative approach using retinal or Schwann cell precursors	Potential to restore damaged retinal or peripheral nerve tissue
Artificial intelligence	AI-assisted retinal image analysis and risk prediction models	Enhances early detection and personalized care pathways
Advanced imaging	Optical coherence tomography (OCT) angiography, corneal confocal microscopy (CCM)	Noninvasive early detection of DR and small-fiber neuropathy
Neuromodulation devices	Spinal cord stimulation, peripheral nerve stimulation	Pain relief and improved nerve function in refractory DPN
Wearable technology	Foot temperature monitors, glucose sensors, retinal scan-enabled apps	Enables real-time monitoring; aids early intervention
Nutraceuticals	Benfotiamine, α-lipoic acid, and combination therapies	Antioxidant and neuroprotective roles; symptom relief in DPN
Novel drug targets	Receptor-interacting protein kinase 1 (RIP1) kinase inhibitors, protein kinase C (PKC) inhibitors (ruboxistaurin), anti-AGEs	Targets inflammation and oxidative stress in DR and DPN

(DPN: diabetic peripheral neuropathy; DR: diabetic retinopathy)

CLINICAL IMPLICATIONS

A multidisciplinary approach, comprising doctors, nurses, dietitians, and other medical staff, would enhance healthcare by improving access to facilities and information, increasing patient satisfaction, facilitating early diagnosis and treatment, providing high-quality clinical care, and offering psychological and social support. As diabetes is a complex disease, multidisciplinary care teams play a pivotal role in managing it.[33] Lifestyle modifications and medications are crucial in preventing DR and DPN. A study revealed that lifestyle modification over 4 years among overweight and obese individuals with impaired glucose tolerance has been shown to decrease the risk of retinal microaneurysms.[34]

Annual eye screenings and maintaining healthy blood sugar, blood pressure, and cholesterol levels are essential in preventing DR. Additionally, maintaining a healthy weight, adopting a balanced diet, and engaging in regular physical activity significantly reduce the risk of DR and its associated complications. Patient education and self-management practices are considered the gold standard in the management of DR. Patient education is essential in encouraging proactive behaviors and fostering self-management in DR. Empowering strategies comprises online education programs for patients to enhance knowledge, improve competency, and strengthen adherence to DR treatment protocols.[35]

Healthcare professionals should adopt a holistic approach to diabetes management, encompassing integrated screening, early diagnosis, prompt intervention, and multidisciplinary care to prevent the progression of complications. Several therapeutic approaches are being explored to address the management of diabetic complications. Furthermore, there is a pressing need for continued research and collaboration to elucidate the pathogenic mechanisms and identify novel therapeutic targets for halting or slowing the onset and progression of diabetic complications.

CONCLUSION

Studies suggest that there is a significant link between DR and DPN, both of which are influenced by the duration of diabetes and contribute to a decline in one's quality of life. These complications arise from prolonged hyperglycemia, leading to vascular and neural damage. Although advanced medical breakthroughs have been helpful in the meticulous evaluation and management of DR and DPN, there is no perfect remedy for retinopathy and neuropathy. Future research may yield numerous new advances in managing DR and DPN. However, prevention measures, lifestyle modifications, and regular annual screenings are essential in preserving both vision and nerve health in individuals with diabetes.

REFERENCES

1. International Diabetes Federation. IDF Diabetes Atlas, 11th edition. Brussels: International Diabetes Federation; 2025.
2. Teo ZL, Tham YC, Yu MC, Chee ML, Rim TH, Cheung N, et al. Global prevalence of diabetic retinopathy and projection of burden through 2045. Ophthalmology. 2021;128(11):1580-91.
3. Wang W, Lo ACY. Diabetic retinopathy: pathophysiology and treatments. Int J Mol Sci. 2018;19(6):1816.
4. Sharma RK, Weldekidan E, Berhane Y, Nathiya D. Diabetic Neuropathy: A Review. Int J Res Pharm Sci. 2015;5(4):24-30.
5. Raman R, Bhende P, Vasconcelos JC, Rajalakshmi R, Prevost AT, Ramasamy K, et al. Prevalence of diabetic retinopathy in India stratified by known and undiagnosed diabetes, urban–rural locations, and socioeconomic indices: results from the SMART India population-based cross-sectional screening study. Lancet Glob Health. 2022;10(12):e1764-73.

6. Pop-Busui R, Boulton AJ, Feldman EL, Bril V, Freeman R, Malik RA, et al. Diabetic Neuropathy: A Position Statement by the American Diabetes Association. Diabetes Care. 2017;40(1):136-54.
7. Dyck PJ, Kratz KM, Karnes JL, Litchy WJ, Klein R, Pach JM, et al. The prevalence by staged severity of various types of diabetic neuropathy, retinopathy, and nephropathy in a population-based cohort: the Rochester Diabetic Neuropathy Study. Neurology. 1993;43(4):817-24.
8. Viswanathan V, Gupta A, Devarajan A, Kumpatla S, Shukla S, Agarwal S, et al. Early screening for foot problems in people with diabetes is the need of the hour: 'Save the Feet and Keep Walking Campaign' in India. BMJ Open Diab Res Care. 2024;12:e004064.
9. Wang Y, Lin Z, Zhai G, Ding XX, Wen L, Li D, et al. Prevalence of and risk factors for diabetic retinopathy and diabetic macular edema in patients with early- and late-onset diabetes mellitus. Ophthalmic Res. 2022;65(3):293-9.
10. Schreur V, van Asten F, Ng H, Weeda J, Groenewoud JMM, Tack CJ, et al. Risk factors for the development and progression of diabetic retinopathy in Dutch patients with type 1 diabetes mellitus. Acta Ophthalmol. 2018;96(5):459-64.
11. Baum P, Toyka KV, Blüher M, Kosacka J, Nowicki M. Inflammatory Mechanisms in the Pathophysiology of Diabetic Peripheral Neuropathy (DN)-New Aspects. Int J Mol Sci. 2021;22(19):10835.
12. Bodman MA, Dreyer MA, Varacallo MA. Diabetic Peripheral Neuropathy. Treasure Island (FL): StatPearls Publishing; 2025.
13. UK Prospective Diabetes Study (UKPDS) Group. Intensive blood-glucose control with sulphonylureas or insulin compared with conventional treatment and risk of complications in patients with type 2 diabetes (UKPDS 33). Lancet. 1998;352(9131):837-53.
14. Behl T, Kotwani A. Exploring the various aspects of the pathological role of vascular endothelial growth factor (VEGF) in diabetic retinopathy. Pharmacol Res. 2015;99:137-48.
15. Ghotaslou R, Memar MY, Alizadeh N. Classification, microbiology and treatment of diabetic foot infections. J Wound Care. 2018;27(7):434-41.
16. Shukla UV, Tripathy K. Diabetic Retinopathy. Treasure Island (FL): StatPearls Publishing; 2025.
17. Wilkinson CP, Ferris FL, Klein RE, Lee PP, Agardh CD, Davis M, et al.; Global Diabetic Retinopathy Project Group. Proposed international clinical diabetic retinopathy and diabetic macular edema disease severity scales. Ophthalmology. 2003;110(9):1677-82.
18. Elafros MA, Andersen H, Bennett DL, Savelieff MG, Viswanathan V, Callaghan BC, et al. Towards prevention of diabetic peripheral neuropathy: clinical presentation, pathogenesis, and new treatments. Lancet Neurol. 2022;21(10):922-36.
19. Sloan G, Selvarajah D, Tesfaye S. Pathogenesis, diagnosis and clinical management of diabetic sensorimotor peripheral neuropathy. Nat Rev Endocrinol. 2021;17(7):400-20.
20. Ruia S, Tripathy K. Fluorescein Angiography. Treasure Island (FL): StatPearls Publishing; 2023.
21. Kansora MB, Goldhardt R. Decision Making in Proliferative Diabetic Retinopathy Treatment. Curr Ophthalmol Rep. 2019;7(1):45-50.
22. Represas-Carrera FJ, Martínez-Ques ÁA, Clavería A. Effectiveness of mobile applications in diabetic patients' healthy lifestyles: a review of systematic reviews. Prim Care Diabetes. 2021;15(6):751-60.
23. Kitsiou S, Paré G, Jaana M. Effects of home telemonitoring interventions on patients with chronic heart failure: an overview of systematic reviews. J Med Internet Res. 2015;17:e63.
24. Ting DSW, Liu Y, Burlina P, Xu X, Bressler NM, Wong TY. AI for medical imaging goes deep. Nat Med 2018; 24:539-40.
25. Gao S, Huang X, Zhang Y, Bao L, Wang X, Zhang M. Investigation on the expression regulation of RIPK1/RIPK3 in the retinal ganglion cells (RGCs) cultured in high glucose. Bioengineered. 2021;12(1):3947-56.
26. Kupis M, Samelska K, Szaflik J, Skopiński P. Novel therapies for diabetic retinopathy. Cent Eur J Immunol. 2022;47:102-8.
27. Ott C, Jumar A, Striepe K, Friedrich S, Karg MV, Bramlage P, et al. A randomised study of the impact of the SGLT2 inhibitor dapagliflozin on microvascular and macrovascular circulation. Cardiovasc Diabetol. 2017;16:26.
28. Cañadas P, Alberquilla García-Velasco M, Hernández Verdejo JL, Teus MA. Update on corneal confocal microscopy imaging. Diagnostics. 2023;13:46.
29. Røikjer J, Borbjerg MK, Andresen T, Giordano R, Hviid CVB, Mørch CD, et al. Diabetic Peripheral Neuropathy: Emerging Treatments of Neuropathic Pain and Novel Diagnostic Methods. J Diabetes Sci Technol. 2024:19322968241279553.
30. Serra J. Microneurography: towards a biomarker of spontaneous pain. Pain. 2012;153:1989-90.
31. Umapathi T, Tan WL, Loke SC, Soon PC, Tavintharan S, Chan YH. Intraepidermal nerve fiber density as a marker of early diabetic neuropathy. Muscle Nerve. 2007;35:591-8.
32. Yang Y, Zhao B, Wang Y, Lan H, Liu X, Hu Y, et al. Diabetic neuropathy: cutting-edge research and future directions. Signal Transduct Target Ther. 2025;10(1):132.

33. Taberna M, Gil Moncayo F, Jané-Salas E, Antonio M, Arribas L, Vilajosana E, et al. The multidisciplinary team (MDT) approach and quality of care. Front Oncol. 2020;10:85.
34. Bryl A, Mrugacz M, Falkowski M, Zorena K. The effect of diet and lifestyle on the course of diabetic retinopathy—a review of the literature. Nutrients. 2022;14(6):1252.
35. Beaser RS, Turell WA, Howson A. Strategies to improve prevention and management in diabetic retinopathy: qualitative insights from a mixed-methods study. Diabetes Spectr. 2018;31(1):65-74.

improvement, and overall enhanced well-being. Limited physical activity frequently resulting from sedentary lifestyles has been associated with the onset of mental health disorders, exacerbating both diabetes and mental state. The everyday requirements of blood glucose tracking, medication schedules, and lifestyle changes contribute to increased psychological strain. Additionally, anxiety stemming from potential diabetes-related complications, such as vision loss, nephropathy, and amputations, further impairs mental well-being.[4]

Furthermore, research clearly indicates that a lack of social support networks and barriers to accessing quality healthcare exacerbate these challenges, increasing the risk of depression and anxiety for PWD. The biopsychosocial model proposed by George and Engel effectively encapsulates the understanding of the critical interconnected factors emphasizing the need for a holistic approaches that address the biological, psychological, and social dimensions to improve mental health outcomes in patients with T2DM.[4]

BURDEN OF A LIFELONG JOURNEY

Managing a chronic illness such as diabetes can have a substantial emotional effect. Meticulous attention to dietary and physiological needs is essential to maintaining optimal glycemic control. PWD must oversee the financial expenditures for medications, equipment, and routine healthcare consultations, including intensive treatment and hospital stays for any potential complications. Beyond the direct medical costs, there are considerable indirect costs associated with diabetes, such as reduced employment due to disability, presentism, and productivity losses arising from premature mortality. These indirect expenses highlight the financial burden of a chronic disease and account for the impact of social determinants of health (SDOH). Disparities in socioeconomic status are a major contributor to the higher rates of diabetes prevalence and its complications. PWD often experience fluctuations in blood glucose levels due to anxiety, exercise, and hormonal changes. The intense fear of hypoglycemia may hinder them from administering enough insulin to keep their blood sugar levels within the prescribed parameters, thereby escalating the vulnerability to complications arising from hyperglycemia.[3]

Stigma surrounding diabetes is pervasive, with over 50% of PWD indicating experiences of discrimination, prejudice or negative attitudes in educational, occupational, and healthcare settings, as well as within their families. Consequently, they might conceal their self-management activities, such as insulin administration in public settings, to mitigate feelings of shame, judgment, and discrimination. Also, weight stigma often intersects with diabetes stigma, as individuals with diabetes frequently encounter misperceptions and biases regarding their condition, especially about obesity and overweight.[3]

Transitioning from pediatric to adult healthcare systems presents another layer of challenge. This period often coincides with heightened concerns about gaining independence and managing increased personal responsibility for one's health. During this vulnerable phase, supportive relationships with family, friends, and healthcare providers become critically crucial to prevent fragmentation of the care team and to sustain self-management abilities.[3]

ASSOCIATION BETWEEN PSYCHOLOGICAL STRESS FACTORS AND CLINICAL SYMPTOMS OF DIABETES

Psychological stress induces a myriad of metabolic changes, including peripheral vasoconstriction, an elevated heart rate, muscle tension, and amplified secretion of stress hormones, all of which ultimately raise blood glucose levels, further complicating the efforts to counteract stress. The impact of stress on blood sugar varies among individuals, particularly those with type 1 diabetes, due to underlying hormonal dysregulation and abnormalities in the autonomic nervous system, as well as individual psychological differences. Several studies have demonstrated that emotional distress in PWD correlates with suboptimal glycemic control, poor self-care practices, and adverse diabetes outcomes. Nonadherence to treatment regimens has been identified as a critical mediator between emotional distress and poor diabetes outcomes. Conversely, reductions in depressive symptoms have shown a positive association with better glycemic control.[1]

It was discovered that key psychological factors, comprising self-efficacy, confidence, strategies to cope with diabetes, and social support, have been linked to enhanced compliance with treatment and effective glycemic management. Typically, the experiences of stressful life events, ongoing environmental pressures, and the challenges of managing diabetes undermine these positive outcomes. Moreover, research indicates that psychological strain can lead to complications in metabolic, gastrointestinal function, sexual health, and neuropathic symptoms in people with the condition.[1]

PSYCHOLOGICAL REACTION IN PATIENTS WITH DIABETES

Managing diabetes is a continuous strain and entails addressing mental health challenges. The emotional responses of patients toward diabetes can be grouped into four fundamental tiers of psychological distress **(Fig. 1)**.[1]

Diabetes Distress

It refers to a unique, often hidden, emotional burden and concerns that patients experience while managing a severe chronic condition such as diabetes.[2] Indicators of DD encompass irritation, exhaustion, rage, depletion, and low spirits. DD differs from major depressive disorder (MDD), as MDD is a clinical psychiatric condition that specifically arises from the emotional challenges associated specifically with diabetes management.[3]

Depression

Adults with diabetes have a depression rate of at least 10% higher than those without diabetes,

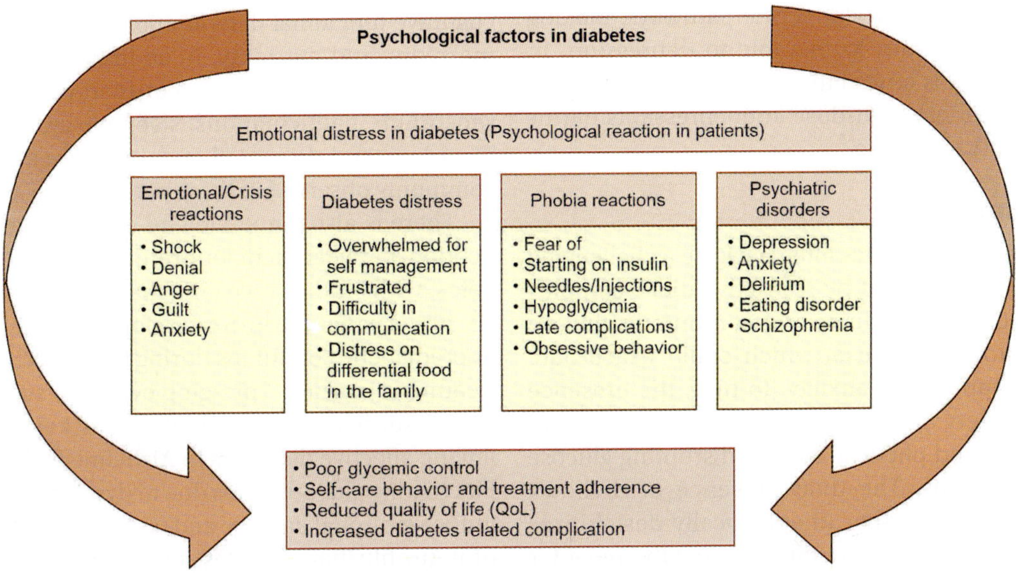

Fig. 1: Psychological elements and adverse effects in patients with diabetes.[1]

with younger adults displaying more depressive symptoms than their older counterparts. Moreover, comorbid depression significantly contributes to underutilization of prescribed medications among adult PWD concerned with financial constraints.[3] Depression may result in obesity and diabetes due to unhealthy lifestyle practices such as sedentary habits, overeating, and neglect of self-care routines. Diabetes, on the other hand, can precipitate depressive symptoms due to the major emotional, social, medical, and economic challenges that accompany managing the condition. Also, the new generation antidepressant drugs can contribute to T2DM by inducing weight gain and insulin resistance.[1] Abnormal fetal development, socioeconomic challenges, and unhealthy lifestyles appear to be causes of both diabetes and depression, triggering the stress response systems. Long-term hypercortisolemia and chronic activation of the sympathetic nervous system cause blood sugar imbalances, known as dysglycemia. Over time, these alterations may contribute to neurodegenerative conditions such as ischemic encephalopathy and cerebral atrophy in the brain. Moreover, diabetes is a state of chronic inflammation that could impair synaptic function and disrupt neuroendocrine pathways, making individuals more vulnerable to depression. In addition, it is crucial to recognize that prolonged use of certain high-dose antidepressants harms glycemic regulation.[5]

Anxiety

People with diabetes often navigate a challenging landscape marked by restrictive diets, complex medication schedules and continuous glucose monitor (CGM) use, which could exacerbate the symptoms of anxiety. In turn, the presence of anxiety may adversely influence dietary choices and physical activity, disrupting glucose homeostasis. The dual presence of diabetes and anxiety further unequivocally destabilizes blood glucose levels, underscoring the need for integrated care approaches.[5]

Eating Disorders

Eating disorders are defined as "a persistent disturbance of eating or eating-related behavior that results in the altered consumption or absorption of food, significantly impairing physical health or psychosocial functioning". The primary triad includes anorexia, bulimia, and binge eating disorder. Research indicates that individuals with diabetes, especially T2DM, are more susceptible to all three disturbances, with binge eating disorder showing a high prevalence within this population. In addition, a unique phenomenon exists particularly in PWD, where they deliberately skip their insulin doses and oral hyperglycemic medications to reduce weight. Regardless of diabetes status, multiple factors that further illuminate these conditions include gender-specific concerns about body weight and shape, abnormal dieting habits, and having a history of depression.[3]

Other Psychiatric Disorders in Diabetes

Delirium, another psychiatric disorder related to diabetes, is often characterized by the occurrence of hypoglycemic episodes or diabetic ketoacidosis. It is associated with prolonged hospital stays, cognitive functional deterioration, and increased morbidity and mortality. In addition, outcomes such as disorientation, confusion, altered sensorium, hallucinations, sleeping–awakening disorders, and disrupted cognitive function are commonly observed in these patients.[1,5]

There is also a notable and concerning connection between schizophrenia (SZ) and diabetes, with studies revealing that approximately 20–30% of patients with SZ develop either diabetes or prediabetic conditions during their psychiatric treatment journey. Emerging evidence suggests that insulin resistance could be a key factor linking affective disorders to Alzheimer's disease. Fluctuating glucose levels due to dysglycemia can induce neuronal damage and foster the formation of neurofibrillary tangles, the characteristic of Alzheimer's disease.[1]

INTERRELATIONSHIP BETWEEN DIABETES MELLITUS AND EMOTIONAL WELL-BEING

Stress is a condition of tension and agitation that emerges when an organism responds suitably to environmental threats. However, chronic stress also exerts a profound influence on overall metabolic health. Activation of the hypothalamic-pituitary-adrenal (HPA) axis and the sympathetic nervous system, triggered by persistent stressors, fosters a cascade of detrimental behaviors like poor nutrition, physical inactivity, smoking, and alcohol consumption **(Flowchart 1 and Fig. 2)**.[5]

HEALTH EFFECTS OF EMOTIONS?

Positive emotions, such as happiness, excitement, and contentment, are correlated with enhanced health behaviors and improved compliance with therapeutic regimens. Physiologically, positive emotions activate the autonomic nervous system, leading to beneficial effects by stimulating the HPA axis, which helps to reduce cortisol levels and enhance immune function through primary (bone marrow and thymus) and secondary (spleen and lymph nodes) lymphoid tissues. Moreover, healthy behaviors, such as engaging in physical activities, trigger the excretion of endorphin, leading to a sense of elation.[6]

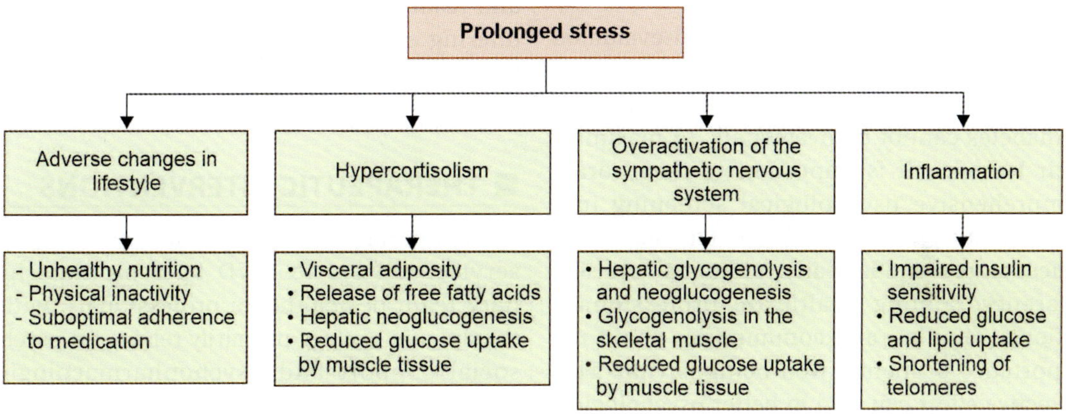

Flowchart 1: The impact of stress-related physiological processes on blood sugar levels.[5]

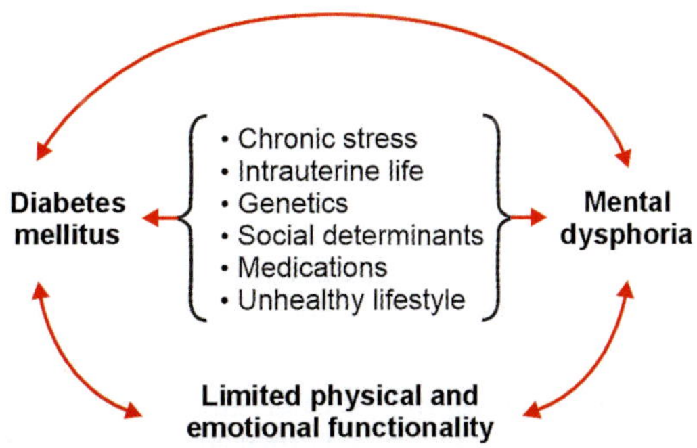

Fig. 2: Diabetes and mental/psychological dysphoria.[5]

In contrast, negative emotions significantly heighten the health risks through stress, anxiety, and depression. These emotional states impair immune responses, making individuals more vulnerable to infections and illnesses. They also increase the production of proinflammatory cytokines, which can promote chronic inflammation that has been linked to a spectrum of age-related conditions, including cardiovascular diseases, osteoporosis, arthritis, Alzheimer's disease, frailty and functional decline, diabetes mellitus, certain cancers, and periodontal diseases.[6]

PSYCHOLOGICAL THERAPIES/ STRATEGIES IN MANAGING DIABETES

The pressing need for effective, well-evaluated psychosocial interventions/therapies to support people dealing with the everyday challenges of diabetes cannot be overstated. To maximize their benefits, it is important to incorporate comprehensive psychological screening into routine diabetes care, ensuring that mental health concerns are identified early. Additionally, raising awareness among healthcare professionals, patients, families, and communities about the importance of mental well-being is vital. This collective effort can lead to better psychological health, enhanced adherence to treatment plans, and ultimately, more successful diabetes management.[1]

GUIDELINES

The American Diabetes Association (ADA) position statement on psychosocial care advocates for screening during the initial visit, at periodic intervals (consultations every 3 months) and whenever there is a change in disease condition, treatment, or life circumstance involving caregivers and family members in these assessments is strongly recommended. However, these best practices are often overlooked in clinical settings due to various reasons, mainly a lack of time and resources. Prompt identification facilitates offering effective treatment for those in need, thereby improving prognosis and ultimately leading to better health outcomes.[7]

THERAPEUTIC INTERVENTIONS

Contemporary care necessitates an integrated service delivery to PWD by a multidisciplinary team of healthcare professionals, with a therapeutic strategy primarily relying on psychosocial support and psychopharmacological interventions **(Table 1)**.[5]

TABLE 1: Psychosocial support and psychopharmacological interventions in patients with diabetes.[5]

Psychosocial support	Guidance on self-care	• Educates on blood glucose monitoring, diet, physical activity, and treatment adherence • Provides individualized instructions to enhance self-care and emotional adjustment
	Cognitive behavioral therapy	• Reorganizes dysfunctional thoughts and changes behaviors • Focuses on optimism and resilience • Improves self-care, mood, and quality of life
	Social supportive networks	• Offers emotional, material, and practical support • Formal (insurance and social services) and informal (family and friends) networks improve outcomes, especially for the vulnerable

Continued

Continued

Psychopharmacological agents	*Antidepressants*: • Antipsychotics • Anxiolytics
Recommendations for clinical practice	• Holistic care includes emotional needs and social circumstances • Diabetes specialists should recognize and manage psychological issues, with psychiatric referrals when necessary • Address both physical and mental health in diabetes management • Psychoeducation: Disease information, acquisition of problem-solving and communication skills, and increase in self-confidence • Education should help patients to accept and manage their condition • State support is essential

CONCLUSION

The interplay between diabetes and psychosocial disorders is multifaceted and cannot be ignored. Their simultaneity can impact glycemic control, self-care routines, and QoL. The emotional and psychological requirements of PWD are often undermined when personal efforts to meet these challenges do not succeed, leading to an increased risk of diabetes-related complications. Consequently, these complications not only diminish QoL but also elevate mortality rates, increase healthcare costs, and diminish productivity. By addressing the psychosocial needs, patients are more likely to adhere to their care plans, which in turn fosters achieving long-term health improvements and better glycemic management. Therefore, a comprehensive understanding of the psychological dimensions affecting PWD will empower Clinicians to formulate strategies that enhance diabetes outcomes and alleviate the overall burden. To facilitate this, ADA strongly recommends ongoing assessment of mental health symptoms for all PWD as part of standard diabetes treatment, ensuring timely referrals to mental health providers as necessary.

REFERENCES

1. Kalra S, Jena BN, Yeravdekar R. Emotional and Psychological needs of People with Diabetes. Indian J Endocr Metab. 2018;22:696-704.
2. Gupta J, Kapoor D, Sood V, Singh S, Sharma N, Kanwar P. Depression Prevalence, its Psychosocial and Clinical predictors, in Diabetes Mellitus Patients attending two Health institutions of North India catering rural Population. Indian J Psychiatry 2020;62:566-71.
3. Tenreiro K, Hatipoglu B. Mind Matters: Mental Health and Diabetes Management. J Clin Endocrinol Metab. 2025;110(Supplement_2):S131-S136.
4. Busili A, Kumar K, Kudrna L, Busaily I. The risk factors for mental health disorders in patients with type 2 diabetes: An umbrella review of systematic reviews with and without meta-analysis. Heliyon. 2024;10(7):e28782.
5. Mangoulia P, Milionis C, Vlachou E, Ilias I. The Interrelationship between Diabetes Mellitus and Emotional Well-Being: Current Concepts and Future Prospects. Healthcare (Basel). 2024;12(14):1457.
6. Chew BH, Shariff-Ghazali S, Fernandez A. Psychological aspects of diabetes care: Effecting behavioral change in patients. World J Diabetes. 2014;5(6):796-808.
7. Snoek FJ. Mental health in diabetes care. Time to step up. Front Clin Diabetes Healthc. 2022;3:1039192.

20 Lifestyle Interventions: Nutrition and Exercise in Diabetes Care

Vanisha S Nambiar, Shonima Venugopal, Sabat Imran Ansari

ABSTRACT

India, with its vast culinary diversity and growing diabetes burden, faces an urgent need for culturally appropriate and sustainable dietary interventions. With type 2 diabetes mellitus reaching epidemic levels, driven by sedentary lifestyles, urbanization, and dietary shifts toward processed foods, there is increasing recognition of the role traditional Indian foods can play in diabetes prevention and management. This chapter explores the therapeutic potential of India's regional diets in managing diabetes through a lifestyle nutrition approach. Emphasis is placed on traditional meals such as the Indian *thaali*, incorporating low-glycemic grains (e.g., millets), legumes, fiber-rich vegetables, fermented foods, and healthy fats, all of which align with evidence-based dietary recommendations for glycemic control, weight management, and metabolic health.

The chapter presents a comprehensive summary of diabetes-friendly food and drink options from various Indian regions—North, South, East, West, Central, North-East, and union territories such as Puducherry—highlighting the role of preparation methods, portion control, and functional ingredients. Key clinical implications include improved patient compliance through culturally tailored counseling, reduction of refined food dependency, and the inclusion of functional beverages and spices with proven antidiabetic properties. Pearls of dietary practice and a food-swap table provide practical guidance for meal planning. By bridging ancestral food knowledge with modern science, this approach promotes an affordable, accessible, and culturally respectful strategy for diabetes care in both rural and urban settings. Ultimately, embracing traditional Indian dietary wisdom can offer a preventive and therapeutic pathway for tackling the diabetes epidemic in India and similar settings worldwide.

Keywords: Traditional foods, Indian *thaali*, Functional ingredients.

INTRODUCTION

Diabetes has emerged as a major global public health concern, with particularly alarming consequences in India. Often referred to as the "second diabetes capital of the world", India has one of the highest rates of type 2 diabetes mellitus, driven by sedentary behavior, rapid urban growth, and increased consumption of processed, calorie-dense foods. There is a high prevalence of prediabetes and diabetes in rural and urban India with a narrowing rural–urban gap. Results from a systematic review and meta-analysis of 1.7 million adults from India revealed that the prevalence of diabetes increased in both urban India and rural India from 3.3% and 2.4%

in 1972 to 19.0% and 15.0%, respectively, in the years 2015–2019. This corresponds to a total of 107 million people with diabetes. The number of adults with prediabetes is probably substantially greater, indicating a significant burden of dysglycemia in the Indian population.[1] Diabetes continues to pose a serious threat to India's social and economic progress, despite being a largely preventable and manageable condition through timely intervention and lifestyle modifications. Reversing this rising trend demands greater awareness, early screening, and long-term lifestyle improvements.

UNDERSTANDING DIABETES AND DIETARY NEEDS

Diabetes mellitus is characterized by elevated blood glucose levels due to insulin dysfunction. Dietary management is crucial in controlling blood sugar levels and preventing complications. It has been shown that diets have multifaceted roles in type 2 diabetes mellitus management. Weight loss and improved cardiometabolic health are two benefits of an energy-restricted diet. People with type 2 diabetes mellitus may benefit from dietary strategies such as plant-based diets, Mediterranean diet, high-protein diets, or low-carbohydrate diets, as well as a higher consumption of omega-3 fatty acids, for cardiometabolic health.[2]

Key dietary goals of nutrition therapy for people with diabetes according to the American Diabetes Association (ADA) 2024[3] include:

- Promoting and supporting healthy eating patterns, emphasizing a variety of nutrient-dense foods in appropriate portion sizes, to improve overall health by:
  - Achieving and maintaining body weight goals
  - Attaining individualized glycemic, blood pressure, and lipid goals
  - Delaying or preventing the complications of diabetes
- Addressing individual nutrition needs based on personal and cultural preferences, health literacy and numeracy, access to healthy foods, willingness and ability to make behavioral changes, and existing barriers to change
- Maintaining the pleasure of eating by providing nonjudgmental messages about food choices while limiting food choices only when indicated by scientific evidence
- Providing individuals with diabetes the practical tools for developing healthy eating patterns rather than focusing on individual macronutrients, micronutrients, or single foods

REGIONAL INDIAN FOODS FOR THE MANAGEMENT OF DIABETES

India has a long way to go and needs to change its course of action if it must reach the targets set by the Sustainable Development Goals. Growing wealth leading to consequent changes in consumption patterns, and ignorance and poverty leading to undernutrition are challenging our food system's ability to provide nutritious food or to contribute to enhanced livelihood opportunities in an environmentally sustainable way. With growing attention to nutrition–agriculture linkages, understanding how to create nutrition-sensitive agriculture and sustainable food systems is an essential task for the future of India.

The diet of Pastoral age, which consisted of small quantities of digestible carbohydrates, large amounts of high-fiber carbohydrates, moderate proteins, and fats, gradually changed over the centuries. From 1775 to 1947, there was a notable decrease in the consumption of fat and protein and an increase in the frequency of intake of high-fiber carbohydrates. The frequency of intake and amounts of fats and low-fiber and refined carbohydrates have increased since 1947, whereas protein intake has only slightly improved.[4] Higher consumption of processed refined staple grains—primarily refined wheat in the Western and Northern parts of India and white rice in the Southern and Eastern regions—has resulted from the nutrition transition brought on by urbanization, strong economic growth rates, and globalization. In addition to this, unhealthy fats; lower quality and quantity of protein; decreased consumption of fruits, vegetables, and fiber; and a sedentary lifestyle are the primary causes of the Indian diabetes epidemic.[5]

Management of diabetes in India, a land of diverse religions and cultures, and varied physiographic regions, is not easy. Food practices reflect cultural identity as well as the social conditions and include methods opted for selection, preparation and serving of food, and all these factors further affect the consumption pattern of food. Indians love to eat diverse food influenced by their regional cuisine which in turn is a result of its political and geographical history (including the influence of invasions from a foreign land, traders of silk route, colonial rule, etc.), variation in the local culture, geographical location (proximity to the sea, desert, or mountains), and economics. Therefore, for management and control of diabetes, it is important to understand the food consumption patterns of Indian population, which are largely influenced by the regional traditional practices and passed on through generations from the primary unit of the family which is influenced by their communities and religion.[6]

Eating customs in India are based on medical and moral beliefs. Ayurveda, the ancient Indian medicinal system emphasizes the idea that "you are what you eat".

DIETARY PRINCIPLES FOR DIABETES PREVENTION AS PER AYURVEDA[7]

Do's (*Pathya*)

- Timely intake of diet
- Intake of old harvested cereals, barley (*yava*), sorghum (*jowar*), whole wheat (*atta*), bitter gourd (*karela*), green leafy vegetables, garlic (*lasuna*), turmeric (*haridra*), and aloe (*kumari*) in vegetables and fruits such as guava, oranges, and Indian blackberry (jamun) may be useful.
- Reduce intake of rice, food rich in carbohydrate, and fried or processed food.

Dont's (*Apathya*)

- Sugarcane juice, jaggery, sugar, and milk products
- Tubers, sweets, soft drinks, fried foods, and sweet fruits such as mango, banana, custard apple, and date are to be avoided
- Staying too long on empty stomach
- Ice cream, burger, pizza, and other fast foods
- Sedentary lifestyle
- Sleeping in the daytime and excessive sleeping
- Alcohol

Methods of preparation of traditional Indian cuisine vary throughout the nation. In India, traditional knowledge regarding food preparation, preservation methods, and medicinal benefits has been developed over many centuries. Due to the presence of functional ingredients including probiotics, dietary fiber, antioxidants, and compounds that can heal the body, Indian traditional foods are also considered as functional foods. These functional ingredients control blood sugar levels and aid in weight management.[8,9]

TRADITIONAL INDIAN *THAALI*: AN ANCIENT MODEL OF A HEALTHY PLATE

Availability of healthy local foods and a balanced diet are the most important factors for maintaining good nutritional status and good health. Food insecurity and imbalanced diets are the root cause of malnutrition and the onset of diseases. The concept of a healthy plate, a visual guide that illustrates the relative proportion of food groups to be included in a balanced healthy diet, has been gaining traction worldwide and is being promoted in India as well to prevent the onset of disease conditions such as diabetes mellitus.[10] India's diverse culinary heritage offers a wealth of traditional foods that can play a pivotal role in managing diabetes **(Table 1)**. The concept of the Indian *"thaali"*—a balanced platter featuring a variety of dishes—embodies the principles of moderation, variety, and nutritional balance. Indian traditional foods, when thoughtfully integrated into the diet, offer a sustainable and culturally resonant approach to managing diabetes. The Indian *thaali* exemplifies a holistic approach to meals, offering a variety of flavors and nutrients **(Table 2)**.

A typical diabetic-friendly *thaali* should include:

- *Grains*: Millets such as bajra, jowar, and ragi have a low glycemic index and are rich in fiber, aiding in blood sugar control. Studies have shown that millets can be beneficial for individuals with diabetes.[11,12]
- *Legumes and pulses* (such as *moong, chana, and urad dal*): Dal (lentils) and legumes provide plant-based protein and fiber and support insulin action which helps in regulating blood glucose levels.[13]
- *Vegetables*: Nonstarchy vegetables such as spinach, bitter gourd (*karela*), [14] and fenugreek

TABLE 1: Diabetes-friendly foods and drinks from various regions of India.

Region	*Examples of foods*	*Key ingredients/methods*	*Diabetes management benefits*
North (J&K, Punjab, Uttar Pradesh and Himachal)	Kalaadi cheese, *moong dal chilla, bajra/missi roti with saag, karela bharta, dalia, nadru monje*, and *siddu*	Whole lentils, mustard greens, bitter gourd, fermented dairy, bajra, low oil, and steamed	High fiber, probiotics, low glycemic index, supports insulin sensitivity, and anti-inflammatory
Central (Madhya Pradesh, Chhattisgarh)	*Bhutte ka kees, chana samosa* (baked), *kadhi, moong dal khichdi, and chana chaat*	Corn, chickpeas, curd, sprouts, lauki, and roasted snacks	Balanced carbs and protein, improved satiety, probiotic-rich, and reduces glucose spikes
West (Gujarat, Maharashtra, Rajasthan, and Goa)	*Methi thepla, handvo, thalipeeth, usal, bajra roti with ker sangri, and modak* (steamed)	Fenugreek, lentils, millets, low-oil cooking, and fermented batters	Blood sugar regulation, anti-inflammatory, fiber-dense, and enhanced insulin function
East (West Bengal, Odisha, Bihar, and Jharkhand)	*Shukto, dalma, pakhala bhata* (light), *sattu paratha, dumbu, and peetha* (savory)	Bitter gourd, red rice, fermented rice, sattu, leafy greens, and low-fat curd	Glycemic index-lowering, gut health, blood sugar stabilization, and protein-rich
North-East (Assam, Manipur, Nagaland, Mizoram, and Tripura)	*Xaak bhaji*, chamthong, galho, bai, mui borok, and jadoh (modified)	Leafy greens, fermented soy/fish, minimal oil, sticky/red rice, and local herbs	High antioxidants, improves gut flora, and reduces insulin resistance
South (Tamil Nadu, Kerala, Karnataka, and Andhra/Telangana)	*Ragi dosa, kootu, avial, saaru, jonna roti, ragi payasam*, and *adai*	Millets, greens, coconut (in moderation), tamarind, and fermented batters	Low glycemic index, high calcium/fiber, probiotic benefit, and controlled carbs
Puducherry and Mahe	Millet risotto, ragi galette, chickpea patties, and quinoa-stuffed peppers	Fusion recipes using millets, legumes, veggies, and olive oil	Low carb, high protein, healthy fats, and portion-controlled

Source: Adapted from Nambiar (2021).[6]

21 Landmark Randomized Controlled Trials in Diabetes: Evidence and Implications

Hemant P Thacker, Shambo Samrat Samajdar, Anuj Maheshwari

ABSTRACT

Over the past four decades, landmark randomized controlled trials (RCTs) have revolutionized diabetes management, evolving from a glucose-centric focus toward an integrated framework that encompasses *metabolic, cardiovascular, and renal protection*. Foundational studies such as the Diabetes Control and Complications Trial (*DCCT)* and United Kingdom Prospective Diabetes Study (*UKPDS)* established the enduring benefits of intensive glycemic control in reducing microvascular complications and introduced the concept of "metabolic memory". Subsequent trials, including *ACCORD (*Action to Control Cardiovascular Risk in Diabetes), *ADVANCE (*Action in Diabetes and Vascular Disease: Preterax and Diamicron MR Controlled Evaluation), and Veterans Affairs Diabetes Trial *(VADT)*, underscored the importance of *individualized glycemic targets* to balance benefits against the risks of hypoglycemia and mortality.

The emergence of *cardiovascular outcome trials (CVOTs)*—notably *EMPA-REG OUTCOME, LEADER, SUSTAIN-6*, and *DECLARE-TIMI 58*—redefined therapeutic priorities by demonstrating that sodium-glucose cotransporter-2 *(SGLT-2) inhibitors* and glucagon-like peptide-1 *receptor agonists* (GLP-1 RAs) reduce cardiovascular and renal events independent of glucose lowering. Parallel renal outcome trials, such as *CREDENCE, DAPA-CKD, FIDELIO-DKD*, and *EMPA-KIDNEY*, established *SGLT-2 inhibition and mineralocorticoid receptor blockade* as dual cornerstones of kidney protection.

Technological innovation through *continuous glucose monitoring (CGM)* and *hybrid closed-loop insulin delivery* has transformed type 1 diabetes care, enabling safer and more precise glycemic control. By 2025, diabetes management has embraced a *multimodal, personalized paradigm* that integrates pharmacologic synergy, precision diabetology, and digital health to optimize outcomes across the cardiorenal–metabolic spectrum.

This synthesis of landmark and emerging evidence affirms that modern diabetes care is anchored in *individualization, prevention, and holistic organ protection*, laying the groundwork for future regenerative and gene-based therapies that aim for durable disease modification or remission.

Keywords: Diabetes mellitus, Randomized controlled trials, Cardiovascular outcomes, SGLT-2 inhibitors, Precision diabetology.

INTRODUCTION

Randomized controlled trials (RCTs) have been instrumental in shaping the management of diabetes mellitus, serving as the cornerstone of evidence-based practice, and transforming therapeutic paradigms. Over the past few decades, these trials have illuminated the intricate relationships between glycemic control, cardiovascular health, and renal outcomes, leading to a more comprehensive understanding of diabetes as a multisystem disease.

Foundational RCTs such as the Diabetes Control and Complications Trial (DCCT) and the United Kingdom Prospective Diabetes Study (UKPDS) provided conclusive evidence that intensive glycemic control significantly reduces the risk of microvascular complications, including retinopathy, nephropathy, and neuropathy.[1] These pivotal studies established the principle of "metabolic memory," demonstrating that early and sustained glucose control yields long-term protective effects. However, subsequent large-scale trials— *ACCORD* (Action to Control Cardiovascular Risk in Diabetes), *ADVANCE* (Action in Diabetes and Vascular Disease: Preterax and Diamicron MR Controlled Evaluation), and Veterans Affairs Diabetes Trial *(VADT)*, —challenged the universality of intensive glucose lowering by revealing limited cardiovascular benefits and, in some cases, increased mortality, emphasizing the importance of individualized treatment goals.[2]

The introduction of cardiovascular outcome trials (CVOTs) following the 2008 US Food and Drug Administration (FDA) mandate marked a paradigm shift from glucose-centric to outcome-driven diabetes care. Trials such as EMPA-REG OUTCOME, and LEADER established that agents like sodium-glucose cotransporter-2 (SGLT-2) inhibitors and glucagon-like peptide-1 receptor agonists (GLP-1 RAs) confer substantial cardiovascular and renal protection beyond glycemic effects.[3] These studies reshaped clinical guidelines and reinforced the need for an integrated approach addressing cardiovascular and renal comorbidities in diabetic patients.

In parallel, landmark studies in diabetic nephropathy and continuous glucose monitoring (CGM) have further refined patient care. Trials assessing renin-angiotensin-aldosterone system (RAAS) blockade and SGLT-2 inhibition have underscored the renoprotective potential of modern therapies,[4] while CGM trials—such as those by the Juvenile Diabetes Research Foundation (JDRF)—have demonstrated improvements in glycemic control and quality of life for individuals with type 1 diabetes.[5]

In summary, landmark RCTs **(Table 1)** have revolutionized diabetes management by evolving

TABLE 1: Landmark trials and clinical lessons in diabetes (1980–2025).

Trial	*Population*	*Key findings*	*Clinical implication*
DCCT (1993)	Type 1 diabetes mellitus (T1DM)	Intensive insulin therapy reduced microvascular complications (retinopathy, nephropathy, and neuropathy) by up to 76%; long-term follow-up (EDIC) confirmed "metabolic memory" benefits	Early intensive glycemic control prevents microvascular disease and offers long-term cardiovascular protection
UKPDS (1998)	Type 2 diabetes mellitus (T2DM)	Intensive therapy with sulfonylureas or insulin reduced microvascular endpoints by 25%; metformin arm showed cardiovascular benefit in overweight individuals	Established the foundation for the "legacy effect" and early intervention in T2DM

Continued

Continued

Trial	*Population*	*Key findings*	*Clinical implication*
ACCORD (2008)	T2DM at high CV risk	Intensive glycemic control (HbA1c <6.0%) increased mortality despite HbA1c improvement	Overly tight glycemic control can be harmful; targets must be individualized
ADVANCE (2008)	T2DM with vascular risk	Intensive control reduced nephropathy by 21% but showed no CV mortality benefit	Reinforced balanced glycemic targets for organ protection
VADT (2009)	T2DM (veterans)	No significant reduction in major cardiovascular events; post-trial legacy benefit observed for microvascular outcomes	Individualized HbA1c goals considering age, duration, and comorbidities
EMPA-REG OUTCOME (2015)	T2DM + established CVD	Empagliflozin reduced CV death by 38% and heart failure hospitalization by 35%	Introduced cardiorenal protection beyond glucose lowering
LEADER (2016)	T2DM + CVD risk	Liraglutide reduced MACE by 13% and CV mortality by 22%	Glucagon-like peptide-1 receptor agonists (GLP-1 RAs) recommended for ASCVD prevention
SUSTAIN-6 (2016)	T2DM + high CV risk	Semaglutide lowered MACE by 26%, improved weight and HbA1c	Validated classwide CV benefit of GLP-1 RAs
DECLARE-TIMI 58 (2019)	T2DM ± CVD	Dapagliflozin reduced HF hospitalizations by 27%; renal benefit observed even without diabetes	Extended SGLT-2 inhibitor indication to broader CKD/HF population
CREDENCE (2019)	T2DM + CKD (eGFR 30–90)	Canagliflozin reduced risk of ESKD, doubling of creatinine, or renal/CV death by 30%	Confirmed renal protection as an independent therapeutic target
DAPA-CKD (2020)	CKD (with or without T2DM)	Dapagliflozin reduced renal composite outcome by 39%; reduced all-cause mortality	Established SGLT-2 inhibitors as standard of care for CKD regardless of diabetes status
FIDELIO-DKD (2021)	T2DM + CKD	Finerenone reduced kidney failure or sustained eGFR decline by 18%; reduced CV events	Introduced MRAs for additive cardiorenal benefit
EMPA-KIDNEY (2023)	CKD (± diabetes)	Empagliflozin lowered risk of kidney disease progression or CV death by 28%; benefit extended to low-albuminuria patients	Expanded SGLT-2 indication to early and nondiabetic CKD
CONFIDENCE (ongoing 2025)	T2DM + CKD	Evaluates dual finerenone + empagliflozin therapy; preliminary data show synergistic albuminuria reduction	Dual pathway modulation expected to redefine CKD standard of care
JDRF CGM trials (2012)	T1DM	Continuous glucose monitoring improved HbA1c, reduced hypoglycemia, and increased treatment satisfaction	Foundation for CGM integration and hybrid closed-loop adoption

Continued

Continued

Trial	*Population*	*Key findings*	*Clinical implication*
FLAIR/ADAPT/ CamAPS FX (2020–2024)	T1DM (youth and adults)	Hybrid closed-loop systems improved time-in-range (+15%) and reduced hypoglycemia events	Automated insulin delivery established as standard in type 1 diabetes management
Dual incretin (SURPASS, 2021–2023)	T2DM + obesity	Tirzepatide (GLP-1/GIP) achieved superior HbA1c and weight loss vs. semaglutide	Dual incretin agonists mark next generation of metabolic therapy
Beta-cell regeneration and gene therapy (2024–2025)	Early T1DM/ T2DM	Preclinical and phase I trials show β-cell neogenesis and functional restoration via gene modulation	Regenerative therapy poised to transition diabetes from chronic control to possible remission

from glycemic-centric approaches to holistic strategies encompassing cardiovascular, renal, and metabolic outcomes. This chapter synthesizes these pivotal contributions and explores their clinical implications for 2025 and beyond, highlighting how evidence from these trials continues to drive the evolution of personalized, outcome-oriented diabetes care.

FOUNDATIONS: INTENSIVE GLYCEMIC CONTROL AND MICROVASCULAR OUTCOMES

Diabetes Control and Complications Trial and the United Kingdom Prospective Diabetes Study

The DCCT and UKPDS remain foundational in establishing the benefits of intensive glycemic control in diabetes. The DCCT, conducted among individuals with type 1 diabetes, demonstrated that intensive insulin therapy—aimed at near-normoglycemia—significantly reduced the incidence and progression of microvascular complications, including retinopathy, nephropathy, and neuropathy, by up to 76% compared with conventional treatment.[6,7] Follow-up data from the Epidemiology of Diabetes Interventions and Complications (EDIC) study extended these findings, demonstrating sustained reductions in cardiovascular events and mortality—a phenomenon termed the "legacy effect" or "metabolic memory".[8,9]

Similarly, the UKPDS—which enrolled patients with newly diagnosed type 2 diabetes—found that intensive glycemic control with sulfonylureas or insulin significantly reduced microvascular complications by 25% compared to conventional therapy.[6] Although the reduction in macrovascular outcomes was modest, the long-term follow-up of UKPDS participants revealed significant benefits in cardiovascular mortality, supporting early intervention in the course of diabetes.[6] Together, these trials established that early and sustained glycemic control is critical in preventing microvascular complications and possibly conferring downstream cardiovascular benefits.

Post-UKPDS Trials: ACCORD, ADVANCE, and VADT

Following the UKPDS, the ACCORD, ADVANCE, and Veterans Affairs Diabetes Trial (VADT) studies evaluated whether more intensive glycemic targets [glycated hemoglobin (HbA1c) <6.0–6.5%] could further reduce cardiovascular morbidity and mortality among patients with type 2 diabetes and higher baseline risk.

challenges such as suboptimal dosing, first-pass metabolism, short half-lives, P-glycoprotein efflux, poor target specificity, and systemic adverse effects. These issues reduce adherence and efficacy. Furthermore, while conventional treatments help control blood glucose, they do not address the complex pathophysiology or complications of diabetes, underscoring the need for improved therapeutic approaches.[1]

EMERGING THERAPEUTIC TARGETS AND MECHANISMS

Drugs for Type 1 Diabetes Mellitus

Type 1 diabetes mellitus (T1DM) is a chronic autoimmune condition that marks the end stage of a multifactorial process involving genetic and environmental factors, leading to immune-mediated destruction of pancreatic β cells and resulting in insulin dependence. A range of clinical trials is currently underway to evaluate novel immunotherapeutic approaches aimed at preventing or modifying the progression of T1DM. These include therapies targeting regulatory T (Treg) cells (e.g., autologous Tregs and CryoTregs), cytokine modulation [e.g., low-dose interleukin 2 (IL-2) and baricitinib], antigen-specific immunotherapies (e.g., Diamyd and peptide vaccine), and immunomodulatory agents [e.g., siplizumab, frexalimab, and Bacillus Calmette–Guérin (BCG) vaccine]. Additional investigational therapies such as UPR21, VX-264, and VCTX-211 are also being studied for their safety and efficacy in T1DM. Details of these ongoing trials, including study design, population, and timelines, are summarized in **Table 1**.[3]

TTP399 (Cadisegliatin)

TTP399 is a novel, oral, liver-selective glucokinase activator under development as an adjunct to insulin therapy in T1DM. It functions by restoring hepatic glucose sensing, promoting glucose uptake and storage, and maintaining a fed-state metabolic profile, thereby reducing ketone production. In the SimpliciT1 phase 2 trial, TTP399 demonstrated a statistically significant improvement in glycated hemoglobin (HbA1c) and a 40% reduction in hypoglycemic episodes compared to placebo, without increasing the risk of diabetic ketoacidosis. A subsequent mechanistic study confirmed no elevation in ketone levels during acute insulin withdrawal and showed improved fasting plasma glucose and reduced hypoglycemia. To date, nearly 600 subjects have been treated with TTP399, which has shown a favorable safety and tolerability profile. Additionally, in a prior phase 2 trial involving T2DM patients, TTP399 significantly reduced HbA1c with minimal incidences of hypoglycemia or hyperlipidemia.[4]

Zimislecel (Formerly VX-880)

Zimislecel is Vertex's investigational, fully differentiated islet cell therapy being evaluated for T1DM patients with severe hypoglycemic events and impaired hypoglycemia awareness. Administered with standard immunosuppression, it is currently in the phase 3 portion of a global phase 1/2/3 trial, expected to complete enrollment and dosing by mid-2025. Zimislecel has received multiple expedited designations, including regenerative medicine advanced therapy (RMAT) and Fast Track from the United States Food and Drug Administration (USFDA), PRIority MEdicines (PRIME) from the European Medicines Agency (EMA), and an Innovation Passport under the UK's Innovative Licensing and Access Pathway (ILAP). Upon anticipated regulatory approvals in 2026, the therapy could initially benefit approximately 60,000 patients with severe T1DM in the United States and Europe.[5]

Monoclonal Antibody

Teplizumab

Teplizumab, an anti-CD3 monoclonal antibody that does not bind to the fragment crystallizable (Fc) receptor, can postpone the onset of clinical (stage 3) T1DM. Teplizumab treatment may yield varying results depending on the stage of T1DM and the β-cell reserve at the time of treatment. In

TABLE 1: Ongoing clinical trials in immunotherapy for type 1 diabetes mellitus (T1DM).

Therapy	*Clinical trials gov ID*	*Official study name*	*Study type*	*Estimated enrollment*	*Eligible age range (years)*	*Start date*	*Estimated completion*
Autologous regulatory T (Treg) cells	NCT 03839462	Clinical safety and therapeutic effects of autologous Tregs in T1DM	Phase II, open-label, single-center	30	8–65	April 2023	December 2027
Bacillus Calmette–Guérin (BCG) vaccinations	NCT02081326	Repeat BCG vaccinations for the treatment of new onset T1DM in children aged 8–18 years	Phase II, randomized, single-center	100	8–18	May 2023	May 2028
BCG vaccinations	NCT02081326	Repeat BCG vaccinations for the treatment of established T1DM	Phase II, randomized, single-center	150	18–65	June 2015	July 2031
CryoTregs in transplantation	NCT05445991	Cryopreserved polyclonal regulatory T cell (CryoTreg) immunotherapy in islet transplantation	Phase I, randomized, single-center	11	18–48	August 2022	May 2025
GSK open	NCT05105170	Clinical and biological responses to repeated administration of low-dose interleukin-2 in patients with T1DM and a residual C-peptide	Phase I, single-center	24	16–45	September 2022	August 2028
Diamyd	NCT05197915	A phase III, randomized, double-blind, placebo-controlled, multicenter trial to evaluate the efficacy and safety of Diamyd® in genetically defined subgroup of patients recently diagnosed with T1DM	Phase III, randomized, multicenter	330	12–28	May 2022	December 2027
Frexalimab	NCT06111956	2-Part randomized, double-blind, placebo-controlled, multicenter phase 2a study with a 52-week and blinded extension assessment	Phase II, randomized, multicenter	192	12–35	December 2023	October 2028

Continued

Continued

Therapy	***Clinical trials gov ID***	***Official study name***	***Study type***	***Estimated enrollment***	***Eligible age range (years)***	***Start date***	***Estimated completion***
JAK inhibitors (baricitinib)	NCT05248324	Multicenter, randomized, double-blind, placebo-controlled study to evaluate efficacy and safety of baricitinib in β-cell function in newly diagnosed T1DM	Phase II, randomized, multicenter	78	12–35	October 2023	June 2027
Siplizumab A	NCT05763453	T cell pathway: Siplizumab dosing in recent onset T1DM	Phase I, open-label, single-center	10	8–45	April 2023	March 2025
Siplizumab B	NCT05951100	A study of siplizumab in children and adolescents with new onset T1DM	Phase I, randomized, multicenter	96	8–14	July 2023	December 2026
UPR21	NCT05782218	A study evaluating safety of UPR21 in participants with autoimmune disease	Phase I, open-label, multicenter	60	18–65	March 2023	June 2026
VCTX-211	NCT05654862	A phase 1/2 study to evaluate the safety, tolerability, and efficacy of VCTX211 in subjects with T1DM	Phase I/II, open-label, single-center	18	18–65	August 2023	August 2026
VX-264	NCT05210530	A phase 1/2 study to evaluate the safety, tolerability, and efficacy of VX-264 in adults with T1DM	Phase I/II, open-label, single-center	17	18–65	March 2021	June 2030

(JAK: Janus kinase)

the phase III PROTECT trial in patients of 8 years of age or older with preclinical (stage 2) disease, teplizumab retained the β-cell function, as measured by stimulated C-peptide levels at week 78. At week 78, patients treated with teplizumab had significantly higher stimulated C-peptide levels than those receiving the placebo [least-squares mean difference, 0.13 pmol/mL; 95% confidence interval (CI) 0.09–0.17; $p < 0.001$]. Additionally, 94.9% (95% CI 89.5–97.6) of patients treated with teplizumab maintained a clinically meaningful peak C-peptide level of 0.2 pmol/mL or higher, compared to 79.2% (95% CI 67.7–87.4) of those receiving placebo. Adverse effects include headache, gastrointestinal problems, rash, lymphopenia, and moderate cytokine release syndrome. Teplizumab shows benefits in preservation of β-cell function.[6]

Drugs for Type 2 Diabetes Mellitus

Oral Glucagon-like Peptide-1 Receptor Agonists

Orforglipron (LY3502970)

Orforglipron is an oral glucagon-like peptide-1 receptor agonist (GLP-1RA) that activates pancreatic β-cell receptors, mimicking endogenous GLP-1. In the phase III ACHIEVE-1 trial in adults with T2DM uncontrolled by diet and exercise, it reduced HbA1c by 1.3–1.6% across doses. At the highest dose, mean weight loss reached 7.9% (16 lbs), and over 65% of population achieved HbA1c ≤ 6.5%, aligning with American Diabetes Association (ADA) targets. The safety profile resembled injectable GLP-1 agonists, mainly with gastrointestinal events. No hepatotoxicity was observed. Orforglipron presents a promising oral option for T2DM treatment.[7]

ECC5004/AZD5004

ECC5004 is a once-daily oral small-molecule GLP-1 receptor agonist for diabetes and obesity. Preclinical studies showed high receptor affinity (IC_{50} = 2.4 nM) with cyclic adenosine monophosphate (cAMP) activation but no β-arrestin-2 recruitment or receptor internalization. In a phase I placebo-controlled trial, healthy volunteers received single doses (1–300 mg) and T2DM patients received multiple doses (5–50 mg) over 28 days. Doses ≥25 mg reduced blood glucose and body weight. The compound exhibited favorable safety and pharmacokinetics, supporting its potential as an oral therapy.[8]

Ecnoglutide Injection

Ecnoglutide (XW003), a GLP-1 analog with cAMP bias, is under development for T2DM and obesity. In a phase III trial in China, patients receiving weekly doses of 0.6 and 1.2 mg had HbA1c reductions of 1.96 and 2.43%, respectively, compared to 0.87% with placebo ($p < 0.0001$). In the 1.2 mg group, 76.1% reached HbA1c ≤ 6.5% and 35.2% reached <5.7%. It was well tolerated, with appetite loss, diarrhea, and nausea as the main mild-to-moderate side effects. Ecnoglutide showed strong efficacy and a safety profile consistent with GLP-1 agonists.[9]

Danuglipron (PF-06882961)

Danuglipron (PF-06882961) is an oral small-molecule GLP-1 receptor agonist under development for T2DM and obesity. In preclinical models, it demonstrated efficacy comparable to injectable GLP-1RAs. A phase 1, placebo-controlled, randomized, double-blind, multiple ascending dose study (NCT03538743) in 98 T2DM patients on metformin showed that danuglipron was generally well tolerated, with mild adverse events such as nausea, dyspepsia, and vomiting. No clinically significant laboratory or electrocardiogram (ECG) abnormalities were observed. Danuglipron led to a modest increase in heart rate and slight reduction in systolic blood pressure, with safety findings consistent with the known GLP-1RA class.[10]

XW014

XW014 is an investigational oral small-molecule GLP-1 receptor agonist in a phase 1 randomized, double-blind, placebo-controlled trial for T2DM

Insulin trial (QWINT), phase 3 trials for T2DM. In QWINT-1 (52 weeks, insulin-naïve adults), efsitora demonstrated noninferior HbA1c reduction compared to daily insulin glargine, with final HbA1c levels of 6.92% versus 6.96% (efficacy estimand) and 7.05% versus 7.08% (treatment-regimen estimand). In QWINT-3 (78 weeks, patients previously on basal insulin), efsitora was noninferior to insulin degludec, achieving HbA1c levels of 6.93% versus 7.03% and 6.99% versus 7.08%, respectively. Efsitora also provided slightly greater time-in-range (70–180 mg/dL) and time-in-tight-range (70–140 mg/dL). Notably, QWINT-1 reported ~40% fewer hypoglycemic events with efsitora than glargine, while QWINT-3 showed comparable safety to degludec. These results highlight efsitora's potential as a convenient and effective once-weekly insulin option in the treatment pipeline.[20]

Insulin Icodec

Insulin icodec is a once-weekly long-acting basal insulin analog for the treatment of T2DM. It is also used for T1DM, In phase 3, a 78-week randomized, open-label trial was conducted in patients with T2DM. Participants were randomized to two groups, group 1: Once-weekly insulin icodec and group 2: Once-daily insulin glargine U100. The mean reduction in HbA1c levels over 52 weeks was more significant with icodec compared to glargine U100 [decreasing from 8.50 to 6.93% for icodec (mean change, –1.55% points), and from 8.44 to 7.12% for glargine U100 (mean change, –1.35% points)]; the estimated difference between the groups (–0.19% points; 95% CI –0.36 to –0.03) established both noninferiority ($p < 0.001$) and superiority ($p = 0.02$) of icodec. Glycemic management showed considerable improvement with once-weekly insulin icodec compared to once-daily insulin glargine U100.[21]

Inhalational Insulin

Insulin Human Inhalational Powder (Technosphere, Afrezza)

Inhaled Technosphere insulin has a more rapid onset of action, which can reduce the postmeal glucose rise as well as rapidly reduce glucose levels when used for corrections. It is used in both T1DM and T2DM. In a 30-week study of people with T1DM utilizing Technosphere insulin (TI) + insulin degludec, the mean HbA1c stayed stable at 7.6% through 17 weeks and then improved slightly to 7.4% at 30 weeks, with a significant drop of 0.21% between weeks 17 and 30 ($p < 0.001$). The percentage of participants with HbA1c < 7.0% increased from 21% at baseline to 42% after 30 weeks. Time spent in range (70–180 mg/dL) increased slightly from 52 to 54%, but time spent in hypoglycemia (<54 mg/dL) remained modest (≤0.6%). In week 30, the average daily TI dose was 53 ± 31 units, nearly double the baseline rapid-acting insulin dose of 24 ± 12 units. Overall, the the TI–degludec regimen maintained stable glucose control with modest improvements and minimal hypoglycemia. HbA1c levels were sustained over 30 weeks using a TI–degludec regimen after switching from automated insulin delivery (AID) or multiple daily insulin injections (MDI).[22]

Amylin (Peptide Hormone)

Amylin, a peptide hormone cosecreted with insulin, plays a critical role in postprandial satiety and energy homeostasis and may act as an adiposity signal by modulating the reward value of food. In individuals with T1DM, the absence of endogenous amylin contributes to impaired appetite regulation and glycemic variability. While GLP-1RAs have demonstrated robust weight loss efficacy in obese and T2DM populations, emerging evidence also supports their utility in T1DM. Amylin analogs, such as pramlintide and cagrilintide, have shown clinical benefits in reducing insulin requirements, improving glycemic control, and promoting weight loss in T1DM. Preclinical studies suggest that combining GLP-1RAs with amylin analogs exerts a synergistic effect on weight reduction, although clinical data remain limited. Early case reports in T1DM patients with obesity treated with pramlintide and GLP-1RA cotherapy have demonstrated encouraging outcomes, including significant weight loss and reduced insulin demand.[23]

Glucagon-like peptide-1 Receptor Agonists and Amylin Analogs

CagriSema (Cagrilintide–Semaglutide)

Cagrilintide is an amylin analog, and semaglutide is a GLP-1 receptor agonist. In a phase 3a (REDEFINE 2) double-blind, randomized, placebo-controlled trial, a total of 1,206 patients were randomly assigned to one of two groups: (1) Cagrilintide-semaglutide (904 patients) or (2) placebo (302 patients). The mean change in body weight from baseline to week 68 was −13.7% in the cagrilintide-semaglutide group and −3.4% in the placebo group (estimated difference: −10.4 percentage points; 95% CI −11.2 to −9.5; $p < 0.001$). More patients in the cagrilintide-semaglutide group than in the placebo group experienced a weight decrease of 5% or more ($p < 0.001$), as well as reductions of at least 10%, 15%, and 20% ($p < 0.001$).

The cagrilintide-semaglutide group had 73.5% of patients with a HbA1c level of 6.5% or below, compared to 15.9% in the placebo group. Gastrointestinal side effects were recorded by 72.5% of patients in the cagrilintide-semaglutide group and 34.4% in the placebo group, most of which were temporary and mild to severe in severity. Once-weekly cagrilintide-semaglutide gives significant results in patients with obesity and T2DM.[24]

Amycretin

Amycretin is a novel, single-molecule dual agonist of the *GLP-1* receptor and the *amylin* receptor, designed to combine glucose-lowering and weight-reduction effects in individuals with overweight, obesity, or type 2 diabetes. In a *first-in-human, phase 1, randomized, double-blind, placebo-controlled, multipart study* conducted in San Antonio, USA, a total of *144 participants* aged *18–55 years* were enrolled. Participants were assigned to receive *single ascending doses* (part A), *multiple ascending doses* (part B), or *dose-escalation regimens* (parts C/D) of oral amycretin, or placebo.

The *primary endpoint* was the incidence of treatment-emergent adverse events (TEAEs), while *secondary endpoints* included pharmacokinetic parameters and exploratory measures of *body weight* and *fasting plasma glucose.* Across all study parts, amycretin demonstrated a favorable *safety and tolerability profile,* with most adverse events being mild to moderate and predominantly *gastrointestinal* in nature.

In part C/D, exploratory pharmacodynamic analyses showed *dose-dependent reductions in body weight and fasting glucose* by day 85. The mean change in *HbA1c* from baseline was *−0.2% with amycretin 50 mg, −0.3% with amycretin 100 mg,* and *−0.3% with 2 × 50 mg,* compared with placebo. Plasma concentrations were consistent with *dose-proportional pharmacokinetics.*

Overall, *amycretin appeared safe, well tolerated, and pharmacologically active,* supporting continued evaluation in *ongoing phase 2 studies* to further characterize its weight-loss efficacy and metabolic benefits.

PERSONALIZED MEDICINE APPROACHES

Personalized medicine integrates biological, clinical, and genetic variability to tailor disease management, recognizing that individual differences influence disease risk, progression, and treatment response. In T2DM, genetic factors significantly contribute to disease development and therapeutic outcomes. Genome-wide association studies (GWAS) have identified over 700 T2DM-associated variants, with key genes such as *SLC30A8, KCNJ11, TCF7L2, ABCC8, SLC2A2,* and *KCNQ1* implicated in insulin secretion and β-cell function. Micro-ribonucleic acid (miRNA), including miR-375, miR-7a, miR-26a-5p, and miR-204, further regulate β-cell activity and insulin secretion, influencing disease course and treatment efficacy.

Epigenetic mechanisms, such as histone modifications and deoxyribonucleic acid (DNA) methylation, also modulate gene expression without altering DNA sequences. Differential methylation in genes such as *TXNIP*, *ABCG1*, and *SOCS3* has been associated with T2DM and may serve as biomarker. Metabolomic profiling using techniques such as LC-MS has revealed altered levels of amino acids, fatty acids, and glycolytic intermediates in T2DM, correlating with complications such as cardiovascular disease and diabetic nephropathy. Furthermore, predictive algorithms are being developed to personalize therapy, stratify risk, and anticipate complications. While not yet widely implemented in clinical practice, the integration of multi-omics data and computational models holds significant promise for advancing precision medicine in T2DM.[27]

FUTURE DIRECTIONS

Future research in diabetes management should prioritize large-scale, long-term clinical trials to validate the efficacy, safety, and durability of novel therapeutic agents, including dual and triple incretin receptor agonists, immunotherapies, glucokinase activators, and islet cell-based interventions. Emphasis should also be placed on integrating personalized medicine approaches using genomic, epigenetic, and metabolomic data to enable individualized treatment strategies. The development of predictive algorithms and multi-omics platforms may further refine patient stratification and therapeutic decision-making. Additionally, optimizing combination regimens, enhancing global access to advanced therapies, and leveraging digital health tools for real-time monitoring and adherence support will be critical for translating these innovations into improved clinical outcomes and broader population-level impact.

CONCLUSION

The evolving landscape of diabetes management reflects significant strides in the development of novel therapeutic agents that target diverse mechanisms underlying both T1DM and T2DM. In T1DM, immunotherapies such as Treg cells, cytokine inhibitors, and antigen-specific vaccines are showing promise in altering disease progression and preserving β-cell function. Adjunctive metabolic agents like TTP399 and islet cell replacement therapies such as Zimislecel offer additional avenues for improving glycemic control and reducing hypoglycemia risk.

For T2DM, emerging treatments including oral GLP-1 receptor agonists, dual/triple incretin agonists, liver-selective glucokinase activators, and long-acting DPP-4 inhibitors address limitations of traditional therapies by enhancing efficacy, tolerability, and patient adherence. The integration of personalized medicine through genetic, epigenetic, and metabolomic insights further supports individualized care strategies. Continued clinical validation and long-term outcome studies will be essential to fully realize the impact of these innovations on global diabetes management.

REFERENCES

1. Dhyani S, Butola M, Sautha V, Jakhmola V. Recent advances in treatment approaches for diabetes mellitus and related complications: a review. Int J Appl Pharm. 2025;17(2):12-30.
2. International Diabetes Federation. The Diabetes Atlas. [online] Available from https://diabetesatlas.org/ [Last accessed September, 2025].
3. Jeun R. Immunotherapies for prevention and treatment of type 1 diabetes. Immunotherapy. 2025;17(3):201-10.
4. Klein KR, Freeman JLR, Dunn I, Dvergsten C, Kirkman MS, Buse JB, et al; SimpliciT1 research group. The SimpliciT1 Study: A randomized, double-blind, placebo-controlled Phase 1b/2 adaptive study of TTP399, a hepatoselective glucokinase activator, for adjunctive treatment of type 1 diabetes. Diabetes Care. 2021;44(4):960-8.
5. Vertex Pharmaceuticals. (2025). Vertex announces program updates for type 1 diabetes portfolio. [online] Available from https://investors.vrtx.com/news-releases/news-release-details/vertex-announces-program-updates-type-1-diabetes-portfolio [Last accessed September, 2025].

6. Ramos EL, Dayan CM, Chatenoud L, Sumnik Z, Simmons KM, Szypowska A, et al; PROTECT Study Investigators. Teplizumab and β-cell function in newly diagnosed type 1 diabetes. N Engl J Med. 2023;389(23):2151-61.
7. Eli Lilly and Company. (2025). Lilly's oral GLP-1, orforglipron, demonstrated statistically significant efficacy results and a safety profile consistent with injectable GLP-1 medicines in successful Phase 3 trial. [online] Available from https://investor.lilly.com/news-releases/news-release-details/lillys-oral-glp-1-orforglipron-demonstrated-statistically [Last accessed September, 2025].
8. Haggag AZ, Xu J, Butcher L, Pagnussat S, Davies G, Lundqvist S, et al. Non-clinical and first-in-human characterization of ECC5004/AZD5004, a novel once-daily, oral small-molecule GLP-1 receptor agonist. Diabetes Obes Metab. 2025;27(2):551-62.
9. Zhu D, Wang W, Tong G, Ma J, Wen B, Zheng X, et al. 742-P: A Phase 3 evaluation of cAMP signaling biased GLP-1 analog Ecnoglutide (XW003) in adults with type 2 diabetes. Diabetes. 2024;73(Suppl_1):742-P.
10. Saxena AR, Gorman DN, Esquejo RM, Bergman A, Chidsey K, Buckeridge C, et al. Danuglipron (PF-06882961) in type 2 diabetes: a randomized, placebo-controlled, multiple ascending-dose Phase 1 trial. Nat Med. 2021;27(6):1079-87.
11. ClinicalTrials.gov. (2024). XW014 in healthy subjects and patients with type 2 diabetes mellitus (T2DM). [online] Available from https://clinicaltrials.gov/study/NCT05579314 [Last accessed September, 2025].
12. Lingvay I, Benamar M, Chen L, Fu A, Jódar E, Nishida T, et al. Once-weekly IcoSema versus once-weekly semaglutide in adults with type 2 diabetes: the COMBINE 2 randomised clinical trial. Diabetologia. 2025;68(4):739-51.
13. Yu N, Xu W, Guo X, Xu M, Zhang W, Yan C, et al. Fotagliptin add-on therapy to metformin in patients with uncontrolled type 2 diabetes: A randomised, multicentre, double-blind, placebo-controlled, Phase 3 trial. Diabetes Obes Metab. 2025;27(7):3933-42.
14. Gao L, Bian F, Pan T, Jiang H, Feng B, Jiang C, et al. Efficacy and safety of cofrogliptin once every 2 weeks in Chinese patients with type 2 diabetes: A randomized, double-blind, placebo-controlled, Phase 3 trial. Diabetes Obes Metab. 2025;27(1): 280-90.
15. Wang W, Yao J, Guo X, Guo Y, Yan C, Liu K, et al. Efficacy and safety of DBPR108 monotherapy in patients with type 2 diabetes: a 12-week, randomized, double-blind, placebo-controlled, Phase II clinical trial. Curr Med Res Opin. 2020;36(7):1107-15.
16. Zhang B, Cheng Z, Chen J, Zhang X, Liu D, Jiang H, et al. Efficacy and safety of Mazdutide in Chinese patients with type 2 diabetes: A randomized, double-blind, placebo-controlled Phase 2 trial. Diabetes Care. 2024;47(1):160-8.
17. De Block C, Bailey C, Wysham C, Hemmingway A, Allen SE, Peleshok J. Tirzepatide for the treatment of adults with type 2 diabetes: An endocrine perspective. Diabetes Obes Metab. 2023;25(1):3-17.
18. Abdul-Rahman T, Roy P, Ahmed FK, Mueller-Gomez JL, Sarkar S, Garg N, et al. The power of three: Retatrutide's role in modern obesity and diabetes therapy. Eur J Pharmacol. 2024;985:177095.
19. Waibel M, Wentworth JM, So M, Couper JJ, Cameron FJ, MacIsaac RJ, et al. Baricitinib and β-cell function in patients with new-onset type 1 diabetes. N Engl J Med. 2023;389(23):2140-50.
20. Eli Lilly and Company. (2024). In a first-of-its-kind fixed dose study, once-weekly insulin efsitora alfa leads to A1C reduction similar to daily insulin. [online] Available from https://investor.lilly.com/news-releases/news-release-details/first-its-kind-fixed-dose-study-once-weekly-insulin-efsitora [Last accessed September, 2025].
21. Rosenstock J, Bain SC, Gowda A, Jódar E, Liang B, Lingvay I, et al. Weekly icodec versus daily glargine U100 in type 2 diabetes without previous insulin. N Engl J Med. 2023;389(4):297-308.
22. Beck RW, Bailey RJ, Klein KR, Aleppo G, Levy CJ, Diner J, et al; INHALE-3 Study Group. Inhaled Technosphere Insulin Plus Insulin Degludec for Adults with Type 1 Diabetes: The INHALE-3 Extension Study. Diabetes Technol Ther. 2025;27(3):170-8.
23. Wong G, Garner EM, Srivastava G. Combined GLP-1 receptor agonist and amylin analogue pharmacotherapy to treat obesity comorbid with type 1 diabetes. JCEM Case Rep. 2023;1(2):luad040.
24. Davies MJ, Bajaj HS, Broholm C, Eliasen A, Garvey WT, le Roux CW, et al; REDEFINE 2 Study Group. Cagrilintide-Semaglutide in Adults with Overweight or Obesity and Type 2 Diabetes. N Engl J Med. 2025;393(7):648-59.
25. Dahl K, Toubro S, Dey S, Duque do Vale R, Flint A, Gasiorek A, et al. Amycretin, a novel, unimolecular GLP-1 and amylin receptor agonist administered subcutaneously: results from a phase 1b/2a randomised controlled study. Lancet. 2025;406(10499):149-62.
26. American Diabetes Association Professional Practice Committee. 8. Obesity and Weight Management for the Prevention and Treatment of Type 2 Diabetes: Standards of Care in Diabetes–2025. Diabetes Care. 2025;48(1 Suppl 1):S167-S180.
27. Nameghi SM. Exploring the recent advancements and future prospects of personalized medicine in type 2 diabetes. Endocr Metab Sci. 2024;16:100193.

23

Diabetes in Special Populations (Pediatric, Elderly, and Gestational)

N Bhavatharini, Sunil S Gupta, VK Sanjeev, ARA Changanidi

ABSTRACT

Diabetes mellitus continues to impose a formidable global health burden, disproportionately affecting physiologically vulnerable groups such as pediatric patients, geriatric individuals, and pregnant women. These populations manifest discrete metabolic profiles, variable clinical trajectories, and distinctive therapeutic exigencies that challenge the applicability of generalized diabetes protocols. In India—where rapid urbanization, nutritional transitions, and shifting epidemiologic patterns converge—the prevalence of diabetes within these cohorts has escalated markedly. The pediatric landscape, historically dominated by type 1 diabetes, now increasingly includes type 2 presentations among urban youth, mandating early detection and assertive insulin-based regimens to forestall acute metabolic decompensation. In older adults, polypharmacy, multimorbidity, and neurocognitive decline potentiate hypoglycemic risk, thereby necessitating individualized glycemic thresholds calibrated to functional and frailty indices. Gestational diabetes mellitus (GDM), with its dual impact on maternal and fetal health, remains insufficiently addressed due to inconsistent screening frameworks and persistently low postpartum surveillance. While transformative advances—such as continuous glucose monitoring (CGM), glucagon-like peptide-1 (GLP-1) receptor agonists, dual incretin therapies, and telemedicine—have redefined diabetes management globally, their diffusion in resource-constrained Indian settings remains uneven. This chapter synthesizes contemporary evidence (2020–2025), contextualized within Indian epidemiological realities, and proposes an integrative clinical paradigm. By emphasizing algorithmic frameworks, comparative treatment matrices, and culturally attuned strategies, it aims to facilitate durable glycemic control and improve long-term outcomes in these high-risk subpopulations.

Keywords: Continuous glucose monitoring, Elderly diabetes, Gestational diabetes mellitus, GLP-1 receptor agonists, Indian epidemiology, Pediatric diabetes.

INTRODUCTION

Diabetes mellitus comprises a group of metabolic cum vascular disorders characterized by chronic hyperglycemia due to defects in insulin secretion, action, or both and various other causes including liver, muscle, brain, gut, kidney, etc. Although more global attention is paid to type 2 diabetes among adults, special populations, children, older adults and pregnant women are underrepresented in terms of surveillance strategies and recommendations. These are the populations of people with unique clinical issues that result in a burden on the healthcare systems, particularly in India, where the epidemic is gaining momentum due to urbanization and changes in lifestyles.

With more than 101 million adults living with diabetes and 136 million with prediabetes, India falls second in the world, prevailed by diabetes.[1] The pediatrics and geriatrics cases are on the rise[2,3] and gestational diabetes mellitus (GDM) is seen in 15–20% of pregnancies and more in urban areas.[4] Type 1 diabetes prevails among children, yet type 2 is increasing among teenagers who are overweight.[5] Elderly diabetes is associated with complications and comorbidities.[6]

Though international frameworks exist, localized strategies are critical. Innovations such as continuous glucose monitoring (CGM), dual incretin therapies, and telemedicine offer promise but face accessibility and implementation barriers.[7,8] This chapter outlines a contextualized, evidence-based approach for India's high-risk diabetic populations.

PEDIATRIC DIABETES

Pediatric diabetes in India is increasingly reported, particularly in urban centers such as Delhi and Mumbai. While type 1 remains predominant, type 2 is rising due to obesity, with 19.3% of urban children projected to be affected by 2024. Genetic factors and undiagnosed monogenic forms such as maturity-onset diabetes of the young (MODY) further complicate detection.[2,3,5] In newly detected diabetes <1 year, always rule out monogenic diabetes since these patients do not require insulin and respond well to sulfonylureas.

Type 1 diabetes mellitus (T1DM) in children typically presents with classical symptoms—polyuria, polydipsia, and unexplained weight loss—and usually diabetic ketoacidosis (DKA), a contributor to pediatric diabetes-related morbidity and mortality. In India, DKA at diagnosis occurs in 30–40% of pediatric cases, markedly higher than in Western nations. This disparity reflects diagnostic delays, limited awareness among caregivers, and constrained access to early healthcare services.[6]

Conversely, type 2 diabetes mellitus (T2DM) in adolescents often presents insidiously, with subtle signs of insulin resistance, including acanthosis nigricans, obesity, hypertension, and polycystic ovary syndrome (PCOS) or with complications itself at diagnosis. Recent data suggest that 11% of obese urban Indian adolescents exhibit impaired glucose tolerance, highlighting the urgency for early risk-based screening.[6]

The 2022 International Society for Pediatric and Adolescent Diabetes (ISPAD) guidelines recommend diagnosis based on plasma glucose, glycated hemoglobin (HbA1c), and oral glucose tolerance test (OGTT)—particularly for suspected T2DM or MODY cases.[8] Fasting hyperglycemia and low C-peptide usually with antibodies is diagnostic for T1DM. C-peptide may be normal or mostly high in T2DM in young patients. The Indian Council of Medical Research (ICMR) 2023 guidelines further advocate CGM use in select pediatric patients, especially those with glycemic variability or poorly controlled T1DM, supporting more precise and individualized diagnosis.

Pediatric diabetes management demands a multidisciplinary team involving endocrinologists, educators, dietitians, psychologists, and caregivers. In T1DM, insulin is mandatory for survival via multiple daily injections (MDI) or continuous subcutaneous insulin infusion (CSII) offering better HbA1c control.[9] T2DM treatment focuses on lifestyle changes, metformin, and insulin for severe hyperglycemia **(Table 1)**.

Recent progress includes wider CGM use, improving glycemic control and reducing hypoglycemia.[8] Hybrid closed-loop systems show potential for near-physiological insulin delivery. Glucagon-like peptide-1 (GLP-1) receptor agonists, such as liraglutide and dulaglutide, are approved for adolescent T2DM.[10] Telemedicine, accelerated by the COVID-19 pandemic, has improved remote glycemic monitoring and continuity of care.[11]

Social stigma, insufficient school-based support, and limited diabetes education hinder

TABLE 1: Comparison of diabetes in special populations.

Characteristic	*Pediatric diabetes*	*Elderly diabetes*	*Gestational diabetes mellitus*
Predominant type	T1DM	T2DM	Glucose intolerance of pregnancy
Common presentations	Polyuria, polydipsia, DKA	*Atypical*: fatigue, or with complications	Asymptomatic, detected via OGTT
Diagnostic challenges	DKA at onset, atypical T2DM	Cognitive impairment, frailty	Paradigm shift in prevalence
Glycemic targets (HbA1c)	<7.5% (ISPAD 2022)	Individualized (7–8% or higher)	FPG <95, 1 hour <140, 2 hour <120 mg/dL
Preferred therapies	Insulin (MDI/CSII), CGM, insulin pump	OADs, GLP-1 RAs, cautious insulin use	MNT, MF insulin if needed

(CGM: continuous glucose monitoring; DKA: diabetic ketoacidosis; FPG: fasting plasma glucose; GLP-1 RAs: glucagon-like peptide-1 receptor agonists; HbA1c: glycated hemoglobin; ISPAD: International Society for Pediatric and Adolescent Diabetes; MF: metformin; OAD: oral antidiabetic drugs; OGTT: oral glucose tolerance test; T1DM: type 1 diabetes mellitus; T2DM: type 2 diabetes mellitus)

adherence. Critically, there is a severe shortage of pediatric endocrinologists and educators, compounded by the lack of standardized growth charts, culturally relevant counseling, and genetic testing infrastructure.[12]

For instance, a 12-year-old girl from Mumbai diagnosed with T1DM [HbA1c 11.2%, blood glucose (BG) 320 mg/dL] began MDI insulin and CGM. A 6-month follow-up showed HbA1c improvement to 7.8%, fewer hypoglycemic episodes, and better academic performance, demonstrating the impact of structured, tech-enabled pediatric diabetes care.

DIABETES IN THE ELDERLY

India's aging population—expected to exceed 192 million by 2030—faces a growing diabetes burden, with prevalence estimates ranging from 25 to 30% among the elderly.[13,14] Atypical presentations, multimorbidity, and physiological decline complicate diagnosis and treatment, increasing the risk of hypoglycemia. Geriatric syndromes such as frailty and sarcopenia intensify complications, yet most guidelines remain adult centric, failing to address the nuanced needs of this vulnerable and underrepresented population. Type 3 diabetes due to insulin resistance in the brain with Alzheimer's disease is also common.

Polypharmacy, which is prevalent in this age group due to multimorbidity, can obscure classic hyperglycemic presentations and increase the risk of drug interactions. Frailty—a syndrome characterized by reduced physiological reserve and heightened vulnerability to stressors—affects up to 40% of elderly Indian diabetics and is strongly associated with increased hospitalization, functional dependence, and mortality.[15] According to the updated recommendations, the 2024 guidelines of the American Diabetes Association (ADA) suggest annual screening of diabetes in the population aged 65 years and older via fasting plasma glucose (FPG), HbA1c, or a 2-hour OGTT.[16] The condition that potentially complicates the accurate diagnostic interpretation of elderly individuals is anemia or chronic kidney disease (CKD), which can produce falsely low HbA1c values. Discordant glucose measurements also contribute to malnutrition and age-related metabolic changes. While underutilized, CGM has shown promise in elderly Indian cohorts by detecting asymptomatic nocturnal hypoglycemia and improving glycemic trend assessment.[17]

International consensus supports the individualization of glycemic targets in older adults. The ADA 2024 recommends an HbA1c goal of 7.0–7.5% for robust, functionally independent elderly; 7.5–8.0% for those with multiple comorbidities or mild cognitive impairment; and up to 8.5% for frail patients with limited life expectancy.[4] Indian expert panels concur with these guidelines but emphasize contextual flexibility, particularly in low-resource environments where intensive glycemic control may pose more harm than benefit.[18]

In elderly individuals with diabetes, pharmacologic strategies should prioritize agents with a low risk of hypoglycemia and demonstrated cardiorenal benefits. Metformin remains the first-line agent when renal function is preserved (eGFR ≥45 mL/min/1.73 m^2). Traditional sulfonylureas such as glibenclamide are generally avoided due to their pronounced hypoglycemic potential. However, newer-generation sulfonylureas such as gliclazide MR may be cautiously employed in select patients. Glipizide, devoid of active metabolites and associated with minimal hypoglycemia, is often preferred in elderly individuals with coexisting CKD.

Repaglinide, with its short action and renal safety, is another suitable option. Dipeptidyl peptidase-4 (DPP-4) inhibitors—such as sitagliptin and vildagliptin—are well tolerated and weight-neutral, making them attractive for geriatric patients. Sodium-glucose cotransporter-2 (SGLT-2) inhibitors, while beneficial for cardiovascular and renal outcomes, must be used cautiously in frail elders due to risks of dehydration, genitourinary infections, and euglycemic ketoacidosis. For advanced disease requiring insulin, basal analogs such as glargine U-300 or degludec are preferred to reduce nocturnal hypoglycemia, though premixed insulin formulations remain common in Indian practice.

Recent advances, including CGM and flash monitoring, have enhanced glycemic control and reduced hospitalizations in elderly diabetics.[19] A 2023 Indian study showed a 36% drop in hypoglycemia-related admissions with CGM-guided insulin use.[20] Tirzepatide shows promise, while telehealth has improved adherence and satisfaction post-COVID-1921 **(Table 2)**.

GESTATIONAL DIABETES MELLITUS

Gestational diabetes mellitus, first diagnosed during pregnancy, poses significant short- and long-term health risks for both mother and child. Its global prevalence ranges from 9 to 26%, with India bearing one of the highest burdens—15 to 20% of pregnancies—marked by urban-rural

TABLE 2: Summary of pharmacotherapy considerations in elderly diabetics.

Drug class	*Advantages*	*Risks/Limitations*
Metformin	Weight-neutral, low hypoglycemia, CV benefits	GI intolerance, contraindicated in CKD
DPP-4 inhibitors	Safe, well-tolerated, no hypoglycemia	Modest efficacy, cost
SGLT-2 inhibitors	CV and renal benefits, weight loss	Genital infections, dehydration
GLP-1 RAs	Weight loss, CV benefits	GI side effects, injectable, costly
Basal insulin analogs	Predictable profile, reduced nocturnal hypoglycemia	Injection burden, monitoring needs
Sulfonylureas (gliclazide and glipizide)	Cost-effective, effective	Hypoglycemia risk, cautious use

(CKD: chronic kidney disease; CV: cardiovascular; DDP-4: dipeptidyl peptidase-4; GI: gastrointestinal; GLP1-RAs: glucagon-like peptide-1 receptor agonists; SGLT-2: sodium-glucose cotransporter-2)

metformin- and insulin-treated GDM cohorts.[11,12] Recent data underscore metformin's safety throughout gestation, with longitudinal studies affirming its role from conception to delivery.[24]

Uncontrolled GDM is associated with a spectrum of adverse obstetric outcomes, including macrosomia, polyhydramnios, preterm delivery, operative births, and shoulder dystocia. Neonates born to mothers with poorly controlled GDM are at higher risk of hypoglycemia, respiratory distress, and subsequent metabolic dysregulation. In India, delays in diagnosis and suboptimal glycemic control significantly contribute to the high incidence of macrosomia.[13] Longitudinal data indicate that 25–35% of Indian women diagnosed with GDM progress to type 2 diabetes within 5 years postpartum,[23] underscoring the critical need for early postpartum surveillance and lifestyle counseling.

Technological advancements are beginning to reshape GDM management in India. Continuous and flash glucose monitoring (CGM and FGM) have been associated with improved glycemic metrics, particularly postprandial control, and reduced rates of macrosomia.[15]

On the research front, novel biomarkers—such as adiponectin, leptin, and placental exosomal microRNAs—are under investigation for their potential in early GDM prediction among high-risk Indian cohorts.[17] Notably, Professor Dr V Seshiah has proposed a paradigm of primordial prevention, advocating a 2-hour postprandial glucose test at the 8th gestational week. Values between 110 and 119 mg/dL prompt early initiation of metformin (500 mg twice daily), continuing through term to mitigate GDM onset.[23]

Perhaps most concerning is the significant gap in postpartum follow-up. Less than 25% of Indian women undergo recommended OGTT testing 6–12 weeks after delivery.[18] Recent data by Dr Geethalakshmi, et al. suggest that an oral glucose challenge test (OGCT) performed on day 3 postpartum predicts future diabetes risk with nearly 80% accuracy, surpassing traditional testing at 6 weeks.[24]

In an instance, a 29-year-old primigravida from Bengaluru, with a BMI of 25.1 kg/m^2, presented at 8 weeks' gestation with a 2-hour postprandial glucose level of 118 mg/dL. She was initiated on metformin 250 mg twice daily, alongside individualized MNT and regular postprandial walking. Serial OGTTs remained within normal limits throughout pregnancy. She delivered a healthy, term neonate weighing 3.1 kg. Postpartum OGTT was normal, highlighting the potential of early intervention and lifestyle optimization in high-risk pregnancies.

RECENT ADVANCES (2020–2025)

The care of diabetes in India has undergone a significant evolution over the last 5 years, as the country has combined pharmacological innovation, digital health, and a shift in the government policy. CGM technology, which was initially limited to tertiary care facilities, is becoming increasingly popular in a wider clinical care environment in India. New research suggests CGM expected efficacy in patients from older age groups, with observed positive increases in time-in-range (TIR) outcomes and a substantial decrease in time below range (TBR), the number of hospital visits due to hypoglycemia events.[1] CGM-guided insulin titration has shown better postprandial glycemic control and a reduction in the incidence of macrosomia in various Indian trials in the context of GDM.[2] Regardless of the cost issue, its affordability has increased, and CGM is slowly becoming a part of insurance benefit coverage, which enhances its full usage outside of big cities.

Examples of such drugs include GLP-1 RAs, such as semaglutide and dulaglutide, which have demonstrated potent cardiovascular and metabolic effects in adults with diabetes and comorbidities.[3] The 2024 Indian observational data indicated a 1.3% average decrease in HbA1c

TABLE 4: Recent advances in diabetes management (2020–2025).

Domain	*Recent advances*	*Key findings/benefits*	*References*
CGM in special populations	Expanded use in elderly and GDM	Reduced hypoglycemia, improved TIR	1, 2
GLP-1 RAs	Semaglutide, dulaglutide in elderly	CV protection, weight loss, and low hypoglycemia risk	3
New insulin analogs	Insulin glargine U-300, degludec	Lower nocturnal hypoglycemia, and flexible dosing	4
Digital health	Smartphone apps, teleconsultation services	Improved HbA1c, adherence, patient satisfaction	5, 6
National guidelines	RSSDI 2025 and ICMR 2023 updates	Focus on individualized targets, CGM, metformin in GDM	7, 8

(CGM: continuous glucose monitoring; CV: cardiovascular; GDM: gestational diabetes; GLP1-RAs: glucagon-like peptide-1 receptor agonists; Hb1Ac: glycated hemoglobin; ICMR: Indian Medical Council of Research; RSSDI: Research Society for the Study of Diabetes in India; TIR: time in range)

with good tolerability and minimal hypoglycemia. In parallel, second-generation basal insulin analogs—specifically insulin glargine U-300 and degludec—offer prolonged duration of action, improved flexibility in dosing, and a lower risk of nocturnal hypoglycemia. Indian registry studies confirm their utility across elderly and frail populations **(Table 4)**.[4]

CLINICAL IMPLICATIONS IN INDIAN PRACTICE

According to a 2023 survey, fewer than 12% of people with diabetes in tier-2 cities and rural areas described CGM or GLP-1 RAs as affordable.[1] Cost is just one aspect of the bigger problem. Drug compliance is especially challenging in the case of elderly patients when the population is forced to deal with polypharmacy, cognitive deterioration, and insufficient support by caregivers, among others.

In addition, despite the considerable potential of digital health platforms, their aggressive growth is hindered by a significant lack of digital literacy, linguistic inequality, and infrastructural deficiencies, at least in nonurban and rural areas. Such systemic disparities risk impairing the connection between technological capacity and real healthcare provision.[2]

Recommendations

The recommended strategies to deal with these acute problems are as follows:

- Embark on the introduction of subsidized CGM gadgets and GLP-1 RA by national health programs that should target high-risk populations.
- Include compulsory screening of diabetes during postpartum in the national antenatal and postnatal care standards.
- Initiate some ways to impart locality-based geriatric diabetes initiatives that involve the population of frailty tests, fingering of the caretakers, and home-based support facilities.

CONCLUSION

Diabetes mellitus is a serious public health problem in India, which is characterized by a growing prevalence rate, younger age of onset, and overlapping genetic, lifestyle, and sociocultural risk factors. Over the last 5 years, therapeutics, digital health, and national guidelines have continued to evolve, resulting in significant improvements in care, primarily for high-risk groups, including children, pregnant women, and the elderly.

New technologies such as second-generation basal insulin analog, GLP-1 receptor agonist,

SGLT-2 inhibitors, gliptins, and CGM have helped achieve better glycemic control and avoid complications. Due to the COVID-19 pandemic, the growth in telemedicine and mobile-based management has expanded care accessibility to underserved areas.

Yet, the following challenges remain crucial, namely insufficient postnatal screening for GDM, inadequate geriatric follow-up, and limited affordability of novel technologies. These gaps should be addressed through policy reform, increased insurance coverage, digital adaptation to cultural needs, and community-based models.

Individualized care driven by technology has recommendations, such as those from the RSSDI 2025 and ICMR 2023. The patient-centered approach and a multidisciplinary approach must continue to be central to mitigating the long-term burden of diabetes in India.

REFERENCES

1. Kalra S, Verma SK, Bhattacharya S. Glycemic guardianship: World Health Organization leads the way. Asian J Diabetol. 2022;23(4):5-6.
2. Rohini HN, Punita P, Santhekadur PK, Ravishankar MV. Gestational Diabetes Mellitus - The Modern Indian Perspective. Indian J Endocrinol Metab. 2023;27(5):387-93
3. Dharmalingam M. Efficacy and tolerability of GLP-1 agonists in patients with type 2 diabetes mellitus: an Indian perspective. Ther Adv Endocrinol Metab. 2014;5(6):159-65.
4. Pi L, Shi X, Wang Z, Zhou Z. Effect of smartphone apps on glycemic control in young patients with type 1 diabetes: A meta-analysis. Front Public Health. 2023;11:1074946.
5. Kalra S. Basal insulin analogues in the treatment of diabetes mellitus: What progress have we made? Indian J Endocrinol Metab. 2015;19(Suppl 1):S71-3.
6. Banerjee M, Chakraborty S, Pal R. Teleconsultation and Diabetes Care Amid COVID-19 Pandemic in India: Scopes and Challenges. J Diabetes Sci Technol. 2020;14(4):714-5.
7. ISPAD. Clinical practice consensus guidelines 2022: Diabetes in children and adolescents. Pediatr Diabetes. 2022;23(Suppl 27):3-9.
8. Roy K, Ghosh S, Samajdar SS, Dey SK, Mukherjee S. Unraveling the interplay between frailty, sarcopenia, and socioeconomic factors in Indian elderly: findings from a tertiary care hospital. J Indian Acad Geriatr. 2025;21(1):46-50.
9. RSSDI 2025 Clinical Practice Recommendations. RSSDI Yearbook 2025, 1st edition. New Delhi: Jaypee Brothers Medical Publishers.
10. Indian Council of Medical Research (ICMR). National Guidelines for Diabetes Management in India, 2023 Update. New Delhi: ICMR; 2023.
11. Ramachandran A, Snehalatha C, Satyavani K, Sivasankari S, Vijay V. Type 2 diabetes in Asian-Indian urban children. Diabetes Care. 2003;26(4):1022-5.
12. Balaji B, Ranjit Mohan A, Rajendra P, Mohan D, Ram U, Viswanathan M. Gestational Diabetes Mellitus Postpartum Follow-Up Testing: Challenges and Solutions. Can J Diabetes. 2019;43(8):641-6.
13. Rizvi AA, Rizzo M. The Emerging Role of Dual GLP-1 and GIP Receptor Agonists in Glycemic Management and Cardiovascular Risk Reduction. Diabetes Metab Syndr Obes. 2022;15:1023-30.
14. Engler R, Routh TL, Lucisano JY. Adoption Barriers for Continuous Glucose Monitoring and Their Potential Reduction With a Fully Implanted System: Results From Patient Preference Surveys. Clin Diabetes. 2018;36(1):50-8.
15. Boureau AS, Guyomarch B, Gourdy P, et al. Nocturnal hypoglycemia is underdiagnosed in older people with insulin-treated type 2 diabetes: The HYPOAGE observational study. J Am Geriatr Soc. 2023;71(7):2107-19.
16. Hills AP, Arena R, Khunti K, et al. Epidemiology and determinants of type 2 diabetes in south Asia. Lancet Diabetes Endocrinol. 2018;6(12):966-78.
17. Rhee JJ, Han J, Montez-Rath ME, Chertow GM. Comparative effectiveness of sodium-glucose cotransporter-2 inhibitors versus glucagon-like peptide-1 receptor agonists in patients with type 2 diabetes and mild/moderate chronic kidney disease. Diabetes Obes Metab. 2024;26(4):1273-81.
18. Rasooly A, Beran D, Ye PP, et al. Digital health for rural diabetes care: Implementation experience from China and India. World J Diabetes. 2025;16(8): 107733.
19. Gupta V. Improvement in Glycemic Metrics With the First and Second Continuous Glucose Monitoring (CGM) Sensor Use in Indian Patients With Type 2 Diabetes Mellitus. Cureus. 2025;17(4):e82061.
20. Dixit JV, Kulkarni RS, Badgujar SY. Diabetes Care in India: A Descriptive Study. Indian J Endocrinol Metab. 2021;25(4):342-7.

21. Seshiah V, Balaji V. Primordial prevention: Maternal health and diabetes. Diabetes Manage. 2013, 3:333-41.
22. Veerasamy S, Balaji V, Chawla R, Sahay R, Divakar H, Das AK, et al. DIPSI 2024—Delhi declaration—A futuristic approach towards primordial prevention of diabetes. J Diabetes Dev Ctries. 2024;44(Suppl 1):S53-601.
23. Seshiah V, Bronson SC, Balaji V, Jain R, Anjalakshi C. Prediction and prevention of gestational diabetes mellitus and its sequelae by administering metformin in the early weeks of pregnancy. Cureus. 2022;14(11):e31532.
24. Geethalakshmi A, Saraswathi S, Kalaivani K, Anjalakshi C, Jain R, Seshiah V. Efficacy of early versus late postpartum DIPSI test in gestational diabetes mellitus women for follow up. Int J Reprod Contracept Obstet Gynecol. 2024;13(4):942-7.

24

Microbiome and Gut Health in Diabetes

Dhruvi Hasnani, Vipul Chavda

ABSTRACT

The gut microbiome has emerged as a critical modulator of immune and metabolic functions relevant to the pathophysiology of diabetes mellitus (DM), encompassing both type 1 (T1D) and type 2 diabetes (T2D). T1D, an autoimmune disorder, is characterized by the destruction of pancreatic β-cells, wherein early-life microbial dysbiosis may contribute to immune activation through impaired gut barrier integrity and reduced production of short-chain fatty acids (SCFAs). In contrast, T2D, driven by insulin resistance and low-grade inflammation, is associated with microbiota-mediated metabolic endotoxemia, diminished SCFA-producing taxa, and elevated proinflammatory microbial species. Recent research highlights functional shifts in microbial metabolic capacity, highlighting the importance of microbial-derived metabolites over taxonomic composition alone. Emerging evidence suggests that microbiota-modulating interventions such as high-fiber diets, probiotics, prebiotics, synbiotics, and fecal microbiota transplantation (FMT) can improve glycemic outcomes and insulin sensitivity. Although the microbiome is not a primary etiological factor, its integration into diabetes care offers promising adjunctive benefits. As clinical applications progress toward personalized strategies, understanding the host–microbiota interface offers a novel paradigm for diabetes prevention and management, requiring rigorous investigation to ensure efficacy, safety, and sustainability in long-term care.

Keywords: Type 1 Diabetes mellitus, Gut microbiota, Type 2 diabetes mellitus, Short-chain fatty acids, Microbiome-targeted therapy.

INTRODUCTION

Diabetes mellitus (DM) is a cluster of metabolic diseases that result from chronic hyperglycemia, which is secondary to malfunction of insulin secretion, or defective insulin action or both. The two major types are type 1 diabetes (T1D) and type 2 diabetes (T2D), with distinct etiologies and pathophysiologies. T1D is an autoimmune disease that generally presents during childhood or adolescence and is characterized by immune-mediated of pancreatic β-cells resulting in an absolute insulin deficiency. Whereas, T2D typically presents in adulthood and is the consequence of insulin resistance and inadequate compensatory insulin release. Although T2D is associated with obesity, physical inactivity, and dietary lifestyle, T1D is a disease that involves complicated interactions between genetic background and environmental triggers, which initiate autoimmune responses.[1] These two types of DM have chronic hyperglycemia as a common feature and long-term complications, but the causes and treatments of the two types are totally different.

Diabetes has become a major public health challenge in the world with an ever-increasing prevalence. As of 2019, the number of diabetics globally was estimated at >460 million and this number is anticipated to increase to 700 million by 2045.[1] It is worth mentioning that roughly 90% of these individuals suffer from T2D, illustrating the international effects of increasing obesity prevalence and abnormal food consumption. T1D, however, is emerging even in several parts of the world.[1] Substantial causes of T2D are excess body weight, sedentary lifestyle, and unhealthy dietary behavior in addition to genetic susceptibility.[2] It is interesting that the marked rise in diabetes incidence, even in groups with little genetic susceptibility, highlights the significant influences of environmental and lifestyle influences. One such environmental factor that has gained increasing attention among the scientists is the gut microbiome, the large collection of microorganisms inhabiting the human gastrointestinal tract and its role in metabolism and immune responses. As illustrated in **Flowchart 1**, alterations in lifestyle and dietary patterns can disrupt the gut microbial ecosystem, impair intestinal barrier integrity, and trigger immunometabolic responses that contribute to the pathogenesis of both type 1 and type 2 diabetes.

The gut microbiome is now understood to function as a crucial metabolic organ, with significant roles in nutrient metabolism, energy extraction, immune modulation, and gut barrier integrity. Commensal gut bacteria assist in the breakdown of complex carbohydrates, synthesize essential vitamins, and produce biologically active metabolites such as short-chain fatty acids (SCFAs), which contribute to the regulation of inflammation and glucose metabolism.[1] Imbalance of the microbiota (dysbiosis) has been associated with several disorders, including obesity, inflammatory bowel diseases, and metabolic syndrome. There is biologic rationale that these changes in the gut microbial ecosystem also could play a role in the pathogenesis or progression of diabetes. Indeed, gut microbiota profiles are different in diabetes from those of healthy subjects and may have an impact on immune regulation, inflammatory status, and insulin sensitivity.[1] However, determining whether these microbial changes are a cause or a consequence of metabolic dysfunction remains a scientific challenge. Nevertheless, the increasing evidence of microbiome association with glucose homeostasis and immune regulation particulate has spurred investigations of modulating the microbiome for therapeutic purposes. The following sections will describe the contribution of gut microbiota to T1D and T2D, recent research findings, and emerging clinical utilities including microbiome-based modalities.

Unhealthy lifestyle behaviors (e.g., smoking, alcohol, inadequate sleep, and physical inactivity) and proinflammatory dietary patterns (rich in saturated fats and refined sugars) contribute to gut microbiota dysbiosis, characterized by microbial imbalance and depletion of beneficial taxa. Dysbiosis impairs intestinal barrier integrity, resulting in increased mucosal permeability and microbial translocation, including lipopolysaccharide (LPS) and other bacterial antigens. These microbial components trigger immune system activation through heightened proinflammatory cytokine release and both innate and adaptive immune responses. This immunological cascade contributes to autoimmune β-cell destruction in T1D, and chronic systemic inflammation, insulin resistance, and hyperglycemia in T2D.

GUT MICROBIOME IN TYPE 1 DIABETES

Type 1 diabetes is an autoimmune condition characterized by the destruction of insulin-producing

in saturated fat and low in dietary fiber can shift the gut microbial composition toward species capable of degrading the intestinal mucus barrier and producing proinflammatory molecules. This shift can compromise gut barrier integrity, allowing endotoxins such as lipopolysaccharide (LPS) from gram-negative bacterial cell walls to enter systemic circulation, a process termed metabolic endotoxemia. Chronic exposure to even low levels of circulating LPS can trigger systemic inflammation and insulin resistance. Pioneering work by Cani et al. demonstrated that a high-fat diet led to increased plasma LPS levels in rodents, and this alone was sufficient to induce T2D-like metabolic features. In parallel, human T2D patients frequently present with elevated serum LPS and markers such as zonulin, which are indicative of increased intestinal permeability and microbial translocation.[1] These findings collectively support the concept that gut dysbiosis contributes to T2D pathogenesis by persistently activating the host's innate immune response.

In terms of taxonomic composition, although studies have yielded heterogeneous results, T2D is generally associated with reduced gut microbial diversity and a relative depletion of SCFA-producing bacteria, such as those that generate butyrate. SCFAs, particularly butyrate, have well-documented roles in enhancing insulin sensitivity and exerting anti-inflammatory effects. Consistently, lower abundances of butyrate-producing species such as *Faecalibacterium prausnitzii, Eubacterium rectale*, and *Roseburia* have been reported in T2D cohorts.[5] For instance, *F. prausnitzii*, a dominant anaerobe in the healthy human colon, is notably depleted in many T2D populations. This species contributes to maintaining gut epithelial integrity and promoting anti-inflammatory responses via butyrate production, and its reduction may further compromise the gut barrier and exacerbate inflammation.

Similarly, *Bifidobacterium* species are frequently found in lower abundance among T2D patients.[1] These beneficial bacteria ferment dietary fibers into acetate and lactate, competitively inhibit pathogenic organisms, and play important roles in immune modulation. A reduction in *Bifidobacteria* may, therefore, contribute to the metabolic dysregulation observed in T2D. Conversely, an increased relative abundance of opportunistic or potentially pathogenic bacteria such as gram-negative Proteobacteria (including certain *Escherichia coli* strains) and sulfate-reducing bacteria has been observed, potentially increasing the endotoxin burden and oxidative stress.[1]

At a more refined taxonomic resolution, changes in the abundance of certain genera such as *Prevotella, Ruminococcus, Collinsella*, and *Lactobacillus* have been reported. These shifts are often accompanied by decreased levels of butyrate-producers. However, these findings are not universally consistent across studies. For example, *Prevotella* has been found to be enriched in some T2D cohorts but depleted in others, depending on geographic and ethnic background. Similarly, *Akkermansia muciniphila*, a mucin-degrading bacterium often considered beneficial, has generally been reported to decrease in T2D and is under investigation as a potential probiotic. Nevertheless, some studies have observed higher levels of *Akkermansia* in diabetic populations, possibly due to the influence of metformin treatment, which is known to increase its abundance.[1] These discrepancies may reflect differences in diet, medication use, patient age, disease stage, or regional factors. For example, the microbiota profile of an elderly insulin-treated T2D patient in Europe may differ substantially from a recently diagnosed, drug-naïve patient in Asia.

Importantly, medication particularly metformin acts as a significant confounder in microbiome studies. Metformin, the most widely used first-line pharmacotherapy for T2D, has pronounced effects on the gut microbiota, enriching beneficial SCFA-producing and mucin-degrading species.[6] Thus, microbiota profiles differ markedly between untreated and metformin-treated patients and must be carefully interpreted in clinical microbiome research.

Despite variability in specific taxa, a recurring pattern in T2D is the presence of a proinflammatory microbiota configuration. Notably, functional shifts in the microbiome may be more informative than mere compositional changes. Shotgun metagenomics has revealed that T2D-associated microbiota have increased potential for producing endotoxins and branched-chain amino acids (BCAAs), while showing decreased capacity for SCFA synthesis.[7] Metabolomic profiles further support these findings, showing elevated levels of circulating BCAAs and aromatic amino acids metabolites linked to insulin resistance and decreased levels of SCFAs and polyphenol-derived metabolites, suggesting impaired fiber fermentation.[8]

Additionally, gut permeability in T2D is moderately elevated, though it is largely attributed to metabolic factors rather than autoimmunity, as is observed in T1D. Chronic hyperglycemia may compromise epithelial tight junctions and shift microbial populations such as high sugar intake can promote the growth of yeast and carbohydrate-fermenting bacteria. Importantly, improved glycemic control has been correlated with restoration of gut barrier integrity in T2D patients,[1] suggesting a bidirectional relationship: Dysbiosis contributes to inflammation and insulin resistance, leading to poor glycemic control, which further deteriorates gut microbiota composition and barrier function. While individual microbial taxa linked with T2D may vary across populations and studies, consistent patterns include reduced microbial diversity, depletion of beneficial taxa such as butyrate producers and *Bifidobacterium*, and enrichment of proinflammatory and potentially pathogenic microbes. These microbial shifts contribute to metabolic endotoxemia, systemic inflammation, and impaired glucose metabolism. Due to the inconsistencies in specific taxa findings, research focus has shifted toward understanding the functional consequences of gut dysbiosis particularly in relation to SCFA production, bile acid metabolism, and endotoxin generation in the pathophysiology of T2D. The subsequent section will explore emerging research that continues to elucidate these complex interactions.

RECENT ADVANCEMENTS

Over the past 5 years, substantial progress has been made in understanding the intricate relationship between the gut microbiome and diabetes. One notable advancement is the emergence of large-cohort studies and meta-analyses aimed at resolving inconsistencies observed in earlier, smaller investigations. A systematic review and meta-analysis published in 2025[9] analyzed 13 studies comparing gut microbiota in adults with T2D versus nondiabetic controls. The analysis revealed no consistent differences in overall microbial diversity between the groups. High heterogeneity among studies was noted, likely due to population variability and methodological discrepancies. Consequently, researchers have advised against overgeneralizing prior results and emphasized the need for standardized methodologies in microbiome research. These observations also highlight the absence of a universal microbial signature in T2D, suggesting that microbial influences on diabetes may be context-specific and function through complex, multifactorial networks rather than through the presence or absence of individual species.

In response to this complexity, the research focus has shifted toward understanding the functional capacity of the gut microbiome. Scientists now emphasize investigating microbial metabolic pathways and end-products such as SCFAs, amino acid derivatives, and proinflammatory molecules rather than specific bacterial taxa. This shift has been facilitated by the growing application of multiomics approaches, including metagenomics, meta-transcriptomics, and metabolomics. From 2020 to 2025, integrated studies employing shotgun metagenomic sequencing with targeted metabolomics have revealed distinct microbial functional profiles in T2D patients. For example, some individuals exhibit enhanced lipopolysaccharide (LPS) biosynthesis, while others show disruptions in bile acid metabolism.[10] Such functional differences may explain variations in disease progression and treatment response. A 2022 study profiling fecal microbiota and serum metabolites in individuals ranging from normoglycemia to prediabetes and T2D demonstrated that diabetes progression is linked with reduced fecal butyrate levels and elevated plasma BCAAs and phenylalanine metabolites associated with insulin resistance.[8]

Another significant advancement involves the interactions between antidiabetic medications and the gut microbiome. Recent findings suggest that several diabetes therapies influence gut microbial composition, directly or indirectly. Among these, metformin has been extensively studied between 2020 and 2023. Metformin administration has been linked to an increased abundance of *Akkermansia muciniphila* and SCFA-producing bacteria in the gut.[11] These microbial changes may enhance metformin's therapeutic effects while also contributing to gastrointestinal side effects. Importantly, baseline microbiota composition might predict an individual's response to metformin therapy. A study published in 2020 reported that individuals with higher baseline levels of Prevotella copri responded less favorably to metformin, whereas those enriched in *Bifidobacterium* adolescentis showed improved glycemic outcomes.[12] This observation indicates that microbiome-tailored personalization of antidiabetic therapy may be achievable. Other categories of drugs, i.e., GLP-1 receptor agonists and sodium-glucose cotransporter-2 (SGLT-2) inhibitors have also demonstrated the ability to modify gut bacteria such as elevations of *Collinsella* and *Akkermansia* that may have implications for production of GLP-1 and SCFA.[1]

In T1D, new discoveries within 2020–2025 changed the view of the immunological connection between the gut microbiota and autoimmunity. It is increasingly apparent that alterations in the gut microbiome in early life, provoked by events such as mode of delivery, exposure to antibiotics, or change in diet, may in turn affect the likelihood of developing autoimmune diabetes. An additional study also demonstrated the importance of microbial metabolites, which derive from tryptophan, in the modulation of immune responses. These metabolites interact with immune cell aryl hydrocarbon receptors, leading to the inhibition of proinflammatory cytokines and potentially providing a protective effect against T1D.[13]

A noteworthy development is the first steps of microbiome research moving from observations to the clinical bedside. Recent clinical trials have tested whether altering the gut microbiome can modify the course of diabetes. In one pivotal randomized controlled trial, fecal microbiota transplantation (FMT) from healthy donors to adults with newly diagnosed T1D led to sustained preservation of C-peptide levels over 1 year, suggesting a potential role for gut modulation in slowing disease progression.[14] Similar efforts in T2D have investigated FMT and defined probiotic formulations as interventions to improve insulin sensitivity. Some trials reported early benefits, such as improved insulin resistance 4 weeks post-FMT.[15] While preliminary, these studies represent a critical shift toward therapeutic application of microbiome science. Together, these recent advancements reflect both a growing clarity with recognizing the microbiome–diabetes connection as a multifaceted and context-specific relationship and a sense of forward momentum, as new tools and early clinical interventions begin to translate mechanistic insights into potential therapeutic strategies.

CLINICAL IMPLICATIONS AND THERAPEUTIC POTENTIALS

Growing evidence supports that the gut microbiome significantly influences metabolic and immune regulation in diabetes mellitus, prompting increasing interest in microbiome-targeted strategies for prevention and adjunctive treatment. These interventions include dietary modifications, probiotics, prebiotics, synbiotics, FMT, and emerging postbiotic therapies. While these modalities are not yet primary treatments, they offer promising complementary benefits in glycemic control and disease modulation.

Dietary management forms the cornerstone of diabetes care and concurrently serves as a powerful modulator of the gut microbiome. Diets high in fiber, such as those incorporating whole grains, legumes, fruits, and vegetables, enhance the abundance of SCFA-producing bacteria, particularly butyrate and propionate producers. In contrast, high-fat and high-sugar diets are associated with microbial dysbiosis. A fiber-rich dietary intervention in T2D patients has been shown to promote microbial diversity and enhance SCFA levels, contributing to improved insulin sensitivity and glycemic outcomes. Furthermore, adherence to dietary patterns such as the Mediterranean diet, known for its high fiber and polyphenol content, has been linked to favorable microbiome composition, including increased *Akkermansia* and *Faecalibacterium* abundance, and reduced T2D risk. Comparable advantages have been reported in the context of DASH and vegetarian diets, which are associated with a decrease in systemic inflammation and an increase in insulin sensitivity, mediated by the gut microbiota. Intermittent fasting, a time-determined feeding pattern, has also shown potential in modulating gut microbial diversity and enriching the abundance of lipid metabolism- and stress resistance-related bacteria, all of which play a role in weight reduction and glycemic control. These results raise the possibility of microbiome intervention as part of dietary management for diabetes. Dietary advice should not be focused on macronutrients, but also on promoting microbiota-supportive foods.[2]

Probiotics are defined as live microorganisms that when administered in adequate amounts confer a benefit to the host and have been studied as to whether they can be used as an adjuvant treatment strategy targeting glycemic control in T2D. The efficacies of certain strains of probiotics in lowering fasting blood glucose and HbA1c are also supported by more than two RCTs or meta-analyses. A recent systematic review reported on the effect of probiotics, which reduced HbA1c by 0.3% and fasting glucose by ~10 mg/dL; the latter was more pronounced following interventions of ≥12 weeks.[16]

Multistrain formulations, incorporating species such as *Lactobacillus acidophilus*, *L. casei*, *L. reuteri*, and *Bifidobacterium bifidum*, have yielded superior outcomes compared to single-strain probiotics. A clinical study using such a combination observed significant reductions of HbA1c and insulin sensitivity in T2D subjects. The mechanisms of these effects are possibly via increased SCFA production, enhanced gut barrier function, decreased systemic endotoxemia, and inflammatory responses.[17] New evidence also suggests the potential role of *Akkermansia muciniphila*, the next-generation probiotic, in enhancing gut barrier function and decreasing adipose inflammation. It is important to note that probiotic efficacy is strain-specific, and not all strains demonstrate uniform benefits. For instance, *Lactobacillus casei Shirota* and *Lactobacillus rhamnosus GG* have shown varying impacts on fasting glucose and insulin sensitivity. Interindividual differences in baseline microbiota may influence colonization and clinical outcomes. Combining probiotics with prebiotics, as in synbiotics, may enhance therapeutic effects. A 2022 meta-analysis indicated that synbiotics provided greater HbA1c reductions than probiotics or prebiotics alone.[18] Given the low dietary fiber intake in many populations, incorporating natural prebiotics through diet or supplements presents a practical microbiome-based strategy for metabolic support.

Fecal microbiota transplantation involves the transfer of stool from a healthy donor to a recipient with the aim of restoring microbial balance. While established in the management of recurrent *Clostridioides difficile* infection, its application in metabolic diseases remains investigational. In a 2023 randomized trial in China, FMT alone significantly improved insulin resistance and BMI in T2D patients, with comparable effects to metformin. The combination of FMT and metformin produced additive benefits.[15] However, durability remains a concern. A 12-week study in Spain reported no sustained improvement in HbA1c post-FMT and even a slight worsening in some cases, possibly due to reversion of the microbiota or dietary nonadherence.[19] In T1D, FMT is still in early exploration. A randomized controlled trial in 2020 demonstrated that repeated FMT preserved β-cell function over 1 year in newly diagnosed T1D patients.[14] Nonetheless, FMT is not currently standard care in diabetes, and safety, donor screening, and long-term outcomes remain key considerations. These microbiota-directed strategies differ in their mechanisms of action but collectively demonstrate improvements in glycemic control and inflammatory markers, as summarized in **Table 1**.

Lifestyle interventions such as regular physical activity are also associated with beneficial microbiome shifts, including increased SCFA-producing bacteria.[20] Postbiotics defined as direct administration of microbial metabolites such as butyrate or propionate are under investigation for their glycemic benefits, though human data remain limited and dose optimization is crucial.

Clinically, integrating microbiome awareness into diabetes care aligns with existing recommendations to enhance fiber intake and reduce unnecessary antibiotic exposure. In the future, personalized microbiome interventions may become part of precision medicine strategies in diabetes management, with tailored probiotics, diet plans, or microbiota-derived diagnostics informing treatment pathways. However, expectations must be tempered. While the microbiome contributes to metabolic regulation, it is not a primary driver of diabetes pathogenesis, and microbiome-targeted therapies provide modest improvements. Nevertheless, these interventions are generally safe, potentially synergistic with pharmacotherapy, and particularly relevant

TABLE 1: Microbiota-directed therapeutic strategies and their impact on glycemic outcomes in diabetes.[20]

Therapeutic strategy	*Mechanism of action*	*Clinical outcomes in diabetic patients*
Probiotics	Introduce beneficial microbial strains to restore gut microbial balance	Reduced fasting blood glucose, HbA1c, HOMA-IR, and proinflammatory markers (e.g., TNF-α, CRP)
Prebiotics	Provide fermentable substrates to selectively nourish beneficial bacteria	Lowered fasting plasma glucose, HbA1c, IL-6, CRP, and TNF-α
Synbiotics	Combine probiotics with supportive prebiotics to enhance synergistic effects	Improved glycemic control and reduced systemic inflammation (e.g., fasting glucose, HbA1c, CRP)
Dietary modifications (e.g., high-fiber diets)	Promote SCFA-producing microbiota via fiber-rich diets	Improved insulin sensitivity and reduced HbA1c, fasting glucose, and HOMA-IR
Fecal microbiota transplantation (FMT)	Restore microbial diversity by transplanting stool from healthy donors	Decreased fasting/postprandial glucose, HbA1c, HOMA-IR, and BMI

(HbA1c: glycated hemoglobin; HOMA-IR: homeostatic model assessment for insulin resistance; TNF-α: tumor necrosis factor-alpha; CRP: C-reactive protein; IL-6: interleukin-6; SCFA: short-chain fatty acids; BMI: body mass index)

for patients with pronounced dysbiosis or early disease stages.

CONCLUSION

The gut microbiome plays a critical role in the pathophysiology of both type 1 and type 2 diabetes, influencing immune tolerance, gut barrier integrity, and metabolic regulation. In T1D, dysbiosis particularly the depletion of butyrate-producing microbes has been linked to increased intestinal permeability and autoimmune activation, while in T2D, diet-induced microbial shifts contribute to inflammation and insulin resistance. Although the microbiome is only one element among genetic and lifestyle factors, emerging interventions such as high-fiber diets, targeted probiotics, and FMT have demonstrated the capacity to modulate glycemic outcomes and delay disease progression. As the field advances, microbiome-informed, personalized strategies may enhance conventional therapies through better prediction of treatment response, early diagnosis, and adjunctive disease management. However, rigorous studies are still required to elucidate causal mechanisms, establish long-term safety, and define clinical guidelines. Overall, understanding diabetes as a disease of disrupted host–microbe interactions represents a paradigm shift that supports integrated approaches to prevention and treatment.

REFERENCES

1. Fliegerová KO, Mahayri TM, Sechovcová H, Mekadim C, Mrázek J, Jarošíková R, et al. Diabetes and gut microbiome. Front Microbiol. 2025;15:1451054.
2. Li SX, Guo Y. Gut microbiome: New perspectives for type 2 diabetes prevention and treatment. World J Clin Cases. 2023;11(31):7508-20.
3. Piccioni A, Rosa F, Mannucci S, Manca F, Merra G, Chiloiro S, et al. Gut Microbiota, LADA, and Type 1 Diabetes Mellitus: An Evolving Relationship. Biomedicines. 2023;11(3):10.3390/biomedicines11030707.
4. Friedlander MSH, Nguyen VM, Kim SK, Bevacqua RJ. Pancreatic Pseudoislets: An Organoid Archetype for Metabolism Research. Diabetes. 2021;70(5):1051-60.
5. Martínez-López YE, Neri-Rosario D, Esquivel-Hernández DA, Padron-Manrique C, Vázquez-Jiménez A, Sánchez-Castañeda JP, et al. Effect of metformin and metformin/linagliptin on gut microbiota in patients with prediabetes. Sci Rep. 2024;14(1):9678.
6. Zhang Q, Hu N. Effects of Metformin on the Gut Microbiota in Obesity and Type 2 Diabetes Mellitus. Diabetes Metab Syndrome Obes. 2020;13:5003-14.
7. Qin J, Li Y, Cai Z, Li S, Zhu J, Zhang F, et al. A metagenome-wide association study of gut microbiota in type 2 diabetes. Nature. 2012;490(7418):55-60.
8. Zhou Z, Sun B, Yu D, Zhu C. Gut Microbiota: An Important Player in Type 2 Diabetes Mellitus. Front Cell Infect Microbiol. 2022;12:834485.
9. Machado JLP, Schaan AP, Mamede I, Fernandes GR. Gut microbiota and type 2 diabetes associations: a meta-analysis of 16S studies and their methodological challenges. Front Microbiomes. 2025;4:10.3389/frmbi.2025.1506387
10. Gurung M, Li Z, You H, Rodrigues R, Jump DB, Morgun A, et al. Role of gut microbiota in type 2 diabetes pathophysiology. EBioMedicine. 2020;51:102590.
11. de la Cuesta-Zuluaga J, Mueller NT, Corrales-Agudelo V, Velásquez-Mejía EP, Carmona JA, Abad JM, et al. Metformin is Associated with Higher Relative Abundance of Mucin-Degrading Akkermansia muciniphila and Several Short-Chain Fatty Acid-Producing Microbiota in the Gut. Diabetes Care. 2017;40(1):54-62.
12. Ezzamouri B, Rosario D, Bidkhori G, Lee S, Uhlen M, Shoaie S. Metabolic modelling of the human gut microbiome in type 2 diabetes patients in response to metformin treatment. NPJ Sys Biol App. 2023;9(1):2.
13. Blok L, Hanssen N, Nieuwdorp M, Rampanelli E. From Microbes to Metabolites: Advances in Gut Microbiome Research in Type 1 Diabetes. Metabolites. 2025;15(2):138.
14. de Groot P, Nikolic T, Pellegrini S, Sordi V, Imangaliyev S, Rampanelli E, et al. Faecal microbiota transplantation halts progression of human new-onset type 1 diabetes in a randomised controlled trial. Gut. 2021;70(1):92-105.
15. Wu Z, Zhang B, Chen F, Xia R, Zhu D, Chen B, et al. Fecal microbiota transplantation reverses insulin resistance in type 2 diabetes: A randomized, controlled, prospective study. Front Cell Infect Microbiol. 2022;12:1089991.

16. Ayesha IE, Monson NR, Klair N, Patel U, Saxena A, Patel D, et al. Probiotics and Their Role in the Management of Type 2 Diabetes Mellitus (Short-Term Versus Long-Term Effect): A Systematic Review and Meta-Analysis. Cureus. 2023;15(10):e46741.
17. Mueller NT, Differding MK, Zhang M, Maruthur NM, Juraschek SP, Miller ER 3rd, et al. Metformin Affects Gut Microbiome Composition and Function and Circulating Short-Chain Fatty Acids: A Randomized Trial. Diabetes Care. 2021;44(7):1462-71.
18. Zhou JR, Yamada R, Huruiti E, Kitahara N, Nakamura H, Fang J, et al. Ripe Tomato Saponin Esculeoside A and Sapogenol Esculeogenin A Suppress CD4+ T Lymphocyte Activation by Modulation of Th2/Th1/Treg Differentiation. Nutrients. 2022;14(10).
19. Gómez-Pérez AM, Muñoz-Garach A, Lasserrot-Cuadrado A, Moreno-Indias I, Tinahones FJ. Microbiota Transplantation in Individuals with Type 2 Diabetes and a High Degree of Insulin Resistance. Nutrients. 2024;16(20).
20. Młynarska E, Wasiak J, Gajewska A, Steć G, Jasińska J, Rysz J, et al. Exploring the Significance of Gut Microbiota in Diabetes Pathogenesis and Management—A Narrative Review. Nutrients. 2024;16(12):1938.

25 Artificial Intelligence and Big Data in Diabetes Research

Alok Modi, Shambo Samrat Samajdar

ABSTRACT

The integration of artificial intelligence (AI) and big-data analytics into diabetes research is transforming the traditional paradigms of prevention, diagnosis, and management. By leveraging large-scale datasets from electronic health records, wearables, imaging, and multi-omics platforms, AI systems now enable early disease detection, individualized risk stratification, and precision therapeutics. Machine-learning algorithms outperform conventional risk calculators, while deep-learning models rival clinicians in retinal and renal prognostication. Reinforcement learning, natural-language processing, and federated frameworks further expand real-time monitoring, clinical decision support, and privacy-preserving collaboration. However, persistent challenges—including data bias, limited interoperability, and the "black-box" opacity of complex models—continue to hinder widespread clinical adoption. Ethical stewardship, robust validation, and cross-sector governance are therefore imperative to ensure trustworthy deployment. As AI and big-data infrastructures mature, their responsible integration promises a future of patient-centric, predictive, and equitable diabetes care.

Keywords: Artificial intelligence, Big-data analytics, Precision diabetology, Machine learning, Predictive healthcare.

INTRODUCTION

Type 2 diabetes mellitus, in particular, ballooned into a global crisis that now touches the lives of at least half a billion people, straining hospitals, families, and national budgets alike.[1,2] Even with an ever-growing toolbox of pills, pumps, and lab tests, routine diabetes care tends to react only after problems erupt and too often treats every patient as if their condition is identical.[1-4] Into this, scene steps the messy but potentially game-changing duet of artificial intelligence (AI) and big-data analytics, technologies that promise to refocus research, Tailor Risk Scores, sharpen clinical judgment, and keep patients in the loop.[5] Machines that learn[3,4] can sift huge piles of numbers to spot odd correlations and twisted curves no human would ever guess were there, often in real time instead of the afterthought that research articles represent. At the same time, big-data toolkits enable hospitals, clinics, wearable device companies, and genomic laboratories to contribute data to a shared analytical framework, allowing population-wide risk assessments that encompass both urban commuters and patients in remote clinics.[6,7] With that kind of plumbing in place, medicine moves from guessing what works for the average man or woman to knowing what will likely pan out for this one person based on their record. Pilot projects are already on the wire. A Taiwanese algorithm trained on 100,000 sliding-window notes now tells nephrologists days ahead of time which diabetics will crash into dialysis.[8] A second system, cleared by the FDA, scans retinal snaps in about as long as it takes a nurse to pour coffee; its positive grades come together with sensitivity levels that run neck-and-neck with seasoned eye doctors.[9]

Artificial intelligence-driven digital platforms are now common in smart-health cities, pre-emptively flagging potential complications, fine-tuning therapeutic protocols, and nudging wide swathes of the population toward healthier habits.

Regardless, the road ahead is littered with obstacles. Varied data vocabularies, stubborn interoperability gaps, and persistent worries about bias all throttle the broader clinical adoption of these models. The opaque inner workings of many algorithms—your typical black box—raise fresh questions about reliability and fairness even before the input noise of everyday practice comes into play. In short, a great many prototypes that shine in controlled silico environments grind to a halt the moment they touch the messy texture of real-world patient records.

The chapter that follows assembles a rigorous, peer-reviewed distillation of big-data interventions in diabetes management, drawing exclusively from 25 cornerstone studies in the field. It takes stock of the underlying technologies, notes where they excel, pinpoints the inevitable cracks, and imagines next steps. The goal is sober yet hopeful—to tell a story in which computation does not eclipse the human element of medicine but instead enlarges its reach. Picture a future where care anticipates need, tailors itself to individuals, and leans resolutely on the weight of credible data.

FOUNDATIONS OF ARTIFICIAL INTELLIGENCE AND BIG DATA IN DIABETES

Big Data Sources in Diabetes Research and Care

- *Electronic health records* decompose into time-stamped lab results, medication logs, and coded diagnoses. Population managers mine those fields for predictive flags while epidemiologists watch for early outbreak signs.[10]
- *A constellation of continuous glucose monitors, insulin pumps, and activity-tracking wearables* pours time-series glucose, movement, and sleep metrics through the cloud every minute. Algorithms sketch customized insulin profiles and warn patients hours before blood sugar crashes.[5,11]
- Genetic variants and circulating biomarkers now sit side-by-side in high-dimensional matrices, inviting machine-learning routines originally designed for image recognition. Researchers dub that overlap precision diabetology and tout it as the next frontier.[12]
- *National health administrations* also wield seemingly pedestrian survey tables. French public insurers ran the SNDS file through gradient-boosting models and staged a country-wide diabetes incidence map, illustrating how fiscal stewardship can double as epidemiological early warning.[13]
- *Apps residing on patients' own phones* offer diaries of meals, mood, pills, and workouts, turning users into passive data exhaust when agreements are signed. Engineers spin those narratives into dashboards that propose nutritional swaps, though sceptics call the merging process sloppy.[5,6-11,14-16]

Obstacles remain. Blank fields multiply, formats drift between vendors, plug-and-play interoperability lags, and the perennial tug-of-war over autonomy and privacy slices the data pool before any clinician ever sees it.[17]

Artificial Intelligence Methodologies in Diabetes: Core Algorithms and Capabilities

Each of these approaches offers distinct strengths and limitations. While predictive accuracy is often high in controlled settings, the lack of transparency in decision-making logic (the "black box" issue) and absence of robust external validation remain major hurdles to clinical adoption.[24]

Scholars have begun to label the application of AI in the management of diabetes an entire ecosystem, one that weaves together disparate computational techniques that share only a broad interest in glycemic control. Diagnostic prediction, therapy recommendation, and later-stage disease interpretation fall under that sprawling rubric **(Fig. 1)**.

- Within the familiar arena of *supervised learning*, classifiers such as support vector machines, decision trees, and bagged random forests have quietly eclipsed heuristic diabetes risk scores once relied upon in outpatient clinics. One regional hospital cohort showed these algorithms could forecast diabetic kidney decline long before crescents appeared in routine urinalysis.[2]
- *Unsupervised methods* have also made their mark by clustering patient data into emergent phenotype groups. These groupings, formed solely on lab values and home glucose readings, reveal striking subtleties in how different subtypes respond to metformin versus newer injectable agents.[3]
- *Deep learning (DL)*: On the imaging side, convolutional neural networks now scan retinal photographs at speeds that far exceed human capacity. That same family of deep architectures, augmented with recurrent and long short-term memory units, also learns to flag impending hypoglycemic dips in streamed CGM traces.[18]
- *Finally, reinforcement learning* has crept into the design of prototype closed-loop insulin pumps, treating each corrective bolus as a trial in an ever-repeating clinical game. The pumps adaptively tighten their dosing schedules based on real-time feedback, edging clinicians closer to wholly automatic glycemic control.[11]
- *Natural language processing (NLP)*: The technology is still finding its footing in diabetes research, yet it has begun lifting meaningful

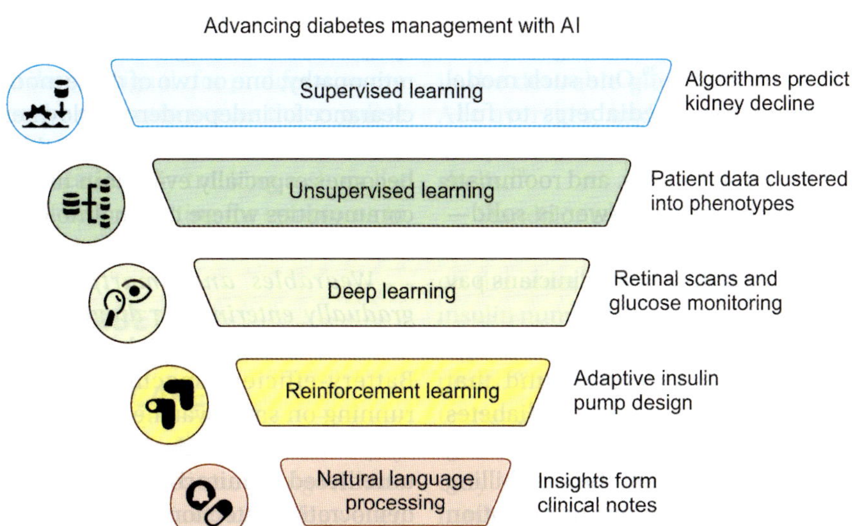

Fig. 1: Types of data.

Lifestyle and Behavioral Interventions

Diabetes management rests largely on the *choices people make each day,* and AI is stepping in to steady those choices with new technology.[5,16] Wearables that log steps, heart rate, and sleep are now paired with mobile health entries that list meals and track mood; the fusion lets the software spit out timely feedback, motivational nudges, and goals that shift as the user shifts. Pattern-recognition routines sift through the merged data, pinpointing the small, stubborn reasons adherence slips and serving bite-sized advice that updates in real time.

Picture a smart-health city where personal devices talk to street sensors measuring smog, heat, and food-market foot traffic. *Algorithms there might tell a resident it is safe to stroll after sunset*[5] because pollution has dropped and blood-sugar readings look steady, or they might nudge someone toward a cheaper, low-glycemic dinner special now posted on a nearby vendor's digital menu.

Natural-language processors also scour patient diaries for keywords and emotional tone, letting doctors see who struggles with *anxiety, fatigue, or outright diabetes distress.* Those findings open the door to customized coaching conversations, extra counseling sessions, or a prompt referral to mental-health professionals trained in chronic disease care.[19]

Medication Optimization and Therapeutic Decision-making

Artificial intelligence has burst onto the *pharmacotherapy stage,* pressing especially hard into the murky territory of polypharmacy among patients who straddle multiple chronic diagnoses. One recent experiment in managing stubborn diabetes grafted a machine-learning apparatus to prescription logs big enough that it no longer had to kneel only to the usual HbA1c number. Instead, renal clearance, heart history, sticking-with-it odds, and the tangled web of possible drug clashes[21] all shared the spotlight, and the emerging combinations nudged both safety and effectiveness in the right direction.

Clinical decision-support shells now circulate both in echoing hospital corridors and in tenacious outpatient clinics, prodding physicians to *reconsider dosages, yank contraindications into daylight,* or even foresee a looming adverse reaction[17] hours before it arrives. Some of the smarter platforms go a step further by fitting the raw clinical advice to the blunt realities of a patient budget or the wiggle-room preferences that emerge during shared decision chats.

None of these digital sparks is meant to elbow the doctor out of the way; the real goal is to handle the grunt work of *sifting risk from reward so human minds* can pay attention where intuition and bedside presence still call the shots. By ranking dangers, laying out flattened options, and juggling trade-offs that fill every corner of a packed clinic hour, the tools give time-pressed clinicians a fighting chance to stay ahead of the perfect storm that modern medication can become.[10]

IMPLEMENTATION CHALLENGES AND ETHICAL CONSIDERATIONS

Advances in AI and big data have sparked considerable optimism about the future of diabetes management, yet the actual shift from laboratory prototypes to hospital workflows is anything but straightforward. Clinicians, policymakers, and patients encounter a tangle of technical glitches, ethical dilemmas, *infrastructural bottlenecks,* and deeply embedded cultural attitudes long before the first algorithm ever lights up an exam-room screen.

Data Quality, Bias, and Generalizability

The gulf between hype and lived experience reminds stakeholders that introducing a novel technology into medicine feels less like plug-and-play and more like asking the entire health system to relearn how it thinks about risk, fairness, and trustworthiness.[20]

A core hurdle lies in the quality of the *datasets* feeding the machine-learning engines; even the sleekest diabetes-prediction tool is still only as solid as the numbers beneath it.[11]

Most high-profile models spring from tightly curated cohorts that, by design or accident, wind up over-representing patients in a single geographic region or a narrow pool of demographics.[11,17] *Internal validation* on those same patients can yield dazzling performance metrics, yet patients met in an outside clinic never see the same reliability.[17]

Embedded biases present an additional danger, because electronic health record tables often carry forward disparities linked to race, income, and access in ways that nobody watching them type knew were happening. A model trained on such lopsided tables can, without malice, amplify age-old inequities and deliver its predictions in a tone that sounds mathematically neutral.[6-16,19,21-25]

Finally, algorithmic overfitting lurks at every turn; systems perfected in quiet test beds may sputter or freeze once the ambient noise of incomplete billing codes and hardware hiccups returns to the ward.

Creating fairer machine-learning systems begins with intentionally recruiting participants from a broad mix of ages, races, and abilities right at the training stage. Researchers must then catalogue dataset quirks in clear, jargon-free language so later users can spot hidden biases before they scale. Even after launch, teams should keep tuning algorithms to reflect shifting social and clinical realities. Commitments to ethics cannot stop at good intentions; they must directly confront the legacy of unequal care so that new tools close, rather than widen, stubborn gaps in public health.

Explainability and Clinical Trust

Artificial intelligence technology in diabetes management frequently stumbles over the so-called *black box hurdle*: The inaccessibility of deep-learning pathways makes it tough for doctors to either verify or dispute its alerts. When the stakes climb, as during insulin dose adjustments or when evaluating signals that might presage a crisis, the absence of a clear rationale can hollow out clinician trust and, by extension, compromise patient safety.[17]

To tackle the transparency gap, researchers have turned to explainable AI plaster: Quick-hit saliency maps, more ponderous feature-attribution tables, and several model-agnostic add-ons that attempt to showcase which variables pulled the most weight. Even so, many of these methods remain in the experimental corridor, so their practicality at the bedside still shows serious cracks and delays. If the visualizations stay nonintuitive or overwhelming, busy clinicians may either overlook the numbers altogether or take them on faith—a gamble that could end badly.[10]

Building reliable bridges of trust demands more than just a slick visualization toolkit. It also calls for extensive validation studies, human-factors tests that capture real nursing workflows, and regulatory guardrails that place *patient safety, ethical transparency, and everyday clinical relevance front and center* **(Fig. 2)**.[17]

Integration with Clinical Workflows and Infrastructure

Most AI applications emerge from university labs or Silicon Valley garages and pay little heed to *on-the-ground hospital life.*[17] Systems rarely talk to one another, interoperability specifications drift, and the constant push-pull of alerts often leaves exhausted providers wondering why yet another gadget was plugged in. Even proven algorithms end up abandoned when they complicate rather than simplify day-to-day rounds.[6-11,14-16]

Real-time deployment means more than writing pretty code; it demands steady data streams, granite-tough servers, ironclad privacy fencing, and an army of 24/7 fixers to nurse the system along. *Cash-strapped district hospitals and rural clinics, already limping along on outdated networks, can lose months* just waiting for the right pipe to open up.[5]

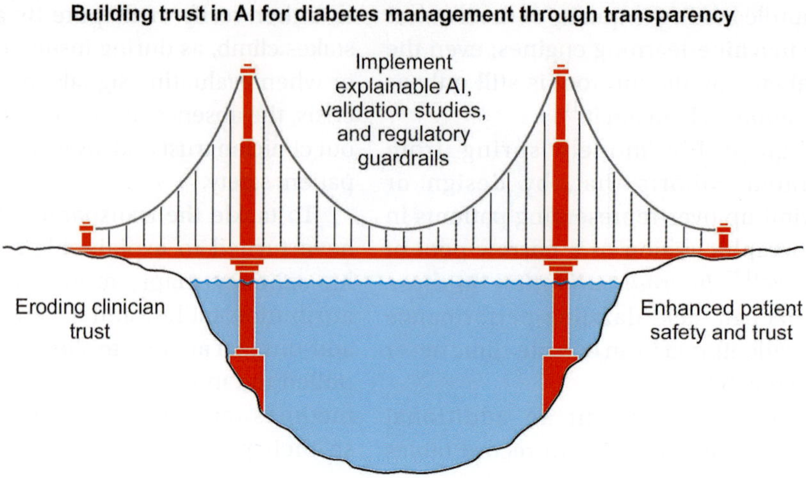

Fig. 2: Building trust in AI transparency.

A smattering of smart-city test beds and flash-in-the-pan pilots shows that seamless handoffs are possible, yet scaling past the demo booth into ordinary practice remains a headache nobody has fully solved. Translating a glamorous demonstration into bread-and-butter workflow, in any geographic setting, is still more promise than protocol.[5-17,19-25]

Data Privacy, Consent, and Governance

Personal health data now flows into devices and databases faster than many patients can comprehend. The *behavioral, geolocation, and genomic slices* of that information turn routine monitoring into a high-resolution portrait of individual lives. Once researchers see such detail, the questions stack up: Who owns this picture, who whispered yes before it was recorded, and how tightly may we draw the curtains around what has been shared? Traditional clinics simply did not gather material of that depth, yet machine learning routines often hunger for exactly that breadth. When new uses appear without upfront notice, the exchange can begin to feel like taking a harvest without offering the farmer fair recompense, and trust drifts away almost overnight.[19]

Technologists sometimes reach for buzzwords such as *blockchain or federated learning,* promising they will mask names while letting algorithms work together. *Those protocols remain experimental, useful more as whiteboard visions than as finished products that routinely protect patient privacy.* Regulators try to keep pace—GDPR cross-examines data flows in Europe while HIPAA writes rules across the United States—yet the rule of law alone will not satisfy a public that now expects co-creation and real-time accountability.[17]

Consent forms first drafted in legalese look even stranger after data has been sliced, diced, and reanalyzed by tools nobody knew existed when the ink dried. Permission thus quickly becomes a museum piece unless institutions redo it, perhaps in discrete bursts, as technologies evolve. Static boxes are being replaced in some trials by rolling disclaimers that patients check or uncheck every few months, though even those feel cumbersome after the fourth or fifth click.[19]

The Human–AI Interface

The human–AI partnership in diabetes clinics ought to leave the physician in charge, with algorithms acting as fast, wide-eyed assistants rather than bossy overlords. Pattern spotting at machine speed is impressive, but it cannot match the warmth of lived experience and midnight spent listening to a worried parent. Making that alliance work will demand fresh training modules that blend statistics, ethics, and a dash of old-fashioned digital courage so doctors do not flinch when a screen flashes unusual blood-glucose predictions.[17]

Patients should be invited, not merely instructed, to work with the AI tools that enter their lives. Apps, chatbots, and watch-based widgets require user-centered design, cultural sensitivity, and clear health messaging if they are to earn that trust. Even the most dazzling algorithm loses its value without a person willing to act on its advice.[5-11,14-16]

The real measure of an AI system will always be its moral compass, not its mathematical elegance. In the end, relevance to clinical practice and a shared sense of humanity will prove far more durable than any temporary spike in technical perfection.

FUTURE DIRECTIONS AND ROADMAP FOR SCALABLE ADOPTION

The field of AI, entwined with big-data analytics, is on the brink of reshaping diabetes management. These innovations risk languishing as little more than laboratory wonders *unless people working in clinics, code, regulation, and ethics align their efforts.* A coherent, patient-centered playbook is, therefore, needed if we hope to move fast while treating both data dignity and public trust with respect.

From Model Development to Real-world Deployment

Much of the enthusiasm around diabetes algorithms has so far rested on datasets collected yesterday, in one narrow spotlight. Tomorrow's tools must survive the cluttered hallways of multiple hospitals filled with patients very different from the ones on the training spreadsheets **(Fig. 3)**.[17]

That demand breaks down into three core tasks:

1. *Robust external validation*: First, researchers must publish results from wide-ranging, prospective cohorts if they want papers to leave the conference center and enter clinicians' daily routines.[17]
2. *Randomized trials*: Second, randomized-controlled trials should measure what people care about: Fewer hypoglycemic events, less phone fretting, and the simple question, Do I trust this alert?[4]
3. *Post-deployment monitoring*: Finally, once an application sits on a monitor in the morning huddle, someone has to catch the drift model will slowly lose its grip and turn fresh data into periodic recalibration.

None of that happens without *engineers, endocrinologists, informatics staff, real patients, and policy writers agreeing, sometimes weekly, on what good enough looks like.*[11]

Interoperability and Infrastructure Reform

Data systems across clinics in many low- and middle-income nations still silo patient information within individual hospitals and laboratories, a fragmentation that undercuts routine use of AI in diabetes management.[5]

Scaling meaningful adoption rests on a set of shared building blocks. Cross-institutional health data standards must permit lab results, ECG waveforms, pharmacy transactions, and smartphone logs to flow without constant manual remapping.[17]

Cloud-centered, pay-as-you-go frameworks can deliver machine-learning pipelines to small clinics that lack dedicated servers or technical support.[9]

National examples such as Frances Service National des Donnees de Sante (SNDS) show how a consolidated repository can empower jurisdiction-wide analyses while protecting patient privacy.[17]

Those structures provide a working playbook for governments eager to run predictive models

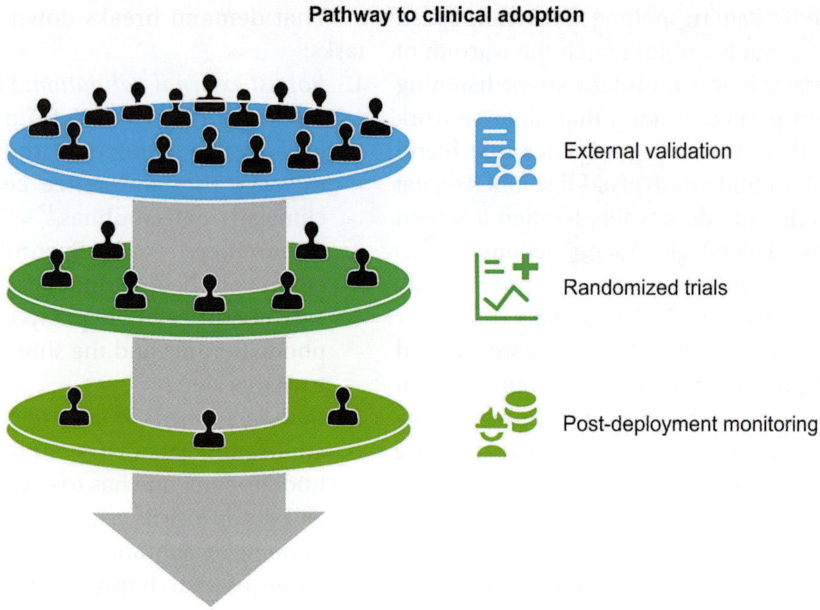

Fig. 3: Pathway to clinical adoption.

on millions of active cases and push actionable insights back to front-line caregivers.[3]

Emerging Technologies and Methodologies

Coming innovations promise to weave *new AI methods* directly into everyday diabetes care. *Federated learning* enables hospitals to fine-tune models collaboratively without shifting highly sensitive patient files to a single cloud domain.[22]

Explainable AI dashboards give clinicians a glimpse of the algorithm's reasoning, a feature increasingly demanded before any system earns long-term trust.[24]

Multi-omics integration: Researchers are mixing genetic, proteomic, and metabolomic profiles into multi-omics frameworks so that therapies can be tailored rather than generalized.[15]

Synthetic datasets are being spun up to cushion rare clinical events like ketoacidosis or extreme hypoglycaemia, thus levelling the training signal for deep-learning code that might otherwise never see those edge cases.[5]

Taken together, these technical shifts target the core bottlenecks of interpretability, scarcity, and privacy that have stalled broader deployment in real-world practice.

Global Equity and Responsible AI

Ethical AI relies on an origin story that is neither exclusive nor unilateral. Systems that aspire to *global equity* must invite citizen input from diverse racial, gender, and income groups, along with people who live beyond traditional urban hubs.[6-17,19-25]

One-size-fits-all algorithms falter when they cross borders; bespoke models are needed for countries that exhibit unique epidemiological profiles and possess varying tiers of technological infrastructure.

Equally important, risk assessments gain relevance only after social determinants of health—such as housing stability, transportation access, and local caregiving networks—have been woven directly into the training data **(Fig. 4)**.[5]

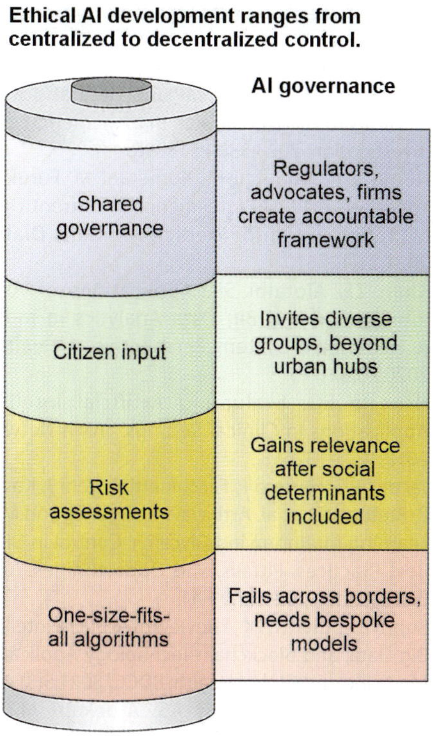

Fig. 4: Ethical AI development.

Shared governance offers the best hedge against runaway algorithms; when regulators, patient advocates, universities, and private firms collaborate, they create a decision-making framework that holds every stakeholder accountable.[3,4]

CONCLUSION

In recent years, AI, big data, and diabetes care have begun to occupy the same conversation almost daily in medical circles. What once felt hypothetical has migrated into clinics and living rooms so quickly that many providers now regard predictive dashboards and smart insulin pens as routine tools. Machine-learning algorithms flag early risk signals, autonomous systems grade diabetic-retinopathy images, and behavioral apps offer in-the-moment nudges that put patient voices back in the foreground. In short, the architecture of diabetes care is bending beneath digital weight.[1-25]

Still, this rapid expansion has unearthed a box of tangled ethical thorns. Questions about transparency, algorithmic bias, data ownership, and simple patient privacy keep legal teams as busy as laboratory staff. Beyond ethics, technical headaches such as interoperability and workflow fit must be resolved if the technology is ever to escape well-funded urban hospitals. And no matter how sophisticated the code, the indispensable human elements—empathy, trust, judgment—remain stubbornly irreplaceable.[6-17,19-25]

Solving diabetes through AI will not come down to perfecting another shiny model; that task is almost dangerously trivial by now. Lasting impact depends on building cohesive systems, crafting sensible policy, and stitching together clinicians, data scientists, patients, and administrators into a working coalition. Only then can the technology hope to alter diabetes's course across entire populations rather than merely servicing individual patients who happen to be early adopters.

Artificial intelligence is entering medicine not as a replacement for clinical judgment, but as an essential extension of it—another layer in the physician's toolkit. Machine learning amplifies human capability rather than supplanting it, taking over the routine and data-intensive tasks so that clinicians can devote greater attention to empathy, foresight, and complex decision-making. When thoughtfully integrated, AI and big data transform diabetes care from reactive disease control to proactive wellness management. The true promise of this technological evolution lies not merely in extending lifespan, but in enhancing the quality of life—empowering both clinicians and patients with deeper insight, shared understanding, and the tools to achieve lasting health.

REFERENCES

1. Musacchio N, Giancaterini A, Guaita G, Ozzello A, Pellegrini MA, Ponzani P, et al. Artificial Intelligence and Big Data in Diabetes Care: A Position Statement of the Italian Association of Medical Diabetologists. J Med Internet Res. 2020;22(6):e16922.
2. Makino M, Yoshimoto R, Ono M, Itoko T, Katsuki T, Koseki A, et al. Artificial intelligence predicts the progression of diabetic kidney disease using big data machine learning. Sci Rep. 2019;9(1):9(1):11862.
3. Rigla M, García-Sáez G, Pons B, Hernando ME. Artificial Intelligence Methodologies and Their Application to Diabetes. J Diabetes Sci Technol. 2018;12(2):303-10.
4. Contreras I, Vehi J. Artificial Intelligence for Diabetes Management and Decision Support: Literature Review. J Med Internet Res. 2018;20(5):e10775.
5. AlZu'bi S, Elbes M, Mughaid A, Bdair N, Abualigah L, Forestiero A, et al. Diabetes Monitoring System in Smart Health Cities Based on Big Data Intelligence. Future Internet. 2023;15(2):85.
6. Guan Z, Li H, Liu R, Cai C, Liu Y, Li J, et al. Artificial intelligence in diabetes management: Advancements, opportunities, and challenges. Cell Reports Medicine. 2023;4(10):101213.
7. Abhari S, Niakan Kalhori SR, Ebrahimi M, Hasannejadasl H, Garavand A. Artificial Intelligence Applications in Type 2 Diabetes Mellitus Care: Focus on Machine Learning Methods. Healthc Inform Res. 2019;25(4):248.
8. Vu GT, Tran BX, McIntyre RS, Pham HQ, Phan HT, Ha GH, et al. Modeling the Research Landscapes of Artificial Intelligence Applications in Diabetes (GAPRESEARCH). IJERPH. 2020;17(6):1982.
9. Rashid MM, Askari MR, Chen C, Liang Y, Shu K, Cinar A. Artificial Intelligence Algorithms for Treatment of Diabetes. Algorithms. 2022;15(9):299.
10. P. et al. Beyond the hype of big data and artificial intelligence: building foundations for knowledge and wisdom. BMC Med. 2019;17. Article number: 143.
11. Kerr D, Klonoff DC. Digital Diabetes Data and Artificial Intelligence: A Time for Humility Not Hubris. J Diabetes Sci Technol. 2019;13(1):123-7.
12. Khalifa M, Albadawy M. Artificial intelligence for diabetes: Enhancing prevention, diagnosis, and effective management. Comp Methods Programs Biomed Update. 2024;5:100141.
13. Haneef R, Kab S, Hrzic R, Fuentes S, Fosse-Edorh S, Cosson E, et al. Use of artificial intelligence for public health surveillance: A case study to develop a machine Learning-algorithm to estimate the incidence of diabetes mellitus in France. Arch Public Health. 2021;79(1):168.
14. Pina AF, Meneses MJ, Sousa-Lima I, Henriques R, Raposo JF, Macedo MP. Big data and machine learning to tackle diabetes management. Eur J Clin Investigation. 2023;53(1):e13890.
15. Nomura A, Noguchi M, Kometani M, Furukawa K, Yoneda T. Artificial Intelligence in Current Diabetes Management and Prediction. Curr Diab Rep. 2021;21(12):61.
16. Khan ZF, Alotaibi SR. Applications of Artificial Intelligence and Big Data Analytics in m-Health: A Healthcare System Perspective. J Health Eng. 2020;2020:1-15.
17. Nsoesie EO. Evaluating Artificial Intelligence Applications in Clinical Settings. JAMA Netw Open. 2018;1(5):e182658.
18. Jacobs PG, Herrero P, Facchinetti A, Vehi J, Kovatchev B, Breton MD, et al. Artificial Intelligence and Machine Learning for Improving Glycemic Control in Diabetes: Best Practices, Pitfalls, and Opportunities. IEEE Rev Biomed Eng. 2024;17:19-41.
19. Supriya M, Chattu VK. A Review of Artificial Intelligence, Big Data, and Blockchain Technology Applications in Medicine and Global Health. BDCC. 2021;5(3):41.
20. Nauman M, Almadhor AS, Albekairi M, Ansari AR, Fayyaz MAB, Nawaz R. The Role of Big Data Analytics in Revolutionizing Diabetes Management and Healthcare Decision-Making. IEEE Access. 2025;13:10767-85.
21. Hosseini MM, Zargoush M, Alemi F, Kheirbek RE. Leveraging machine learning and big data for optimizing medication prescriptions in complex diseases: A case study in diabetes management. J Big Data. 2020;7(1):1-24.
22. Mohsen F, Al-Absi HRH, Yousri NA, El Hajj N, Shah Z. A scoping review of artificial intelligence-based methods for diabetes risk prediction. NPJ Digit Med. 2023;6(1):197.
23. Huang J, Yeung AM, Armstrong DG, Battarbee AN, Cuadros J, Espinoza JC, et al. Artificial Intelligence for Predicting and Diagnosing Complications of Diabetes. J Diabetes Sci Technol. 2023;17(1):224-38.
24. Mehta N, Pandit A, Shukla S. Transforming healthcare with big data analytics and artificial intelligence: A systematic mapping study. J Biomed Informatics. 2019;100:103311.
25. Kong X, Peng R, Dai H, Li Y, Lu Y, Sun X, et al. Disease-specific data processing: An intelligent digital platform for diabetes based on model prediction and data analysis utilizing big data technology. Front Public Health. 2022;10:1053269.

26

Diabetes and Cancer Risk

Jayanta Kumar Panda, Narsingh Verma

ABSTRACT

Diabetes mellitus (DM) is one of the most significant global health challenges, affecting millions of individuals and imposing a substantial burden on healthcare systems. Over the past few decades, an increasing body of epidemiological and experimental evidence has indicated a strong link between diabetes and the development of various malignancies. This association appears to be multifactorial, involving shared risk factors such as obesity and sedentary lifestyle, as well as biological pathways inherent to the diabetic state itself. Understanding the mechanisms behind this relationship is crucial for early prevention and management of cancer in diabetic populations.

Keywords: Diabetes mellitus, Type 2 diabetes mellitus, Cancer risk, Diabetic retinopathy, Hyperinsulinemia, Hyperglycemia, Insulin resistance, Oxidative stress, Inflammation, Insulin-like growth factor, Epidemiology, Metformin, Glycemic control, Cancer prevention, Public health.

INTRODUCTION

Diabetes mellitus—especially type 2 diabetes mellitus—is one of the most widespread chronic health problems globally. Likewise, cancer remains a leading cause of morbidity and mortality. Over many decades researchers have observed that people with diabetes appear to have a higher risk of developing various cancers, and worse cancer outcomes. But, how strong is that risk? What mechanisms may underlie it? And what can people with diabetes (or those caring for them) do to reduce those risks? This article reviews recent evidence on the association between diabetes and cancer risk, the underlying biological mechanisms, clinical implications, and recommendations **(Fig. 1)**.

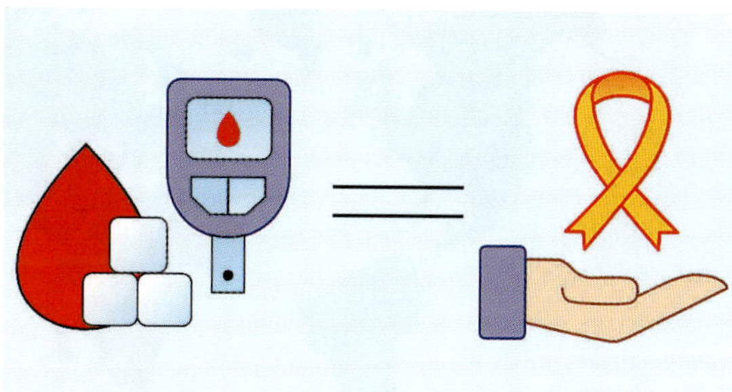

Fig. 1: Diabetes and cancer—two diseases, one metabolic link.

EPIDEMIOLOGY: WHAT STUDIES SHOW

Multiple epidemiological studies, including large cohort, meta-analysis, and population-based registry studies, show that diabetes is associated with a higher incidence of many types of cancer. Key findings from your provided sources.

Nationwide Cohort Study from Taiwan[1]

- A large retrospective cohort study compared >1.75 million people with diabetes versus matched nondiabetes controls over 12 years.
- Overall, people with diabetes had ~20% higher risk of any new cancer than those without.
- Particularly high risks were for *liver* (HR ≈ 1.69) and *pancreas* (HR ≈ 1.87) cancers. Moderate increased risks for colon, kidney, female reproductive organs, gallbladder, brain cancers, etc. There were also borderline increases for stomach, skin, soft-tissue, female breast, urinary tract (excluding kidney), and lymphatic/hematopoietic cancers.
- The study also examined diabetic retinopathy (DR), a microvascular complication of diabetes. They found that people with DR had even higher cancer risk: ~31% higher cancer incidence than diabetic persons without DR. Among those with DR, proliferative retinopathy (PDR) had somewhat higher risk again compared to nonproliferative DR (NPDR) **(Fig. 2)**.

Review: The Relationship between Diabetes Mellitus and Cancers[2-6]

- In this review, the authors summarized evidence, both epidemiological and mechanistic, for cancer risk in *both* type 1 diabetes mellitus (T1DM) and type 2 diabetes mellitus (T2DM).

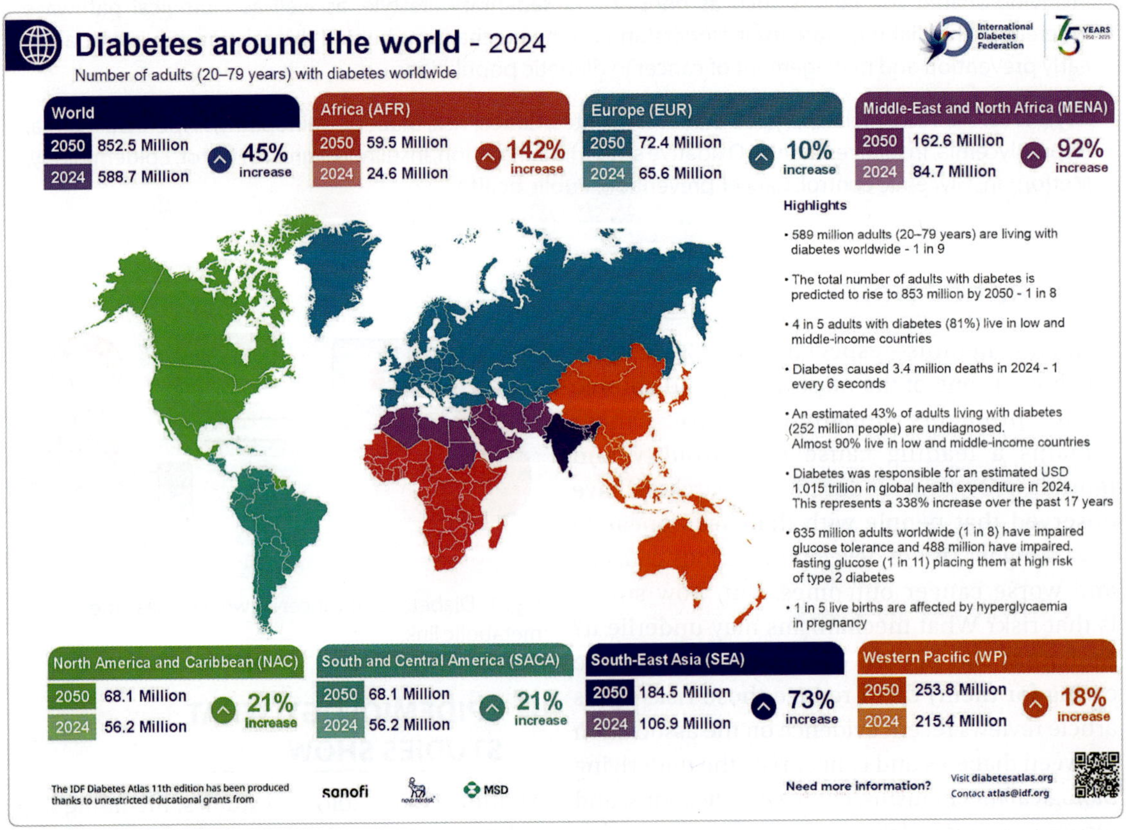

Fig. 2: *Global diabetes surge*: A growing concern for cancer risk worldwide.

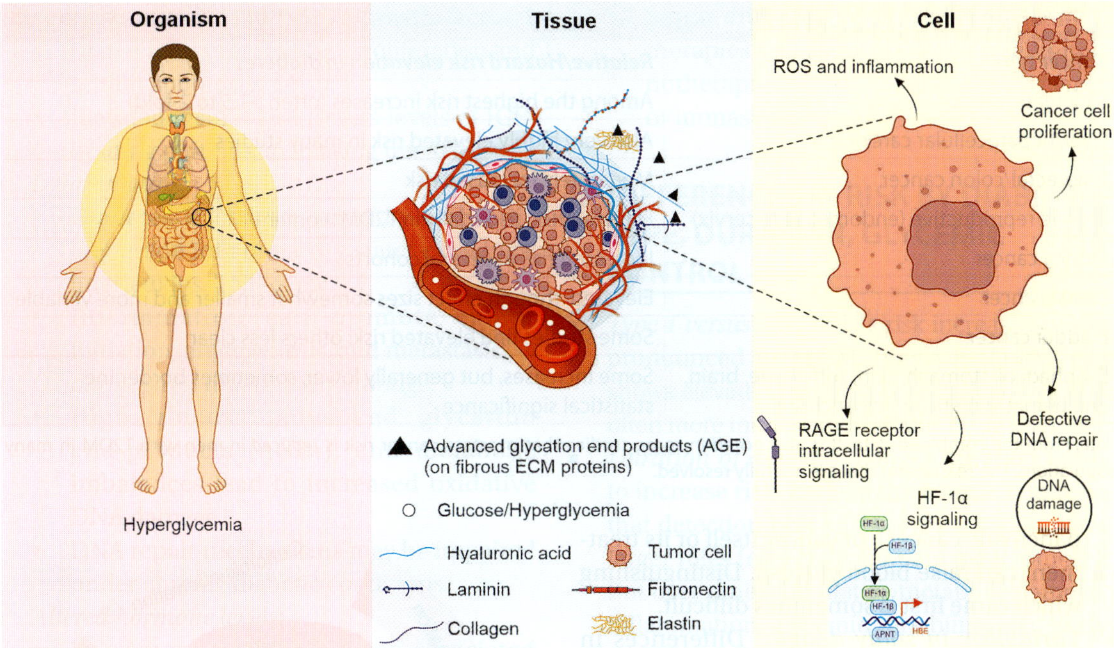

Fig. 3: The relationship between diabetes mellitus and cancers.

(ECM: extracellular matrix; HIF: hypoxia-inducible factor; RAGE: receptor for advanced glycation end products)

- They note increased incidence in many cancer types in people with diabetes, and elevated cancer mortality **(Fig. 3)**.

Consensus Report[4]

This older article also outlines cancers most robustly associated with diabetes: Liver, pancreas, endometrium, colon and rectum, breast, and bladder. Increased risks are especially pronounced for T2DM.

Other Studies

- A Chinese retrospective cohort (Nan-Hu district, Zhejiang) found increased overall cancer incidence among T2DM patients. Women with T2DM had elevated risk of breast cancer and leukemia; men had increased risk of pancreatic, liver, and kidney cancers.
- Studies show that even prediabetic elevations of fasting glucose are associated with higher risk of certain cancers.

Patterns and Cancer Types

Refer to **Table 1**.

Strengths, Weaknesses, and Confounders

Several caveats are important when interpreting the data:

- *Shared risk factors*: Obesity, older age, low physical activity, poor diet, alcohol use, and smoking are risk factors for both diabetes and cancer. Unless adjusted for, they can confound observed associations. Many studies adjust for some of these, but not always all.
- *Detection/surveillance bias*: People with diabetes have more frequent contact with healthcare systems, possibly leading to earlier detection of some cancers that might otherwise go unnoticed. This could inflate incidence somewhat.
- *Reverse causation*: Diabetes may sometimes be diagnosed because of early cancer (especially

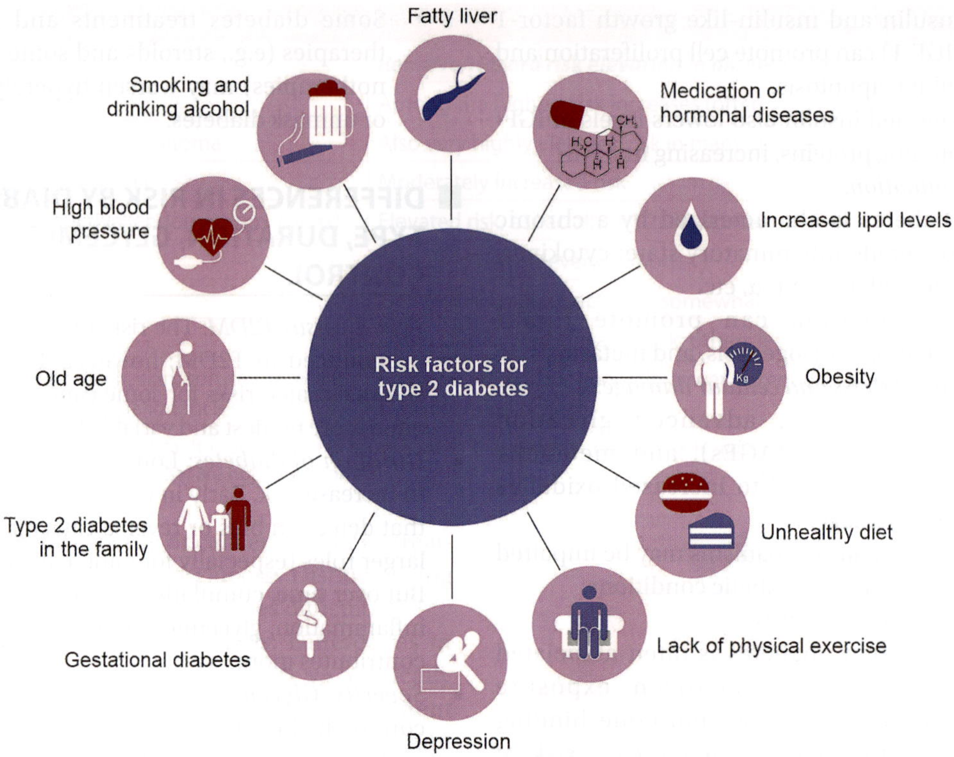

Fig. 5: Major risk factors contributing to the development of type 2 diabetes mellitus.

Source: Landgraf R, Aberle J, Birkenfeld AL, et al. Therapie des Typ-2-Diabetes. In: Diabetologie und Stoffwechsel. 2018;S83-290.

Glycemic Control and Lifestyle Interventions

- Maintaining good glycemic control may reduce cancer risk. The Taiwan study's finding around retinopathy suggests that interventions to prevent complications may also reduce cancer risk.
- *Lifestyle measures*: Weight management, healthy diet (low in processed sugars and saturated fats, and high in fiber), physical activity, avoiding tobacco and excess alcohol.

Choice of Diabetes Therapies

- There has been discussion (and concern) over whether some antidiabetic medications (especially those that increase insulin levels) could increase cancer risk. Few studies show the evidence but few other studies disagree.

Some medications (e.g., metformin) have been associated in observational studies with potentially lower cancer risk. However, causality is not established **(Fig. 6)**.

Monitoring and Managing Comorbidities

- *Diabetes often comes with other risk factors*: Nonalcoholic fatty liver disease (NAFLD), obesity, dyslipidemia—these also contribute to cancer risk. Managing these conditions may reduce risk.

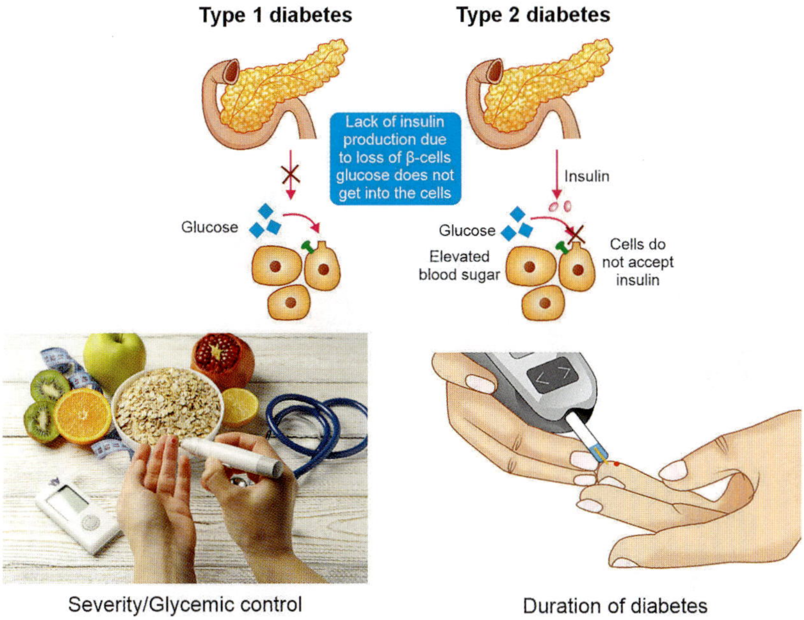

Fig. 6: Factors influencing diabetes-related complications—type, duration, and severity of glycemic control.

- Monitoring for signs of cancer or cancer risk factors in diabetic care (e.g., elevated liver enzymes, abdominal imaging in selected cases, etc.) may be warranted in some populations.

Psychological and Health System Aspects

- Diabetes management is challenging enough; adding cancer risk to the conversation may increase anxiety among patients. Clear communication and patient's education are essential.
- Health systems need integrated care pathways, so oncologists and diabetologists/endocrinologists can collaborate.

RECENT ADVANCES AND NEW INSIGHTS

- The large Taiwan study is relatively new (2024) and adds important data on how diabetic complications (retinopathy) further stratify risk. This is novel in showing that microvascular complications correlate with cancer risk.
- "Review" updates on both types of diabetes, and highlights that not only incidence, but cancer mortality is higher in diabetic populations.
- Some studies are examining glycemic variability (not just average blood sugar or HbA1c) as a risk factor. Also, research is ongoing into biomarkers [e.g., vascular endothelial growth factor (VEGF) and inflammatory mediators] that may help to clarify risk and mechanisms **(Fig. 7)**.

SUMMARY: HOW MUCH IS THE RISK?

Putting all this together, what is a rough quantification of risk?

- Overall, risk of developing *any* cancer in people with diabetes is increased by somewhere around *10–30%* compared to people

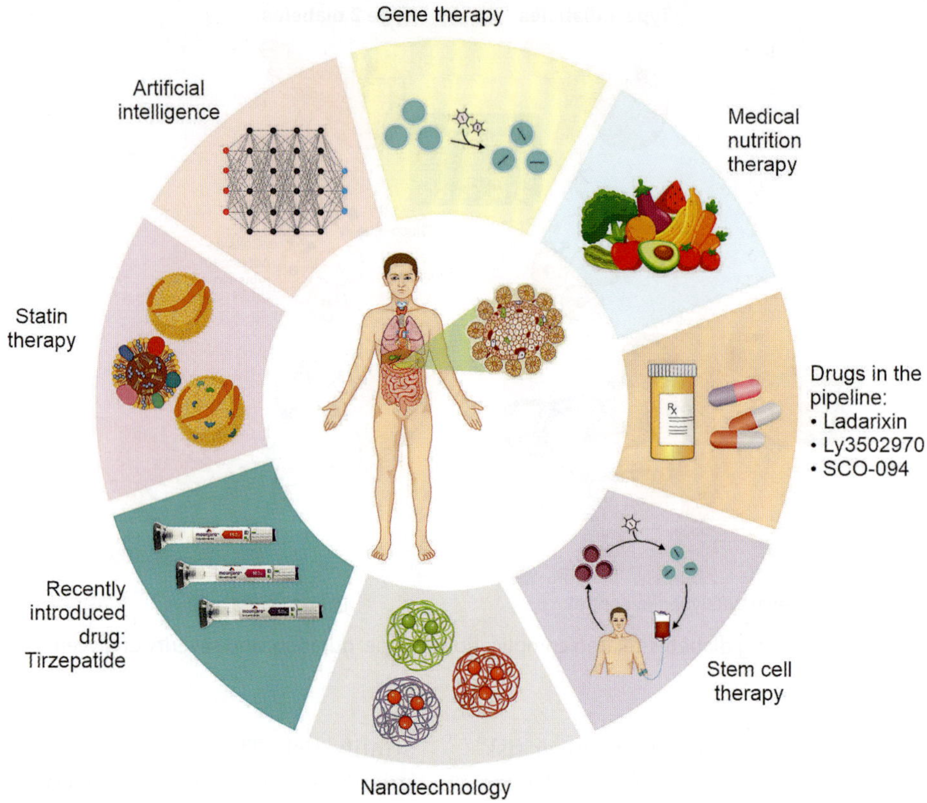

Fig. 7: Emerging therapeutic approaches in diabetes management, including gene therapy, AI, nanotechnology, and novel pharmacologic and nutritional interventions.

without diabetes, depending on population, control of confounding factors, etc.

- For specific cancers such as liver, pancreas, endometrium, and risk elevation may be much higher—often 1.5–2.5× or more.
- For cancers such as colon, breast, kidney, and moderate increase.
- Some cancers (like prostate) show decreased or neutral risk in many studies.

AREAS OF UNCERTAINTY

- Exactly how much of the observed risk is due to diabetes itself versus shared risk factors (like obesity, diet, and inactivity) versus complications versus treatments.
- How different diabetes therapies modulate cancer risk (both positively and negatively)?
- The role of glycemic variability and newer biomarkers in risk prediction
- Interactions with genetics, ethnicity, and environmental exposures
- *Optimal screening strategies*: which cancers, when to start screening, how frequently, cost-effectiveness **(Fig. 8)**.

PRACTICAL RECOMMENDATIONS

For people with diabetes, clinicians, and public health authorities, the following are practical steps based on current evidence:

1. *Good glycemic control*:
    - Aim for target HbA1c appropriate to patient's age and comorbidities.
    - Avoid prolonged periods of hyperglycemia and large glycemic swings.

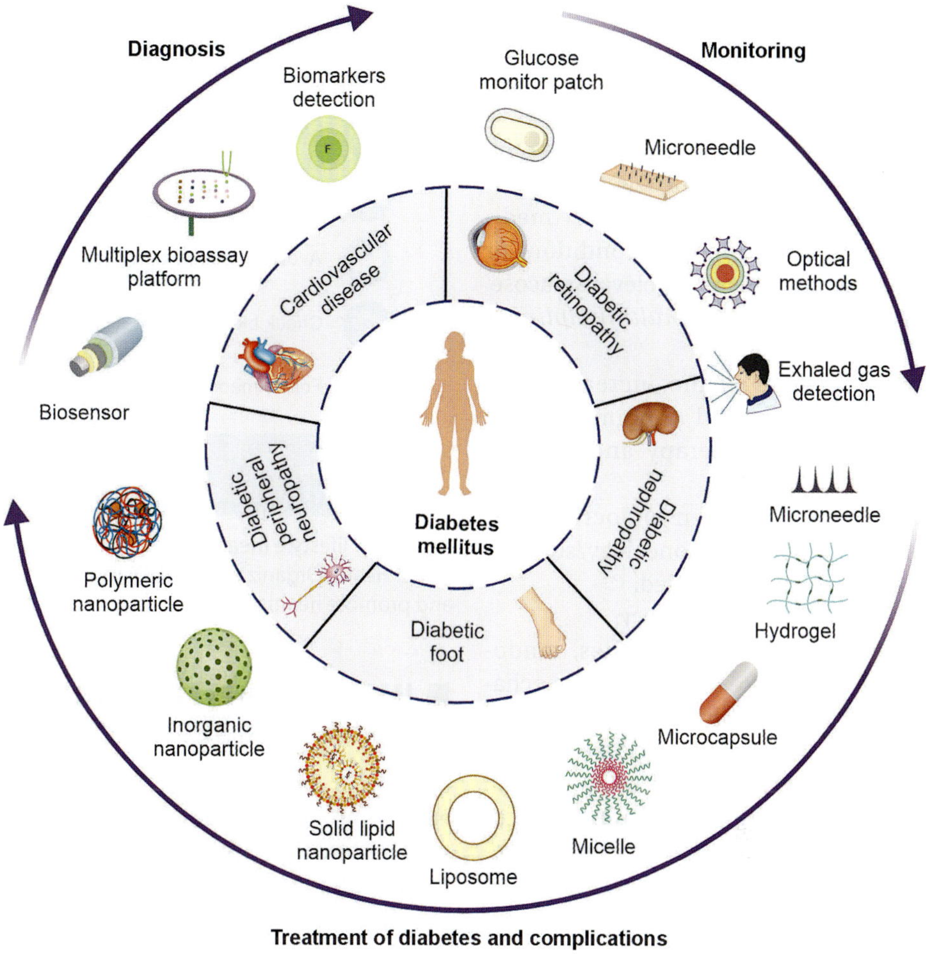

Fig. 8: Overview of diagnostic, monitoring, and treatment strategies for diabetes and its complications.

2. *Lifestyle interventions*:
   - Maintain healthy weight; if overweight or obese, lose weight gradually.
   - *Eat a balanced diet*: Emphasize fiber, vegetables, limit processed carbohydrates and red/processed meats, and unhealthy fats.
   - Regular physical activity.
3. *Monitoring for complications*:
   - Regular screening for diabetic complications (retinopathy, nephropathy, etc.)—those may be markers of higher cancer risk.
   - *Routine health checks*: Liver function, imaging as needed if suspicion arises (especially in people with risk factors for liver cancer, e.g., fatty liver disease).
4. *Cancer screening as per guidelines, possibly enhanced for high risk*:
   - Follow standard screening (colorectal, breast, endometrium, etc.).
   - For persons with diabetes and additional risk factors, consider earlier or more frequent screening for certain cancers (this should be informed by national/local guidelines).

5. *Choice of diabetic medications*:
   - Use medications that do not excessively raise insulin levels if possible and appropriate.
   - Consider metformin, which has some observational evidence of benefit.
   - Monitor effects of steroids, other medications used for comorbid conditions or cancer therapy which may elevate glucose.
6. *Patient's education and multidisciplinary care*:
   - Inform patients of the increased risk so they understand the importance of adherence to therapy and lifestyle change.
   - Collaboration between endocrinology/diabetes specialists and oncology/surgery/general medicine as needed.
7. *Research participation and policy*:
   - Support further cohort studies, randomized trials (where feasible), and mechanistic studies to clarify causation.
   - Public health policies to reduce obesity, promote healthy lifestyle at population level will serve dual purpose (diabetes prevention and potentially cancer prevention) **(Fig. 9)**.

CASE STUDY/EXAMPLE: DEMONSTRATIVE STUDY (TAIWAN STUDY)

To ground these more abstract findings, the Taiwan retrospective cohort gives a clear example:

- ~1.75 million adults with diabetes matched to ~1.75 million without, followed over 12 years.
- Diabetes associated with *20% higher risk* of overall cancer
- Strongest increased risks: *Pancreas* (~87% higher) and *liver* (~69%).
- Presence of DR increased risk further (~31% more risk compared to diabetics without DR). Proliferative DR had still higher risk than nonproliferative. This suggests that diabetic vascular damage (a proxy of disease severity) is an additional risk marker.

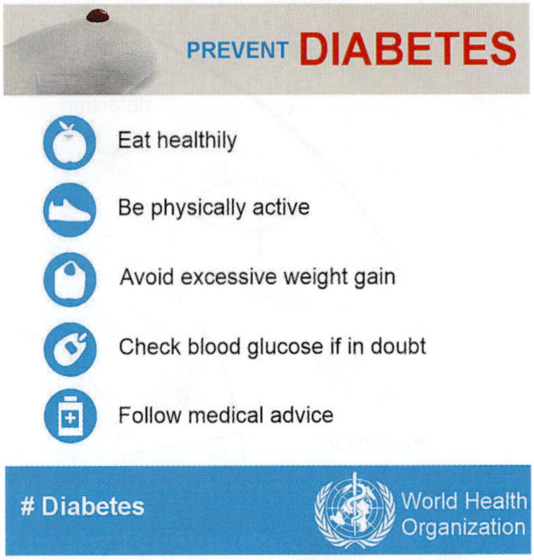
PREVENT DIABETES
Eat healthily
Be physically active
Avoid excessive weight gain
Check blood glucose if in doubt
Follow medical advice
Diabetes
World Health Organization

Fig. 9: Key lifestyle measures recommended by the World Health Organization (WHO) to prevent diabetes and promote healthy living.

IMPLICATIONS FOR INDIA (OR SIMILAR SETTINGS)

Given your location (India/Odisha environment, etc.), some specific implications:

- The burden of diabetes is growing rapidly in India. Many people are diagnosed late, often have poorer glycemic control, and complications are more common. This could mean higher relative risk of cancer in diabetic populations in India.
- *Liver cancer risk*: Given rates of hepatitis B, hepatitis C, and rising NAFLD, the interplay with diabetes may make liver cancer a more pressing concern.
- Pancreatic cancer is harder to screen for but possibly more common with rising diabetes prevalence.
- *Need for increased awareness among both doctors and patients*: Cancer risk is less known among many patients with diabetes, and early detection often delayed.
- *Resource constraints*: Specialized cancer screening is expensive; thus, need cost-effective prioritization (which cancer types and which populations) is key.

CONCLUSION

The weight of evidence indicates that *DM* (especially T2DM) is associated with increased risk of many cancers—particularly liver, pancreas, colon, endometrium, breast, and kidney. The risk is amplified by poor control, longer duration, presence of complications (e.g., retinopathy), obesity, and other metabolic disturbances. While shared risk factors complicate the picture, there are plausible biological mechanisms linking diabetes to cancer initiation, promotion, and progression.

From a public health and clinical standpoint, the critical messages are:

- Improve glycemic control and prevent or delay diabetic complications.
- Promote patient's lifestyle changes (diet, exercise, and weight management).
- Consider enhanced cancer screening strategies for high-risk diabetic populations.
- Monitor effects of diabetes therapies on cancer risk, but do not withhold needed treatment.
- Foster collaboration between specialties and integrate cancer risk discussions in diabetes care.

Given the rising prevalence of diabetes globally and especially in low- and middle-income countries, the interplay between diabetes and cancer risk is a serious emerging issue. More research is needed to refine risk estimation in specific populations, discern causality more clearly, identify biomarkers, and establish evidence-based screening guidelines tailored for people with diabetes.

REFERENCES

1. Chang CH, Hsu CC, Hsieh CY, et al. Association between diabetic retinopathy and cancer risk: a nationwide population-based cohort study. BMC Medicine. 2024;22(1):3430.
2. MD Anderson Cancer Center. (2024). Diabetes management during cancer care. [online] Available from https://www.mdanderson.org/patients-family/diagnosis-treatment/emotional-physical-effects/diabetes-management.html [Last accessed Oct., 2025].
3. Zeng Y, Liu X, Wang J, et al. Diabetes mellitus and cancer risk: epidemiological evidence and mechanistic insights. Digestive and Liver Disease. 2024;56(8):1142-50.
4. Giovannucci E, Harlan DM, Archer MC, Bergenstal RM, Gapstur SM, Habel LA, et al. Diabetes and cancer: A consensus report. Diabetes Care. 2010;33(7):1674-85.
5. Cancer Treatment Centers of America. (2024). What to know about diabetes and cancer. [online] Available from https://www.cancercenter.com/community/blog/2024/12/diabetes-and-cancer [Last accessed Oct., 2025].
6. Zhu B, Qu S. The relationship between diabetes mellitus and cancers and its underlying mechanisms. Endocrinology. 2022;13:800995.

27

Diabetes Remission: Strategies, Evidence, and Long-term Outcomes

Krishnadev Jothydev, Mohamed Abdul Khader M, Jothydev Kesavadev

ABSTRACT

Type 2 diabetes mellitus (T2DM), traditionally considered a chronic and progressive condition, is now recognized as a potentially reversible metabolic state under certain circumstances. Growing evidence from randomized clinical trials and real-world data has shown that sustained normoglycemia, achieved through intensive lifestyle intervention, pharmacotherapy, or metabolic surgery, can lead to diabetes remission in a subset of individuals. This chapter traces the historical evolution of the remission concept, from the first [American Diabetes Association (ADA) consensus in 2009 to the 2021 joint ADA–European Association for the Study of Diabetes (EASD)–Endocrine Society–Diabetes UK definition], which describes remission as maintenance of glycated hemoglobin (HbA1c) < 6.5% for at least 3 months without glucose-lowering therapy. The mechanisms underlying remission include reversal of hepatic and pancreatic steatosis, restoration of insulin sensitivity, and partial β-cell recovery. Predictors such as short disease duration, preserved β-cell function, and substantial weight loss (≥ 10–15%) strongly influence outcomes. Beyond caloric restriction and bariatric surgery, pharmacologic innovations, especially glucagon-like peptide-1 (GLP-1) receptor agonists, dual and triple agonists, and early insulin initiation, have expanded the possibilities for remission. Continuous glucose monitoring (CGM), digital health tools, and structured counseling with SMART goals further support durable metabolic control. Nevertheless, socioeconomic barriers, limited access to multidisciplinary care, and the challenge of sustaining weight loss remain major obstacles. Remission represents a new paradigm in diabetes management, one emphasizing early, individualized, and technology-enabled interventions aimed at restoring metabolic health rather than merely controlling hyperglycemia.

Keywords: Type 2 diabetes mellitus (T2DM), diabetes remission, glycemic control weight loss, lifestyle intervention.

INTRODUCTION

Diabetes is a chronic metabolic disorder defined by the body's inability to produce sufficient insulin, respond to it effectively, or both, culminating in persistent hyperglycemia and a cascade of complications across multiple organ systems. Among its various forms, type 2 diabetes mellitus (T2DM) is the most widespread, intricately linked to modern lifestyles, genetic predisposition, and the metabolic shifts of aging.[1] However, this long-standing notion of diabetes as an inevitably progressive disease is now being challenged. In recent years, a confluence of clinical trial evidence and real-world outcomes has illuminated a new paradigm, that remission once deemed improbable is in fact, attainable. It is now well-established that, through intensive lifestyle interventions (ILIs), significant weight management, or bariatric surgery, some individuals with type 2 diabetes (T2D) can achieve and maintain blood glucose levels below the diagnostic threshold for diabetes, without the use of glucose-lowering medications, for extended periods.

EVOLUTION OF DEFINITION OF REMISSION IN TYPE 2 DIABETES MELLITUS

The concept of remission in T2DM has evolved significantly over the past decade, reflecting both advances in metabolic research and a growing recognition of the clinical relevance of sustained normoglycemia without pharmacologic intervention. As the focus in diabetes care gradually shifts from lifelong management to potential reversal of disease processes, the need for standardized, consensus-based definitions of remission has become increasingly important.

The first formal definition of remission was proposed in 2009 by Buse and colleagues through a consensus statement issued by the American Diabetes Association (ADA). This framework introduced three categories of remission, all characterized by achieving and maintaining glycemic targets without the use of glucose-lowering medications or surgical interventions. (1) Partial remission is defined as maintaining an HbA1c below 6.5% and fasting plasma glucose between 100 and 125 mg/dL for at least 12 months without pharmacologic therapy, while (2) complete remission requires normoglycemia with an HbA1c < 6.0% and fasting glucose < 100 mg/dL sustained for 1 year, and (3) prolonged remission refers to the continuation of complete remission for over 5 years, all without the use of glucose-lowering medications.

Subsequently, pragmatic proposals—aimed at simplifying measurement burden—suggested using HbA1c < 6.5% maintained for ≥ 6–12 months off therapy. In the Indian context, expert commentaries have argued for practical definitions that recognize the foundational role of lifestyle measures (and, in some proposals, ongoing metformin) while prioritizing objective glycemic thresholds and sustained follow-up.

A major step was the 2021 joint consensus of the ADA, European Association for the Study of Diabetes (EASD), the Endocrine Society, and Diabetes UK, which defined remission as HbA1c < 6.5% for ≥ 3 months in the absence of glucose-lowering therapy. Where HbA1c is unreliable (e.g., hemoglobinopathies), fasting plasma glucose (FPG) < 126 mg/dL or continuous glucose monitor (CGM)-derived glucose management indicator (GMI) may be used. The consensus emphasizes that remission is a transient state requiring ongoing surveillance.

CURRENT DEFINITION

The 2021 international consensus remains the most widely adopted: HbA1c < 6.5% for ≥ 3 months without glucose-lowering therapy, with confirmation ≥ 3 months after therapy withdrawal and at least annual reassessment thereafter. In individuals with unreliable HbA1c, FPG < 126 mg/dL or GMI may substitute. The ADA Standards of Care 2025 do not redefine remission but strongly emphasize strategies (e.g., ≥ 10–15% weight loss when feasible, and the broader use of CGM) that improve glycemia and cardiometabolic risk. Remission is not a cure; relapse can occur with weight regain or progressive β-cell dysfunction, so continued complication screening remains essential.[2,3]

In essence, remission refers to a phase during which blood glucose levels remain within the nondiabetes range without the aid of glucose-lowering medications. However, it is crucial to distinguish remission from a definitive cure, as diabetes remains a chronic and irreversible condition. The term "remission" is preferred over "reversal" in scientific literature, as it more accurately reflects the temporary nature

TABLE 1: Evolution of remission definitions in type 2 diabetes mellitus.

Year	*Proponent(s)*	*Type of remission*	*Definition summary*
2009	ADA (Buse et al.)	Partial	HbA1c < 6.5% and FPG 100–125 mg/dL for ≥1 year without medication
		Complete	HbA1c < 6.0% and FPG <100 mg/dL for ≥ 1 year without medication
		Prolonged	Complete remission sustained > 5 years without medication
2019	Nagi et al.	General	Glycemia below diagnostic threshold for ≥ 6 months without medication
2021	Kalra et al.	General	Glycemia below diagnostic threshold for ≥ 6 months with or without lifestyle/metformin
	Joint Consensus (ADA, EASD, Endocrine Society, Diabetes UK)	Standardized Definition	HbA1c < 6.5% for ≥ 3 months without glucose-lowering therapy; annual monitoring advised

(ADA: American Diabetes Association; EASD: European Association for the Study of Diabetes; HbA1c: glycated hemoglobin)

of glycemic normalization without implying permanent resolution. Remission is a medically defined state borrowed from oncology indicating the absence of active disease progression, but not necessarily its complete eradication. In contrast, the term "reversal" is less precise and may misleadingly suggest a permanent cure, which is not supported by current evidence in the context of T2D. Remission acknowledges the possibility of relapse, the ongoing need for monitoring, and the potential return of hyperglycemia under adverse conditions such as weight regain or β-cell decline **(Table 1)**.[4]

PREVALENCE OF REMISSION

Although remission of T2D has significant clinical implications, its prevalence and determinants in community-based populations remain inadequately understood. A study by Karter et al. reported that remission is relatively uncommon. In their large cohort, the incidence rates per 1,000 person-years were 2.8 for partial remission, 0.24 for complete remission, and 0.04 for prolonged remission. Over a 7-year follow-up period, the cumulative incidence was 1.47% for partial remission, 0.14% for complete remission, and 0.007% for prolonged remission. Overall, approximately 1.6% of the cohort achieved any form of remission, with higher rates (4.6%) observed among individuals diagnosed within the previous 2 years. Factors positively associated with remission included older age (> 65 years), shorter duration of diabetes and absence of glucose-lowering therapy at baseline.[5] Building on this, Thom et al. reported that in their intervention group [n = 149; mean age 53 years; mean body mass index (BMI) 35 kg/m^2], both baseline characteristics and weight changes during the study influenced remission outcomes. Participants with higher baseline HbA1c were less likely to achieve remission at 12 months, highlighting that lower initial HbA1c favors remission. Men and those on fewer antidiabetic medications at baseline were more likely to achieve remission, largely due to greater weight loss, whereas participants with anxiety or depression were less likely, reflecting smaller reductions in weight.[6] Individuals with higher baseline body weight tend to achieve greater weight loss and exhibit a higher frequency of T2D remission. In contrast, those with lower initial weight have less potential for weight reduction, leading to smaller declines in HbA1c and consequently a lower likelihood of remission. This relationship underscores the critical role of weight loss in managing T2D. A systematic review and meta-regression analysis by Kanbour et al. (2025) demonstrated a robust dose-response relationship between bodyweight loss and diabetes remission, independent of factors such as age, diabetes duration, HbA1c, BMI, and type of intervention. The study found that for every 1% decrease in body weight, the probability of achieving complete remission increased by 2.17%, and partial remission by 2.74%. Notably, participants who lost 30% or more of their body weight had a 79.1% chance of complete remission and an 89.5% chance of partial remission.[7]

PATHOPHYSIOLOGICAL REVERSAL AND REMISSION IN TYPE 2 DIABETES MELLITUS

T2DM is a progressive metabolic disorder characterized by an initial phase of insulin resistance and compensatory hyperinsulinemia, followed by gradual deterioration of pancreatic β-cell function and eventual insulin deficiency. According to the twin cycle hypothesis, chronic caloric excess promotes ectopic fat accumulation in the liver and pancreas. Hepatic fat contributes to insulin resistance, whereas pancreatic fat impairs insulin secretion. When this ectopic fat accumulation exceeds an individual's *personal fat threshold*, the balance of glucose regulation is disrupted, leading to the manifestation of T2DM. Therapeutic interventions that reduce insulin resistance or enhance insulin secretion can improve glycemic control and, in some cases, enable remission **(Fig. 1)**.

Reduced Insulin Resistance

Insulin resistance, particularly at the hepatic level, plays a central role in the pathogenesis of T2DM. Hepatic steatosis impairs insulin's ability to suppress gluconeogenesis, primarily due to the accumulation of intrahepatic diacylglycerol

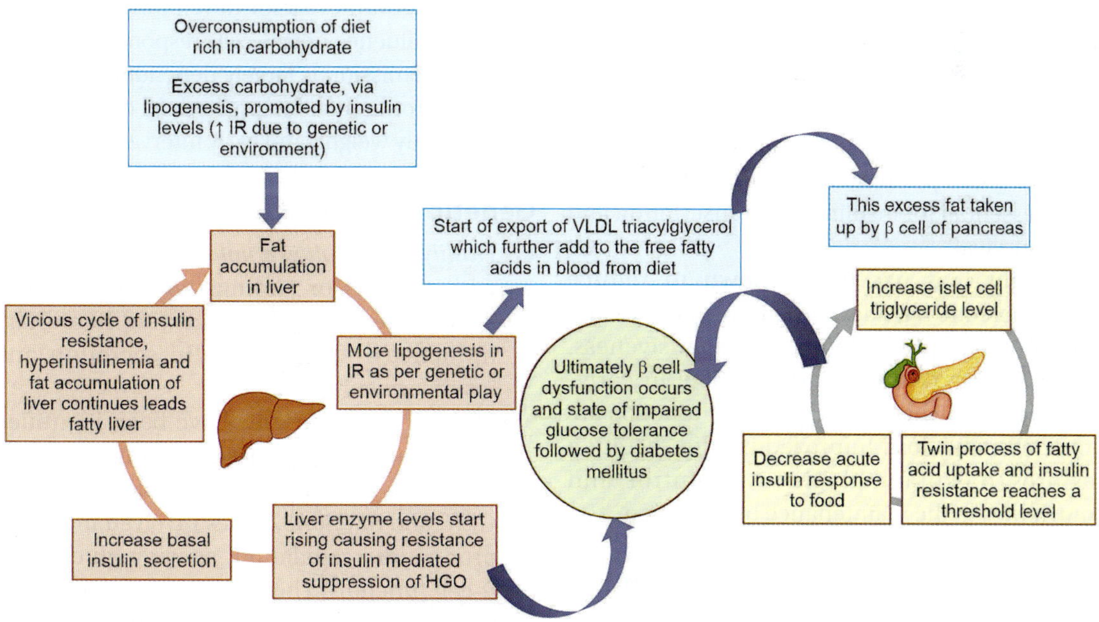

Fig. 1: Twin cycle hypothesis.

(IR: insulin resistance; HGO: hepatic glucose output; VLDL: very-low-density lipoprotein)

Source: Kumar et al., 2023.[11]

(DAG), which activates protein kinase C epsilon (PKCε). This activation inhibits insulin receptor substrate-2 (IRS-2) signaling and reduces downstream activation of phosphoinositide 3-kinase (PI3K) and Akt, thereby impairing insulin-mediated suppression of hepatic glucose output. Weight loss reduces hepatic lipid content, reversing DAG accumulation and restoring insulin signaling through improved IRS-2–PI3K–Akt pathway function. In peripheral tissues such as skeletal muscle and adipose tissue, weight reduction improves insulin sensitivity via enhanced GLUT4 translocation and increased mitochondrial oxidative capacity, promoting better glucose uptake and utilization. These changes collectively lower fasting plasma glucose levels and contribute significantly to metabolic normalization.[8,9]

β-cell Functional Recovery

Alongside insulin resistance, progressive β-cell dysfunction contributes to hyperglycemia in T2DM. Accumulation of triglycerides and toxic lipid intermediates (e.g., ceramides) within pancreatic islets induces lipotoxicity, which disrupts β-cell function through oxidative stress, mitochondrial dysfunction, and endoplasmic reticulum (ER) stress. This impairs the expression of key transcription factors such as PDX1 and MafA, essential for insulin gene transcription and β-cell survival.[9,10]

Weight loss has been shown to reduce intrapancreatic fat, alleviating lipotoxic pressure and enhancing β-cell glucose responsiveness. This recovery is particularly feasible in early-stage diabetes when β-cell mass and function are not irreversibly lost. Improved insulin secretion restores postprandial glucose control and contributes to the maintenance of remission.

Effects of Weight Loss on Remission

Substantial weight reduction, typically in the range of 10–15 kg, has emerged as a key predictor of diabetes remission. Such weight loss leads to marked improvements in both insulin sensitivity and β-cell function through the reduction of ectopic fat in the liver and pancreas. Clinical trials and real-world studies have consistently demonstrated that individuals achieving this level of weight loss are more likely to attain and sustain remission, particularly when weight loss occurs early in the disease course. Importantly, remission is not merely a reflection of normal blood glucose levels but a physiological restoration of metabolic health. However, the long-term maintenance of remission is contingent upon the sustained adherence to lifestyle interventions that preserve the improvements in tissue-level insulin dynamics.[9]

GENETIC AND ENVIRONMENTAL DETERMINANTS OF DIABETES REMISSION

Genetic and environmental (or lifestyle) factors interact significantly to influence the likelihood of remission in T2DM. While genetic predisposition sets a background risk for developing T2DM and may also influence how β-cells respond to stress or recovery, remission is largely dependent on modifiable environmental factors such as diet, physical activity, body weight, and early intervention.

Genetic Factors

- *Family history plays a notable role*: Individuals with parents or siblings who have T2DM have increased risk, suggesting hereditary influences on both insulin secretion and insulin sensitivity.
- Multiple gene variants have been identified that affect diabetes risk. Among these are *TCF7L2, ABCC8, CAPN10, GLUT2, GCGR, GCK*, and *SLC30A8*, genes involved in insulin production, regulation, sensing glucose, or β-cell function. These genes show that some people may be genetically more vulnerable to damage, affecting insulin secretion or to challenges in glucose metabolism.

- However, each individual genetic variant generally has a small effect; the cumulative burden of several such variants plus interactions among them is what contributes to overall predisposition. Genetic predisposition alone is rarely sufficient without environmental triggers.

Environmental/Lifestyle Factors

- Obesity, sedentary behavior, poor diet, and other modifiable lifestyle factors are essential determinants: they not only contribute to development of T2DM but critically influence the potential for remission. For example, weight loss and increased physical activity are among the strongest predictors of remission.
- Early diagnosis and intervention (i.e., shorter duration of diabetes) amplify the chances that lifestyle modifications will reverse metabolic derangements. The earlier that interventions begin, the more likely insulin secretion and insulin sensitivity can be restored before irreversible β-cell loss occurs.
- Environmental exposures also include socioeconomic factors, access to healthcare, food quality, physical environment, and support for sustained behavior change.[12]

Interplay between Genetics and Environment

- The potential for remission is often shaped by the interaction between genetic background and environmental modifiability. Someone with moderate genetic predisposition but who undertakes early, effective lifestyle interventions (weight loss, diet, exercise) may have a better chance of remission than someone with stronger genetic risk who delays intervention.
- Genetic predisposition may determine the threshold at which environmental stress (e.g., adiposity, lipotoxicity) begins to impair β-cell function or insulin sensitivity.

Epigenetics

Environmental stimuli can lead to epigenetic changes (heritable alterations in gene expression) that impact gene function and contribute to the development of diabetes later in life.

PREDICTORS OF REMISSION

The prediction of T2D remission following metabolic surgery has garnered considerable scientific and clinical attention. Schauer et al. (2003) were among the first to report that longer diabetes duration, insulin dependence, and limited postoperative weight loss were associated with lower remission rates after Roux-en-Y gastric bypass (RYGB). In subsequent years, predictive models such as the DiaRem, ABCD, and IMS scores have been developed to estimate remission likelihood based on preoperative clinical variables. These tools aid in individualized risk assessment and guide surgical decision-making by incorporating factors like age, BMI, C-peptide levels, diabetes duration, insulin use, and baseline glycemic control.[12,13]

DiaRem Score (for Roux-en-Y Gastric Bypass)

The DiaRem score uses preoperative parameters HbA1c, insulin use, and number of glucose-lowering medications to estimate remission probability following RYGB. Lower scores are associated with higher chances of remission:

- Score *0–2*: 87% remission
- Score *3–7*: 66% remission
- Score *8–12*: 32% remission
- Score *13–17*: 16% remission
- Score *18–22*: 5% remission

Patients with better glycemic control and no insulin use have the greatest remission potential.

ABCD Score

The ABCD score includes Age, BMI, C-peptide levels, and diabetes duration. Each is scored

> 40 kg/m^2 or > 35 kg/m^2 when accompanied by obesity-related comorbidities such as T2DM. Substantial evidence indicates that metabolic surgery can lead to remission of T2DM in a significant proportion of patients, typically more than one-third. Furthermore, the likelihood of achieving remission is closely associated with the extent of postoperative weight loss, with greater weight reductions correlating with improved glycemic outcomes and sustained metabolic control.[11]

Among the available surgical options, RYGB and SG are the most commonly performed procedures for weight loss and diabetes remission. RYGB involves creating a small gastric pouch and rerouting food directly to the jejunum, bypassing most of the stomach, the duodenum, and part of the proximal jejunum. In contrast, SG removes about 75% of the stomach, including the ghrelin-producing fundus, resulting in a crescent shaped stomach. SG is technically simpler than RYGB and is associated with fewer complications and nutritional deficiencies, while still offering effective metabolic benefits. Less commonly used procedures such as adjustable gastric banding (AGB) and biliopancreatic diversion (BPD) have declined in popularity. AGB has shown limited weight loss effectiveness, and BPD, although potent, carries a higher risk of long-term nutritional deficiencies.[20]

The metabolic benefits of bariatric surgery extend beyond weight loss. Calorie restriction after surgery quickly lowers glucose levels by reducing insulin demand and improving hepatic insulin sensitivity. Interestingly, glycemic improvements often occur within days, before significant weight loss, suggesting other mechanisms are involved. These include hormonal changes such as increased GLP-1, GIP, and PYY, and reduced ghrelin, which improve insulin secretion and satiety. The proximal bowel hypothesis proposes that bypassing the upper intestine alters gut signals that may otherwise impair glucose control. Additional factors such as changes in bile acid metabolism, the gut microbiome, and even taste perception may also contribute to improved glucose homeostasis and diabetes remission.[20]

The STAMPEDE Trial: Evidence for Diabetes Remission through Metabolic Surgery

The STAMPEDE (Surgical Therapy and Medications Potentially Eradicate Diabetes Efficiently) trial was a landmark randomized controlled study that evaluated the potential of metabolic surgery to induce remission of T2DM. Conducted at the Cleveland Clinic, the trial enrolled 150 adults with poorly controlled T2DM and a BMI between 27 and 43 kg/m^2, including individuals below traditional surgical BMI thresholds. Participants were assigned to one of three groups: advanced medical therapy (AMT) alone, AMT plus SG, or AMT plus RYGB. At 3 years, rates of diabetes remission were significantly higher in both surgical groups compared to medical therapy alone. Many surgical patients discontinued insulin and other antidiabetes medications entirely, and these improvements were sustained over time. Surgery also led to improved quality of life and reduced reliance on cardiovascular medications.

These findings provided compelling evidence that metabolic surgery is not only effective for glycemic control but can also induce durable remission of T2DM, even in patients with moderate obesity.[21]

Pharmacotherapy

Pharmacological therapy serves as a critical non-surgical approach in achieving remission of T2DM. Broadly, glucose-lowering agents can be categorized into three functional classes: *Insulin sensitizers, nutrient load reducers*, and *insulin secretagogues* **(Table 2)**.[11]

Beyond their glucose-lowering effects, certain pharmacologic agents also promote weight loss and enhance insulin sensitivity, both of which are key determinants in achieving T2DM remission. Pharmacotherapy has therefore become central to sustaining remission, with GLP-1 receptor

TABLE 2: Functional classification of diabetes medications: Implications for remission and metabolic health.[11]

Functional class	*Mechanism of action*	*Representative agents*	*Calorie restriction/energy modulation effect*
Insulin sensitizers	Enhance peripheral insulin sensitivity	• *Direct:* Metformin, pioglitazone • *Indirect:* Pramlintide, bromocriptine	Improve glucose utilization; may indirectly support weight loss (especially metformin)
Nutrient load reducers	Limit glucose availability or enhance glucose elimination	• *α-glucosidase inhibitors (AGIs):* Acarbose, miglitol • *SGLT-2 inhibitors:* Dapagliflozin, empagliflozin	• AGIs delay carbohydrate absorption, reducing postprandial glucose • SGLT-2i promote glycosuria → glucose/energy loss → mimic caloric restriction
Insulin secretagogues	Stimulate insulin secretion from pancreatic β-cells	• *Sulfonylureas* (gliclazide, glimepiride) • *Meglitinides* (repaglinide, nateglinide)	Mainly glucose-lowering; less direct effect on energy restriction
Calorie restriction mimetics (emerging concept)	Replicate metabolic benefits of caloric restriction and weight loss	• SGLT-2i (glucose-wasting) • GLP-1 receptor agonists (e.g., Liraglutide, Semaglutide)- • AGIs	Reduce appetite, caloric intake, or induce energy loss → potential adjunct in diabetes remission

(SGLT-2: sodium-glucose cotransporter-2; GLP-1: glucagon-like peptide-1)

agonists and sodium-glucose cotransporter-2 (SGLT-2) inhibitors demonstrating notable efficacy in improving glycemic control while reducing body weight.

Glucagon-like Peptide-1 Receptor Agonist: Liraglutide

Liraglutide, a glucagon-like peptide-1 (GLP-1) receptor agonist, has demonstrated significant therapeutic potential in T2D by improving glycemic control, supporting β-cell function, enhancing endogenous insulin secretion, and promoting weight reduction, thereby contributing to the achievement of glycemic remission. Kesavadev et al. (2012) reported that 24 weeks of liraglutide therapy in Indian patients with T2D resulted in significant improvements in glycemic and metabolic parameters. Fasting plasma glucose decreased by 48.5 mg/dL, postprandial glucose by 66.7 mg/dL, and HbA1c by 2.26% ($p < 0.001$). Patients also experienced an average weight loss of 8.65 kg and a reduction in body mass index of 3.26 kg/m^2. Additionally, systolic blood pressure, lipid profile, and serum creatinine levels improved, and no serious adverse events or hypoglycemic episodes were reported.[22]

Furthermore, in a prospective 24-week observational study of 195 Indian patients, Kesavadev et al. (2015) demonstrated that liraglutide therapy added to existing antidiabetic treatment significantly lowered fasting plasma glucose from 163.8 mg/dL to 111.6 mg/dL ($p < 0.001$) and reduced HbA1c from 8.14% to 6.96% ($p = 0.006$), with 41% of patients achieving HbA1c ≤ 6.5%. Patients also experienced a mean weight reduction of 4 kg, alongside improvements in blood pressure and serum cholesterol, with only mild and transient adverse events.[23]

Collectively, these findings indicate that liraglutide not only improves glycemic control and cardiometabolic parameters but also, by reducing glucotoxicity, enhancing β-cell function, and promoting weight loss, can support the achievement and maintenance of diabetes

TABLE 3: Trial-based outcomes with GLP-1 RAs: Glycemic targets, remission potential, and weight reduction.

Study	*GLP-1 RAs/Regimen*	*Key outcome*
DiaRem-1 (India)[24]	• Liraglutide + dapagliflozin + metformin (intervention) vs. • Vildagliptin + glimepiride + metformin (control)	• ~31% achieved remission—HbA1c < 6.5% (total) • 28.6% (intervention) • 33.3% (control)
Metabolic intervention + insulin degludec/ liraglutide (2024)[25]	Intensive lifestyle + metformin + fixed-ratio degludec/liraglutide (16-week intervention)	• *12 weeks postinduction*: 17.7% remission; • *52 weeks:* 6.3% maintained remission
Semaglutide—STEP-2[26]	• Once-weekly semaglutide 2.4 mg and 1.0 mg + lifestyle • (68 week intervention)	*≥ 5% weight loss:* • *68.8%* (semaglutide 2.4 mg) • *28.5%* on placebo
Semaglutide—STEP-10 (Prediabetes)[27]	Semaglutide 2.4 mg weekly + lifestyle intervention	At 52 weeks, ~81% achieved normoglycemia vs. 14% placebo (on-drug)
Liraglutide after glucotoxicity resolution[28]	Insulin first to control hyperglycemia → switch to liraglutide monotherapy	Maintained ~6.2% HbA1c after 24 weeks on liraglutide

(GLP-1 RAs: glucagon-like peptide-1 receptor agonists)

remission in appropriately selected patients. Several recent studies have evaluated the potential of GLP-1 receptor agonists, either alone or in combination with other agents, to induce glycemic remission in T2D. Key trials highlighting varying strategies and outcomes are summarized in **Table 3**.

Glucagon-like Peptide-1/GIP Dual Agonists: Tirzepatide

Tirzepatide, a dual GLP-1 and GIP receptor agonist, has demonstrated substantial efficacy in both weight reduction and glycemic control. Clinical trials indicate that participants receiving tirzepatide achieved significant weight loss, with a proportion attaining near-normal blood glucose levels, suggesting the potential for diabetes remission. Notably, the study by Fitch et al. reported that patients in the tirzepatide group were more likely to achieve weight reductions of ≥ 10%, ≥ 15%, ≥ 20%, and ≥ 25%, underscoring the agent's robust and dose-dependent impact on body weight and metabolic outcomes, thereby potential for remission.[14] Further supporting these findings, a study by Popovic et al. demonstrated that treatment with tirzepatide increased the odds of achieving normoglycemia by > 16 times compared to control, indicating significant progress toward attaining diabetes remission.[29,30] These studies collectively underscore the potential of tirzepatide in not only managing T2D but also in inducing remission in a significant proportion of patients.

Triple Receptor Agonists: Retatrutide

Retatrutide, a triple receptor agonist targeting GLP-1, GIP, and glucagon receptors, has shown substantial and dose-dependent weight loss, supporting its potential role in T2D remission. In a 48-week phase 2 obesity study, participants receiving retatrutide 8 mg and 12 mg achieved weight reductions of 22.8% and 24.2%, respectively, highlighting both the magnitude and durability of its effect. Such significant weight loss is closely linked to improvements in insulin sensitivity and glycemic control, thereby enhancing the likelihood of diabetes remission.[31]

Role of α-glucosidase Inhibitors in Diabetes Remission

α-glucosidase inhibitors (AGIs) reduce postprandial hyperglycemia by slowing the digestion and absorption of carbohydrates in the gut, minimizing the need for insulin secretagogues. When combined with metformin, AGIs have been shown in randomized controlled trials to support meaningful weight loss and improved glycemic control.[11] Additionally, observational studies in high-risk populations, such as individuals with impaired glucose tolerance, have shown that AGI therapy can lower the progression to T2D. A meta-analysis of five trials involving acarbose indicated a reduction in the incidence of T2D, with a number needed to treat (NNT) of 10, and a decrease in BMI by 0.3 kg/m^2.[32]

Combination Therapy

Combination therapy with SGLT-2 inhibitors not only enhances glycemic control, body weight reduction, and cardiovascular outcomes compared with monotherapy but also supports T2DM remission. A patient with newly diagnosed T2DM, baseline BMI of 26.0 kg/m^2, HbA1c of 10.3%, insulin resistance, β-cell dysfunction, and fatty liver achieved drug-free remission after 18 months of SGLT-2 inhibitor and metformin therapy, with HbA1c normalizing to 5.3% and BMI reduced to 21.3 kg/m^2. This illustrates the potential of SGLT-2 inhibitor–based combination therapy to induce weight loss and metabolic restoration in real-world clinical practice.[33]

Clinical Evidence for Pharmacotherapy: Insights from the SURPASS Trials

The 40-week, multi-center, randomized, placebo-controlled *SURPASS-1 trial* (NCT03954834) evaluated tirzepatide monotherapy in 478 adults with T2D inadequately controlled by diet and exercise. Participants (mean HbA1c 7–9.5%, BMI ≥ 23 kg/m^2) were naïve to injectable or recent oral antidiabetes therapy. Tirzepatide doses (5, 10, 15 mg) were titrated from 2.5 mg weekly in 4-week increments to optimize efficacy and tolerability. The 15 mg dose produced a mean HbA1c reduction of –2.07% and weight loss of 11.0%, with up to 51% achieving normoglycemia (HbA1c < 5.7%), suggesting potential drug-free diabetes remission.[34]

In SURPASS-2, tirzepatide outperformed semaglutide 1 mg in both glycemic and weight outcomes, with mean HbA1c reduction up to 2.3% and weight loss reaching 11.2 kg. These findings support tirzepatide's role in facilitating remission through simultaneous improvements in glycemic control, insulin sensitivity, and weight reduction.[35]

Role of Insulin in Diabetes Remission

Early intensive insulin (EII) therapy entails a short-term, aggressive insulin regimen in newly diagnosed T2D patients, aiming to rapidly restore normoglycemia, enhance β-cell function, and reduce glucotoxicity. Evidence indicates that short-term intensive insulin therapy administered during the early stages of T2D (preferably within the first 2 years of diagnosis) can promote glycemic remission. A meta-analysis reported that remission was achieved in approximately 46% of patients at 1 year and 42% at 2 years following a brief course of intensive insulin treatment, highlighting its potential to restore β-cell function and improve metabolic control when initiated early in the disease course.[11]

Kesavadev et al. (2017) demonstrated that early insulin initiation in patients with newly diagnosed T2D led to sustained improvements in glycemic control over a 10-year period. Mean HbA1c declined from 10.9 to 7.56%, with significant reductions in fasting and postprandial glucose levels. Notably, insulin requirements remained stable without dose escalation, suggesting preserved insulin sensitivity. The study supports early insulin use as a strategy to improve long-term outcomes, delay complications, and potentially support diabetes remission.[36] These findings suggest that early insulin initiation not only improves glycemic outcomes and delays the onset of complications but may also support diabetes remission by reducing glucotoxicity, preserving β-cell function, and minimizing long-term insulin requirements, thereby establishing a cost-effective and durable foundation for diabetes care.

In a related observational cohort study, patients who initiated insulin therapy within 7–8 years of T2D onset were compared with those who began insulin treatment after > 8 years. The findings indicated that early insulin initiators maintained glycemic control with a substantially lower total daily insulin dose (mean 9 units/day) compared with late initiators (LII), who required an average of 30 units/day. Furthermore, while the LII group experienced a significant decline in estimated glomerular filtration rate (eGFR), renal function remained stable in the EII group. These results suggest that early initiation of insulin may not only help preserve kidney function but also support durable glycemic remission by alleviating β-cell stress and minimizing long-term insulin requirements.[37]

Teplizumab in Delaying the Onset of Type 1 Diabetes

Type 1 diabetes (T1D) is an autoimmune disease marked by progressive β-cell destruction, leading to absolute insulin deficiency. Since β-cell loss is largely irreversible once clinical symptoms appear, interventions that delay disease onset are critical. Teplizumab, a humanized anti-CD3 monoclonal antibody, has been FDA-approved to postpone T1D in high-risk individuals.[38] The *PROTECT trial*, a phase 3, randomized, placebo-controlled study, demonstrated that two 12-day courses of teplizumab, administered 26 weeks apart, significantly preserved β-cell function in children and adolescents with newly diagnosed T1D. At week 78, teplizumab-treated patients maintained higher stimulated C-peptide levels, with 94.9% achieving clinically meaningful preservation (≥ 0.2 pmol/mL) versus 79.2% in the placebo group. By sustaining endogenous insulin production, teplizumab exemplifies a preventive approach analogous to remission, maintaining metabolic function before irreversible β-cell loss occurs.[39]

IMPACT OF CONTINUOUS GLUCOSE MONITORING ON LONG-TERM DIABETES REMISSION

Continuous glucose monitoring (CGM) has emerged as a pivotal tool in facilitating and sustaining diabetes remission, particularly in T2D. By providing real-time, comprehensive glucose data, CGM enables precise management of glycemic variability, a critical factor in β-cell preservation and overall metabolic stability. Its utility is now being extended to prediabetes as well. Kesavadev et al. (ADA 2023) investigated its clinical value in this population and found that CGM uncovered significant postprandial glycemic excursions and variability that routine self-monitoring of blood glucose (SMBG) failed to detect. Following a 3-month program of lifestyle changes informed by CGM feedback, participants demonstrated meaningful improvements, including reductions in fasting glucose (from 110.8 to 91 mg/dL), HbA1c (from 5.9 to 5.4%), and glycemic fluctuations, accompanied by an average weight loss of 2.35 kg.[40] These results support the role of CGM not only in enhancing metabolic monitoring but also in motivating behavioral changes that may delay or prevent the onset of T2D. Studies have also demonstrated that early intervention using CGM, combined with intensive lifestyle modifications, can significantly enhance the likelihood of achieving and maintaining T2D remission. For instance, a randomized clinical trial involving 475 hospitalized patients with diabetes utilized structured real-time CGM programs alongside continuous subcutaneous insulin infusion (CSII). This approach led to improved glycemic control without the hypoglycemic risk and increased rates of diabetes remission.[41] Furthermore, postoperative CGM recordings have been shown to predict diabetes remission 1 year after bariatric surgery, with specific metrics such as time spent above range and glucose variability serving as strong indicators.[42] These findings underscore the critical role of CGM in not only achieving remission but also in providing the necessary data to tailor and optimize treatment strategies for long-term success.

ROLE OF DIGITAL HEALTH AND TELEMEDICINE IN SUSTAINED DIABETES REMISSION

Digital health and telemedicine encompass a broad array of technologies including mobile applications, wearable devices, remote monitoring tools, and teleconsultation platforms, designed to optimize healthcare delivery. These solutions aim to enhance the efficiency, accessibility, and overall quality of care, while also empowering individuals to take an active role in managing their health.[43] In the context of diabetes, such technologies support sustained remission by enabling real-time monitoring of blood glucose, physical activity, and medication adherence. Moreover, continuous virtual engagement with healthcare providers facilitates timely interventions and reinforces behavioral changes essential for long-term glycemic control. Collectively, these innovations create a supportive digital ecosystem that strengthens self-management and aids in maintaining diabetes remission.

A recent review of nine studies assessing digital health interventions found that more than half (56%) demonstrated clinically significant improvements in at least one metabolic outcome, including reductions in body weight (22%), HbA1c levels (22%), or incidence of T2D (11%). Among these, two out of three computer-based programs (67%) demonstrated significant reductions in both HbA1c levels and body weight. Similarly, half of the mobile-based strategies including SMS messaging, app-based support, and telehealth were effective in lowering either HbA1c or the incidence of T2D. These findings underscore the growing clinical relevance of digital platforms in facilitating diabetes remission through improved glycemic control and weight management.[43]

Innovative Digital Health Approaches for Sustained Diabetes Remission

- *BT001: Digital CBT App + standard care*—A randomized trial (n = 669) tested a cognitivebehavioral therapy-based app (BT001) versus a control app, both in addition to usual care. Over 90 days, the BT001 group saw a mean HbA1c reduction of approximately -0.28%, whereas the control group saw a slight increase; the treatment group difference was 0.39% ($p < 0.0001$). The more app modules completed, the greater the HbA1c reduction.[44]
- *Integrated digital health platform with artificial intelligence (AI) driven dietary management*: In a 48-week, open-label, randomized multicenter trial involving adults with T2D (HbA1c 7.0–8.5%, BMI ≥ 23 kg/m^2), the use of a digital health platform, integrating AI-driven dietary recommendations, intermittent personal CGM use, and clinician feedback, resulted in significantly greater HbA1c reductions and weight loss compared to standard care. These improvements were observed as early as 24 weeks and sustained through 48 weeks, without an increase in hypoglycemic episodes. The findings highlight the platform's potential to enhance long-term glycemic and weight outcomes in routine diabetes management.[45]
- *Digital therapeutic intervention in India*: A 12-week, single-arm study evaluated a mobile app based digital therapeutic program in 128 adults with T2D. Participants used the app alongside standard antidiabetes therapy, achieved reductions in HbA1c (–0.84%), fasting glucose (–8.39 mg/dL), postprandial glucose (–14.97 mg/dL), and modest BMI loss (–0.24 kg/m^2). Greater improvements were associated with higher baseline HbA1c (≥ 7.5%), absence of smoking behavior, no

history of COVID-19 infection, and higher engagement with the digital program. These results indicate that structured digital interventions can improve glycemic control and support modest weight reduction, highlighting their potential role in sustaining diabetes remission.[46]

- *Digital twin technology trial [18-month randomized controlled trial (RCT)]*: An 18-month randomized trial investigated the efficacy of Digital Twin (DT) technology integrating wearable sensors with AI-guided dietary and activity recommendations in adults with T2D (mean age 44 years; mean disease duration 3.7 years). Among 207 participants who completed at least 6 months and were eligible for remission evaluation, 64.3% achieved sustained diabetes remission at 18 months. Significant improvements were observed: HbA1c decreased from 8.9 to 6.4%, body weight from 78.1 to 72.8 kg, BMI from 27.2 to 25.2, waist circumference from 97.4 to 88.1 cm, HOMA2IR from 1.9 to 1.5, and HOMA2B from 51.9 to 70.9. Standard care participants showed minimal changes. These findings demonstrate DT technology's potential to support sustained diabetes remission through real-time monitoring, personalized feedback, and AI-driven guidance.[36]
- *App-based lifestyle intervention (Asia): D'LITE study:* In a randomized clinical trial involving 204 adults with T2D, a smartphone-based intervention integrating personal health tracking with behavioral modification strategies resulted in significantly greater reductions in body weight and HbA1c compared with standard care over 6 months. Participants using the app also demonstrated a higher likelihood of reducing their diabetes medication dosages. These results indicate that mobile health driven lifestyle interventions can effectively enhance glycemic control and promote weight loss in overweight or obese individuals with T2D in an Asian population.[47,48]

Collectively, such digital interventions may contribute to achieving and sustaining diabetes remission by supporting long-term lifestyle adherence and metabolic improvements.

ROLE OF COUNSELING PROGRAMS AND SMART GOALS IN FACILITATING DIABETES REMISSION

Structured counseling initiatives play a vital role in assisting individuals with T2D to attain and sustain remission. Such programs generally integrate patient education, behavior change techniques, and continuous support to promote lasting lifestyle modifications. Incorporating SMART (Specific, Measurable, Achievable, Relevant, Time-bound) goals offers a systematic framework that enables patients to convert general lifestyle guidance into concrete, actionable strategies.[49]

The American College of Lifestyle Medicine's (ACLM) clinical practice guidelines advocate for the use of SMART goals in lifestyle interventions for T2D. These guidelines emphasize the importance of establishing priorities for lifestyle change through shared decision-making and utilizing SMART goals to support positive lifestyle changes. This approach has been associated with improved patient outcomes, including weight loss and better glycemic control.[50] Evidence suggests that structured counseling programs incorporating SMART goal setting can significantly enhance adherence to dietary changes, increase physical activity, and optimize medication use all of which are critical components for achieving and sustaining T2D remission. When reinforced with regular follow-up and professional support, SMART goals empower patients by breaking down broad health recommendations into clear, manageable actions that improve clinical outcomes. In particular, SMART goal-setting has proven effective as a behavioral strategy for promoting physical activity among individuals with diabetes. The integration of technology such as mobile health applications and wearable devices further strengthens this approach by facilitating real-time feedback, self-monitoring, and tailored guidance. A systematic review demonstrated that computer-based interventions, with or without wearable support, led to increased physical activity, weight loss, and reductions in HbA1c when paired with behavioral coaching.[51]

Similarly, in diabetes care, a 2022 study published in the *Journal of Pharmacy Practice* reported that patients who engaged in SMART goal-setting experienced clinically meaningful improvements in glycemic control. These patients demonstrated an average HbA1c reduction, required fewer medication adjustments, and showed enhanced overall disease management, with an average of 1.5 individualized goals set per participant. Collectively, these findings highlight the role of SMART goals not only in facilitating behavior change but also in translating generalized health guidance into practical, outcome-driven actions. Such approaches are instrumental in supporting durable diabetes remission and promoting long-term self-management.[52] Collectively, these findings underscore the critical role of structured counseling programs and SMART goal frameworks in empowering patients, optimizing lifestyle interventions, and supporting long-term metabolic improvement. By integrating these strategies, healthcare providers can enhance the likelihood of achieving durable remission in individuals with T2D.

CHALLENGES IN ACHIEVING TYPE 2 DIABETES REMISSION

Despite growing evidence supporting the feasibility of T2D remission, numerous systemic, socioeconomic, and individual-level barriers impede its widespread implementation and sustainability. A primary challenge lies in the limited accessibility of multidisciplinary care, which includes structured dietary counseling, supervised physical activity, psychological support, and continuous clinical monitoring. Such comprehensive care models are often unavailable or underutilized in resource-limited settings, where health systems may lack the requisite infrastructure, trained personnel, and integrated care pathways necessary to support long-term remission strategies.

Economic constraints further compound the problem, as many of the evidence-based interventions associated with remission such as very-low-calorie diets, CGM, and newer pharmacotherapies including GLP-1 receptor agonists and SGLT-2 inhibitors remain financially inaccessible to large segments of the population, particularly in low- and middle-income countries. The cost effectiveness and scalability of such interventions remain critical concerns, especially in publicly funded healthcare systems. A large observational study of 61,907 adults initiating GLP-1 receptor agonists found that patients facing higher 30-day out-of-pocket (OOP) costs were significantly less likely to stick with treatment (nonadherence). Higher costs were also associated with greater rates of diabetes-related hospitalizations and emergency department visits.[53]

Furthermore, sociocultural and behavioral factors present significant obstacles. The global rise in the availability and consumption of energy-dense, ultra-processed foods, coupled with sedentary lifestyles, undermines efforts to achieve the caloric restriction and weight loss necessary for remission. In many contexts, environmental determinants of health, such as food insecurity, lack of access to safe exercise spaces, and deeply entrenched cultural dietary practices, further complicate adherence to therapeutic lifestyle changes. Low health literacy, limited patient engagement, and psychosocial comorbidities such as depression, anxiety, or diabetes distress may also negatively impact adherence to remission-oriented interventions.

On the clinical front, the absence of standardized remission protocols, inadequate provider training, and the lack of consensus on long-term follow-up frameworks limit the integration of remission strategies into routine diabetes care. Moreover, remission may not be biologically attainable in all individuals particularly those with long-standing disease duration, marked β-cell failure, or significant comorbidities emphasizing the need for personalized approaches that account for disease heterogeneity.

In summary, the pursuit of diabetes remission must be contextualized within the broader challenges of healthcare access, affordability, cultural relevance, and patient engagement. Addressing these multifactorial barriers requires the development of equitable, culturally tailored, and evidence-informed strategies that can be feasibly implemented across diverse clinical and socioeconomic settings.

FUTURE DIRECTIONS IN ADVANCING DIABETES REMISSION

The pursuit of sustained remission in T2D necessitates the integration of personalized, technology-enabled, and system-level approaches. Future strategies should prioritize the following:

- *Integration of precision medicine:* Tailoring therapeutic interventions to individual genetic, metabolic, and behavioral profiles holds promise for optimizing remission outcomes. Precision approaches may identify subgroups most likely to benefit from specific dietary, pharmacological, or surgical interventions, thereby enhancing treatment efficacy and sustainability.
- *Application of AI:* AI enabled analytics can assist in early identification of candidates for remission, predict therapeutic responses, and optimize clinical decision-making through real-time data integration. Such technologies offer scalable tools to support individualized care pathways and proactive management.
- *Advancement of digital health technologies:* The adoption of CGM, telemedicine platforms, mobile applications, and digital therapeutics enables real-time monitoring, enhances patient engagement, and reinforces behavior change, all of which are essential for maintaining glycemic control and preventing relapse.
- *Establishment of structured follow-up systems:* Long-term remission is contingent upon ongoing surveillance and support. The development of standardized postremission monitoring frameworks, including both digital and in-person components, is vital to detect early signs of metabolic deterioration and facilitate timely interventions.
- *Addressing health equity and accessibility:* Ensuring equitable access to remission-focused care remains a critical challenge, particularly in low and middle-income countries. Efforts should include cost-reduction initiatives, integration of remission targets into public health policies, and expansion of infrastructure to deliver multidisciplinary care across diverse healthcare settings.

CONCLUSION

Diabetes remission represents a transformative approach in the management of T2D, shifting the focus from mere glycemic control to the restoration of metabolic health. Achieving and sustaining remission requires a multifaceted strategy, incorporating lifestyle modification, pharmacologic therapy, structured counseling, and digital health technologies. Advances in precision medicine and artificial intelligence offer the potential to individualize treatment, anticipate patient responses, and optimize long-term outcomes. Digital platforms and remote monitoring tools further enhance patient engagement, support behavior change, and enable timely clinical interventions. Despite these advances, barriers such as limited access, high costs, and resource constraints, particularly in low and middle-income settings, remain significant challenges. Addressing these issues through integrated, evidence-based, and technology enabled strategies is essential for realizing the potential of diabetes remission as a durable and achievable clinical goal.

REFERENCES

1. World Health Organization. Diabetes [Online] Available from https://www.who.int/news-room/fact-sheets/detail/diabetes [Last accessed October, 2025].
2. Riddle MC, Cefalu WT, Evans PH, Gerstein HC, Nauck MA, Oh WK, et al. Consensus Report: Definition and Interpretation of Remission in Type 2 Diabetes. Diabetes Care. 2021;44(10):2438-44.
3. Wisconsin Academy of Family physicians. 2025 ADA Standards of Medical Care in Diabetes: Updates! [Online] Available from https://www.wafp.org/assets/files/2025_ADA_Updates_All_Sections_95.pdf?utm [Last accessed October, 2025].
4. Diabetes UK. Diabetes UK. [Online] Available from https://www.diabetes.org.uk/about-diabetes/type-2-diabetes/remission/what-is-type-2-diabetes-remission [Last accessed October, 2025].
5. Karter AJ, Nundy S, Parker MM, Moffet HH, Huang ES. Incidence of Remission in Adults With Type 2 Diabetes: The Diabetes & Aging Study. Diabetes Care. 2014;37(12):3188-95.
6. Thom G, Messow C-M, Leslie WS, Barnes AC, Brosnahan N, McCombie L, et al. Predictors of type 2 diabetes remission in the Diabetes Remission Clinical Trial (DiRECT). Diabet Med. 2021;38(8):e14395.
7. Kanbour S, Ageeb RA, Malik RA, Abu-Raddad LJ. Impact of bodyweight loss on type 2 diabetes remission: a systematic review and meta-regression analysis of randomised controlled trials. Lancet Diabetes Endocrinol. 2025;13(4):294-306.
8. Jornayvaz FR, Shulman GI. Diacylglycerol Activation of Protein Kinase Cε and Hepatic Insulin Resistance. Cell Metab. 2012;15(5):574-84.
9. Raveendran AV. Remission of type 2 diabetes mellitus: Emerging concepts and proposed diagnostic criteria. World J Methodol. 2024;14(4):95210.
10. Vilas-Boas EA, Almeida DC, Roma LP, Ortis F, Carpinelli AR. Lipotoxicity and β-Cell Failure in Type 2 Diabetes: Oxidative Stress Linked to NADPH Oxidase and ER Stress. Cells. 2021;10(12):3328.
11. Kumar A, Margekar SL, Kumar R. Diabetes Remission: Myth or Reality? Indian J Med Spec. 2023;14(1):3-8.
12. Healthline. Is type 2 diabetes genetic? [Online] Available from https://www.healthline.com/health/type-2-diabetes/genetics [Last accessed October, 2025].
13. Aminian A, Brethauer SA, Kashyap SR, Kirwan JP, Schauer PR. DiaRem score: external validation. Lancet Diabetes Endocrinol. 2014;2(1):12-3.
14. Goldenberg JZ, Day A, Brinkworth GD, Sato J, Yamada S, Jönsson T, et al. Efficacy and safety of low and very low carbohydrate diets for type 2 diabetes remission: systematic review and meta-analysis of published and unpublished randomized trial data. BMJ. 2021;372:m4743.
15. Gower BA, Goss AM, Yurchishin ML, Deemer SE, Sunil B, Garvey WT. Effects of a carbohydrate-restricted diet on β-cell response in adults with type 2 diabetes. J Clin Endocrinol Metab. 2025;110(7):1811-7.
16. Kim J, Kim B, Kim MK, Baek KH, Song KH, Han K, et al. Lifestyle changes and remission in patients with new-onset type 2 diabetes: A Nationwide Cohort Study. J Korean Med Sci. 2025;40(7):e24.
17. Lean ME, Leslie WS, Barnes AC, Brosnahan N, Thom G, McCombie L, et al. Primary care-led weight management for remission of type 2 diabetes (DiRECT): an open-label, cluster-randomised trial. The Lancet. 2018;391(10120):541-51.
18. Diabetes UK. Weight loss can put type 2 diabetes into remission for at least 5 years, DiRECT study reveals. [Online] Available from https://www.diabetes.org.uk/about-us/news-and-views/weight-loss-can-put-type-2-diabetes-remission-least-five-years-reveal-latest-findings [Last accessed October, 2025].
19. Salvia MG. The Look AHEAD Trial: Translating lessons learned into clinical practice and further study. Diabetes Spectr. 2017;30(3):166-70.
20. Jackson HT, Anekwe C, Chang J, Haskins IN, Stanford FC. The role of bariatric surgery on diabetes and diabetic care compliance. Curr Diab Rep. 2019;19(11):125.
21. STAMPEDE Study. Cleveland Clinic. [Online] Available from https://my.clevelandclinic.org/departments/bariatric/medical-professionals/stampede [Last accessed October, 2025].
22. Kesavadev J, Shankar A, Krishnan G, Jothydev S. Liraglutide therapy beyond glycemic control: An observational study in Indian patients with type 2 diabetes in real world setting. Int J Gen Med. 2012;5:317-22.
23. Kesavadev J, Shankar A, Gopalakrishnan G, Jothydev S. Efficacy and safety of liraglutide therapy in 195 Indian patients with type 2 diabetes in real world setting. Diabetes Metab Syndr Clin Res Rev. 2015;9(1):30-3.
24. Sudhayakumar A, Arjunan D, Bhansali S, Bhujade H, Bhadada SK, Malhotra S, et al. Realisation of Remission of Diabetes Using Pharmacotherapy (DiaRem-1). Indian J Endocrinol Metab. 2025;29(2):217-23.
25. Punthakee Z, Hall S, McInnes N, Sherifali D, Tsiplova K, Kirabo FR, et al. Evaluating remission of type 2 diabetes using a metabolic intervention including fixed-ratio insulin degludec and liraglutide: A randomized controlled trial. Diabetes Obes Metab. 2024;26(12):5600-8.

26. Davies M, Færch L, Jeppesen OK, Pakseresht A, Pedersen SD, Perreault L, et al. Semaglutide 2·4 mg once a week in adults with overweight or obesity, and type 2 diabetes (STEP 2): a randomised, double-blind, double-dummy, placebo-controlled, phase 3 trial. The Lancet. 2021;397(10278):971-84.
27. McGowan BM, Bruun JM, Capehorn M, Pedersen SD, Pietiläinen KH, Muniraju HAK, et al. Efficacy and safety of once-weekly semaglutide 2·4 mg versus placebo in people with obesity and prediabetes (STEP 10): a randomised, double-blind, placebo-controlled, multicentre phase 3 trial. Lancet Diabetes Endocrinol. 2024;12(9):631-42.
28. Arakawa M, Ebato C. Efficacy of liraglutide as a follow-up therapy after resolution of glucotoxicity with intensive insulin therapy. Diabetes Metab Syndr Clin Res Rev. 2013;7(4):223-5.
29. Aronne LJ, Horn DB, Le Roux CW, Ho W, Falcon BL, Gomez Valderas E, et al. Tirzepatide as compared with semaglutide for the treatment of obesity. N Engl J Med. 2025;393(1):26-36.
30. Popovic DS, Patoulias D, Koufakis T, Stavropoulos K, Karakasis P, Ruža I, et al. Achievement of normoglycemia with tirzepatide in type 2 diabetes mellitus: A step closer to drug-induced diabetes remission? J Diabetes Complications. 2024;38(8):108800.
31. Sanyal AJ, Kaplan LM, Frias JP, Brouwers B, Wu Q, Thomas MK, et al. Triple hormone receptor agonist retatrutide for metabolic dysfunction-associated steatotic liver disease: a randomized phase 2a trial. Nat Med. 2024;30(7):2037-48.
32. Van De Laar FA, Lucassen PL, Akkermans RP, Van De Lisdonk EH, De Grauw WJ. (2006) Alpha-glucosidase inhibitors for people with impaired glucose tolerance or impaired fasting blood glucose. [Online] Available from https://doi.wiley.com/10.1002/14651858.CD005061.pub2 [Last accessed October, 2025].
33. Sugiyama S, Jinnouchi H, Hieshima K, Kurinami N, Jinnouchi K. (2020). Type 2 Diabetes Remission and Substantial Body Weight Reduction Achieved with Metformin and a Sodium-Glucose Cotransporter 2 Inhibitor. [Online] Available from https://www.cureus.com/articles/27508-type-2-diabetes-remission-and-substantial-body-weight-reduction-achieved-with-metformin-and-a-sodium-glucose-cotransporter-2-inhibitor [Last accessed October, 2025].
34. Rosenstock J, Wysham C, Frías JP, Kaneko S, Lee CJ, Fernández Landó L, et al. Efficacy and safety of a novel dual GIP and GLP-1 receptor agonist tirzepatide in patients with type 2 diabetes (SURPASS-1): a double-blind, randomised, phase 3 trial. The Lancet. 2021;398(10295):143-55.
35. Frías JP, Davies MJ, Rosenstock J, Pérez Manghi FC, Fernández Landó L, Bergman BK, et al. Tirzepatide versus semaglutide once weekly in patients with type 2 diabetes. N Engl J Med. 2021;385(6):503-15.
36. Kesavadev J, Joshi S, Saboo B, Thacker H, Shankar A, David A, et al. Abstract #238: Improved short term and long term outcomes of early insulin initiation in type 2 diabetes over 10 years. Endocr Pract. 2017; 23:50.
37. Kesavadev J, Warrier R, Ramachandran L, Shankar A, David A, Ajai NA, et al. 530-P: Early Insulin Initiation in T2DM Is Associated with Prevention of eGFR Decline and Lower Insulin Dose Requirements. Diabetes. 2019;68(Supplement_1):530-P.
38. Novograd J, Frishman WH. Teplizumab therapy to delay the onset of type 1 diabetes. Cardiol Rev. 2024;32(6):572-6.
39. Ramos EL, Dayan CM, Chatenoud L, Sumnik Z, Simmons KM, Szypowska A, et al. Teplizumab and β-Cell function in newly diagnosed type 1 diabetes. N Engl J Med. 2023;389(23):2151-61.
40. Abstracts from ATTD 20147th International Conference on AdvancedTechnologies & Treatments for Diabetes Vienna, Austria, February 5–8, 2014. Diabetes Technol Ther. 2014;16(S1):A-1-A-162.
41. Wang Y, Lu J, Wang M, Ni J, Yu J, Wang S, et al. Real-time continuous glucose monitoring-guided glucose management in inpatients with diabetes receiving short-term continuous subcutaneous insulin infusion: a randomized clinical trial. Lancet Reg Health - West Pac. 2024;48:101067.
42. Turquetil A, Morello R, Joubert M, Le Roux Y, Reznik Y. Early continuous glucose monitoring for predicting remission of type 2 diabetes 1 year after bariatric surgery. Diabetes Metab. 2021;47(6):101255.
43. Nguyen V, Ara P, Simmons D, Osuagwu UL. The role of digital health technology interventions in the prevention of type 2 diabetes mellitus: A systematic review. Clin Med Insights Endocrinol Diabetes. 2024;17:11795514241246419.
44. Hsia J, Guthrie NL, Lupinacci P, Gubbi A, Denham D, Berman MA, et al. Randomized, controlled trial of a digital behavioral therapeutic application to improve glycemic control in adults with type 2 diabetes. Diabetes Care. 2022;45(12):2976-81.
45. Lee YB, Kim G, Jun JE, Park H, Lee WJ, Hwang YC, et al. An integrated digital health care platform for diabetes management with AI-based dietary management: 48-week results from a randomized controlled trial. Diabetes Care. 2023;46(5):959-66.
46. Chawla R, Jaggi S, Gupta A, Bantwal G, Patil S. Clinical utility of a digital therapeutic intervention in Indian

patients with type 2 diabetes mellitus: 12-week prospective single-Arm Intervention Study. JMIR Diabetes. 2022;7(4):e41401.

47. Shamanna P, Dharmalingam M, Vadavi A, Keshavamurthy A, Bhonsley S, Thajudeen M, et al. 20-OR: Digital twin (DT) technology in type 2 diabetes remission and glycemic improvement—eighteen months results from a randomized controlled trial. Diabetes. 2024;73(Supplement_1):20-OR.
48. Lim SL, Ong KW, Johal J, Han CY, Yap QV, Chan YH, et al. Effect of a smartphone app on weight change and metabolic outcomes in Asian adults with type 2 diabetes: A randomized clinical trial. JAMA Netw Open. 2021;4(6):e2112417.
49. Thorough Care. SMART Goals: A Collaborative and Patient-centered Approach to Health. [Online] Available from https://www.thoroughcare.net/blog/smart-goals-patient-centered-care-coordination?utm [Last accessed October, 2025].
50. Rosenfeld RM. American College of Lifestyle Medicine. 2025. New clinical practice guideline puts lifestyle interventions at forefront of diabetes care. [Online] Available from https://lifestylemedicine.org/lifestyle-medicine-and-the-path-to-type-2-diabetes-remission/ [Last accessed October, 2025].
51. Takahashi PY, Quigg SM, Croghan IT, Schroeder DR, Ebbert JO. SMART goals setting and biometric changes in obese adults with multimorbidity: Secondary analysis of a randomized controlled trial. SAGE Open Med. 2019;7:2050312119858042.
52. Cook HE, Garris LA, Gulum AH, Steber CJ. Impact of SMART goals on diabetes management in a pharmacist-led telehealth clinic. J Pharm Pract. 2024;37(1):54-9.
53. Zhang D, Gencerliler N, Mukhopadhyay A, Blecker S, Grams ME, Wright DR, et al. Association of patient cost sharing with adherence to GLP-1RA and Adverse health outcomes. Diabetes Care. 2025;48(8):1329-36.

28

Diabetes Mellitus and Sports Medicine

Kenjom Ngomdir, Abhinav Verma

ABSTRACT

Diabetes mellitus, once viewed as a constraint to athletic participation, is now increasingly recognized as a condition that can be effectively managed to support optimal performance. This chapter explores the intersection of diabetes mellitus and sports medicine, focusing on both the physiological implications of exercise in individuals with type 1 and type 2 diabetes mellitus, and the necessary clinical, nutritional, and pharmacological adaptations. It addresses essential screening protocols, risk management strategies, and the impact of physical activity on glycemic control and overall health outcomes. The discussion further integrates recent technological advancements—such as continuous glucose monitoring, automated insulin delivery systems, and precision nutrition—into practical frameworks for athletic participation. Through a multidisciplinary approach, the chapter provides evidence-based guidance to healthcare professionals supporting individuals with diabetes mellitus in both recreational and competitive sports, emphasizing safety, performance, and long-term metabolic health.

Keywords: Diabetes mellitus, Sports medicine, Exercise physiology, Glycemic control, Insulin management.

"When the whistle blows, the clock ticks, and the crowd roars, the real opponent isn't the rival team—it's the condition inside your own body. For Kapil Dev, Anil Kumble, Wasim Akram, Alexander Zverev and a growing roster of Indian athletes, diabetes became the silent teammate that forced them to rewrite the playbook on health, discipline, and triumph."

INTRODUCTION

This chapter delves into how renowned athletes have transformed the challenge of diabetes mellitus into an opportunity to adopt performance-boosting lifestyle habits. The discipline of *sports medicine* plays a critical role in exploring two major dimensions of this connection: How athletes manage diabetes mellitus while engaging in physical activity, and the potential short- and long-term effects of exercise on individuals with diabetes mellitus.[1,2]

Athletes diagnosed with diabetes mellitus often need to make specific modifications to their routines in order to safely participate in training and competition. In return, physical activity may offer therapeutic benefits, provided that it is approached with proper medical oversight.

Numerous accomplished athletes have demonstrated that a diabetes mellitus diagnosis is not a barrier to success. A notable example is Sir Steve Redgrave, the British rower, who was diagnosed with diabetes mellitus at 35 after already securing four Olympic gold medals. Despite this diagnosis, he continued his career and remarkably secured a fifth gold medal at the 2000 Sydney Olympics.

In India, several high-level athletes have also defied diabetes mellitus and achieved success, including cricket legends Kapil Dev and Anil Kumble, as well as tennis player Kyra Shroff. On the global stage, celebrated figures such as swimmer Gary Hall (winner of 10 Olympic medals), fast bowler Wasim Akram, and tennis star Alexander Zverev (Olympic gold medalist and former world number two) stand as testaments to what can be accomplished despite living with this condition.

CLINICAL IMPLICATIONS

Diagnosis

Type 1 and type 2 diabetes mellitus are typically diagnosed through specific blood glucose criteria. A fasting plasma glucose level taken after at least 8 hours without food that is above 7 mmol/L (126 mg/dL), or a reading exceeding 11 mmol/L (200 mg/dL) 2 hours following an oral glucose tolerance test, are indicative of diabetes mellitus. In addition, the emergence of characteristic symptoms may also support the diagnosis.[3]

Pre-participation Medical Screening

It is now standard practice—especially in contact sports—to conduct a comprehensive medical evaluation for all athletes prior to the season, training, or competition. This includes screening for metabolic conditions such as diabetes mellitus.

Diabetes Mellitus Screening in Athletes

Before beginning or intensifying an exercise regimen, diabetic individuals should undergo a full medical evaluation. Special focus should be placed on examining potential diabetic complications, particularly in the cardiovascular system, lower extremities, and eyes.

To ensure safe participation in sports, the athlete's blood sugar must be reasonably controlled. Long-term glycemic markers like glycated hemoglobin (HbA1c) and fructosamine provide valuable insight. HbA1c reflects control over the past 2–3 months, whereas fructosamine covers a shorter span of roughly 3 weeks. Laboratory reference ranges may vary, but in general, an HbA1c of 7% or less is considered acceptable.

Patients are encouraged to maintain a diary of blood glucose measurements taken at different times of the day. It is also advisable to assess cholesterol and triglycerides, as well as kidney function, which includes evaluating levels of urea, creatinine, and electrolytes. Further tests may involve checking for protein in the urine and calculating creatinine clearance.

Key Areas for Physical Examination

- *Cardiovascular*: This includes monitoring blood pressure (including changes on standing), checking heart sounds, peripheral pulses, and listening for carotid bruits.
- *Ophthalmologic*: Screening for diabetic eye complications such as retinopathy, cataracts, and glaucoma
- *Neurologic*: Evaluating for signs of peripheral neuropathy

CARDIAC RISK ASSESSMENT PRIOR TO EXERCISE

A thorough cardiovascular evaluation is vital before starting exercise, especially because ischemic heart disease affects up to 50% of individuals with type 2 diabetes mellitus at diagnosis. Due to autonomic neuropathy, many diabetics may not experience chest pain even during cardiac events, making screening essential.

Exercise stress testing is advised in individuals who meet any of the following criteria:

- Engage in high-intensity physical activity (above 60% of predicted maximum heart rate)
- Have had type 2 diabetes mellitus for >10 years
- Have had type 1 diabetes mellitus for over 15 years
- Are older than 25 years
- Exhibit any cardiovascular disease risk factors
- Have evidence of microvascular or macrovascular complications
- Have diagnosed peripheral arterial disease

DIABETES MELLITUS AND ITS COMPLICATIONS

Both type 1 and type 2 diabetes mellitus can contribute to a range of complications that impact several organ systems. A major concern is the acceleration of atherosclerosis, significantly raising the chances of acute heart attacks—by approximately two to three times. Similarly, peripheral artery disease becomes more prevalent, and the likelihood of stroke nearly doubles. Additionally, diabetes mellitus may lead to damage in the eyes (retinopathy), kidneys (nephropathy), and nerves (autonomic neuropathy), which can result in delayed stomach emptying, impaired sweating mechanisms, and even asymptomatic heart ischemia. These complications are especially critical for those engaging in physical activity. The probability of developing such issues increases with the duration of the disease and poor glucose regulation. Statistically, individuals living with diabetes mellitus have a life expectancy about two-thirds that of those without the condition.[4]

TREATMENT OPTIONS IN DIABETES MELLITUS

Managing diabetes mellitus, whether type 1 or type 2, revolves around keeping blood sugar levels as close to normal as possible. For individuals with T1DM, external insulin administration is essential, complemented by dietary regulation and frequent glucose monitoring. In contrast, insulin is typically prescribed only when lifestyle management fails in people with type 2 diabetes mellitus. Most type 2 diabetics can manage their condition through structured exercise, dietary changes, and weight reduction.

However, if these interventions prove insufficient, oral hypoglycemic medications may be introduced. These drugs are generally used before resorting to insulin, which is reserved for patients who cannot achieve control otherwise. Regardless of diabetes mellitus type, a diet low in fat and rich in complex carbohydrates, while limiting simple sugars, is highly recommended for effective management.

Diabetes Mellitus and Its Pharmacotherapy

There are four main categories of insulin based on how quickly they act and how long they last:

1. *Rapid-acting insulin*: This form begins working within 5–15 minutes, peaks at around 1 hour, and remains effective for 3–5 hours. Examples are insulin lispro and insulin aspart.
2. *Short-acting insulin*: Onset occurs in about 30 minutes, with a peak effect between 2 and 3 hours and a duration of action lasting 5–8 hours. Common types include regular insulin such as Actrapid and Humulin R.
3. *Intermediate-acting insulin*: These have a delayed onset of 1–2 hours, reach peak activity between 4 and 10 hours, and offer extended effects for 6–18 hours. Examples include Protophane and Monotard.
4. *Long-acting insulin*: These begin acting after >2 hours and can maintain basal insulin levels for a full 24 hours. Glargine is one such example. Insulin Degludec is another long-acting option that does not have a sharp peak; it typically starts working within 1.5 hours and maintains effectiveness for 11–24 hours.

Insulin Therapy in Physically Active Individuals

For diabetic individuals who exercise, insulin regimens can be customized. A typical routine may involve taking rapid-acting insulin before meals and a longer-acting dose at bedtime. Alternatively, some may use continuous subcutaneous insulin infusion (CSII), where a pump delivers small, controlled doses throughout the day and larger boluses before food intake. The device's infusion set is usually changed every 2–3 days. However, these pumps can malfunction or become blocked, and their upkeep can be expensive.

Oral Hypoglycemic Agents in Type 2 Diabetes Mellitus

Patients with type 2 diabetes mellitus who do not respond well to lifestyle adjustments over a 2- to 3-month period may be prescribed oral hypoglycemics. If exercise leads to weight reduction, the dosage of these medications might be lowered or discontinued altogether. *Metformin* is generally the first-line therapy, improving insulin sensitivity and decreasing glucose production in the liver.

Sulfonylureas, another class of medications, work by stimulating the pancreas to release more insulin. However, they carry a risk of causing hypoglycemia and should be used carefully during intense exercise. If, after 3 months of using a single medication (monotherapy), HbA1c levels are still above 7%, healthcare providers may recommend combining drugs for better control.

Pump Therapy: Continuous Subcutaneous Insulin Delivery

Continuous subcutaneous insulin infusions (or pump therapy) are being used to tighten control and increase flexibility of treatment. Benefits include fewer erratic swings in blood glucose and decreased risk of hypoglycemia, more appropriate matching of insulin to food intake, and improved targeting of the dawn phenomena.

There are two main components to insulin delivery in pump therapy:

1. *Basal insulin* is delivered as a continuous infusion of small increments of rapidly acting insulin over 24 hours to meet requirements during fasting and sleep. This generally comprises 40–50% of total daily insulin use.
2. *Bolus insulin* is patient-activated doses given with meals to correct hyperglycemic excursions. Mealtime boluses can be delivered in one of two ways. The standard single wave bolus delivers the entire dose within 1–2 minutes, while a dual wave bolus gives part of the dose immediately with the remainder being infused slowly over a predetermined time. The infusion set is replaced every 2–3 days with a new subcutaneous infusion site. Some circulating insulin is required to maintain glycemic control during exercise, which may be facilitated by an insulin pump.

NUTRITION AND HYDRATION MANAGEMENT FOR THE DIABETIC ATHLETE

The significance of a diet rich in carbohydrates and low in fat for optimal glycemic control is now well-recognized.

Fortunately, this aligns with the established recommendations aimed at enhancing athletic performance. Some individuals, particularly older adults with type 2 diabetes mellitus, may have previously followed a low-carbohydrate diet, which could lead to depleted glycogen reserves and diminished physical output. The carbohydrate needs of athletes can differ significantly, so it is vital that individuals regularly track their blood glucose to tailor carbohydrate intake before, during, and after physical activity.

Responses to physical exertion differ greatly among individuals. Accurate determination of personal carbohydrate needs can only be achieved through regular glucose monitoring at various stages of exercise. **Table 1** can serve as an initial reference but should not be relied

TABLE 1: Meal timing and frequency.			
Pretraining	30–60 g carbs + 15–20 g protein	30–60 minutes before exercise	For example, banana with peanut butter
During prolonged activity (>60 minutes)	30–60 g easily digestible carbs	Every hour	Sports drinks, glucose gels, or fruit
Post-training	1.0–1.2 g carbs/kg + 20–25 g protein	Within 30 minutes for glycogen replenishment	For example, roti + lentils + curd
Regular meals	4–6 small meals/snacks	Daily to avoid large glucose fluctuations	Regular normal meals

upon exclusively. Endurance athletes engaging in carbohydrate loading before an event might need to increase insulin dosage to compensate for the elevated carbohydrate consumption. Ensuring proper insulin-carbohydrate balance before, during, and after the event is critical.

It is recommended that insulin-dependent athletes receive tailored advice from a healthcare team, including a sports dietitian and physician, to design an individualized nutrition and training plan. Key considerations for diabetic athletes include:

- Understanding how various forms of exercise and environmental conditions affect their blood glucose response
- Always carrying fast-acting carbohydrate sources—such as fruits, fruit juices, barley sugar, or biscuits—especially when exercising away from home
- After strenuous activity, glucose levels may remain low for several hours. It is crucial to replenish glycogen by consuming carbohydrates postexercise to avoid hypoglycemia.
- Dehydration can mimic low blood sugar symptoms. Athletes should stay hydrated by drinking adequate fluids before, during, and after workouts.
- Alcohol should be avoided after exercise, as it can both reduce blood sugar and worsen dehydration.
- The optimal time for training is when blood sugar is slightly elevated but not too high—typically 1–2 hours after eating.
- During intermittent exercises, carbohydrate intake during breaks is essential to stabilize glucose levels and manage hunger.
- For long-duration physical activities, consistent intake of food or fluids containing carbohydrates is essential to maintain glucose availability.
- Lastly, insulin absorption from limbs may increase during physical exertion. To manage this, it may be helpful to inject insulin into areas of the body less affected by muscular activity, such as the abdomen.

Nutritional Tweaks for Diabetic Athletes

"Food is fuel, but for athletes with diabetes, it's also a finely tuned medication."

Nutrition for diabetic athletes is not about restriction, it is about precision. By mastering the timing, quality, and balance of every bite, athletes can keep their blood sugar in the sweet spot while powering through every sprint, jump, and swing **(Tables 2 and 3)**.

Why Nutrition Matters?

- *Stabilizes blood glucose*: Keeps levels steady before, during, and after training/competition
- *Optimizes performance*: Provides sustained energy without spikes or crashes
- *Supports recovery*: Aids muscle repair, glycogen restoration, and overall health

TABLE 2: Hydration and electrolytes for diabetics undertaking sports and exercises.

Water	500 mL to 1 L per hour of activity; more in hot/humid conditions
Electrolytes	Add natural sources like coconut water, lemon juice, or salted buttermilk to prevent hyponatremia.

TABLE 3: Sample diabetic (2,500 kcal) athlete meal plan.

Meal timing	*What's on the plate?—Carbs, protein, fats*
Breakfast 7:00 AM	1 cup rolled oats cooked with 1 cup skim milk + 1 tsp ghee + 1 banana + 2 almonds—*Carbs 55 g, protein 15 g, fats 8 g*
Midmorning 10:00 AM	1 small apple + 1 cup low-fat Greek yogurt—*Carbs 25 g, protein 12 g, fats 3 g*
Lunch 12:30 PM	1 cup brown rice + 1 cup mixed dal + 1 cup sautéed veggies + 1 tsp olive oil + 1 cup cucumber raita—*Carbs 70 g, protein 18 g, fats 10 g*
Afternoon snack 3:30 PM	1 cup roasted chana + 1 orange—*Carbs 30 g, protein 10 g, fats 5 g*
Pre-workout 5:00 PM	1 slice whole wheat bread + 1 tbsp peanut butter + ½ cup low-fat milk—*Carbs 30 g, protein 15 g, fats 10 g*
Post-workout 7:00 PM	1 cup sweet potato mash + 100 g grilled fish + ½ cup steamed broccoli—*Carbs 45 g, protein 25 g, fats 8 g*
Dinner 8:30 PM	2 rotis + 1 cup mixed vegetable curry + 1 cup low-fat paneer cubes + ½ cup curd—*Carbs 55 g, protein 20 g, fats 12 g*
Night snack 10:00 PM	½ cup warm milk + 1 tsp honey (optional)—*Carbs 15 g, protein 5 g, fats 3 g*

Key Principles

- *Balanced macronutrients*:
  - *Carbohydrates*: 45–60% of total calories, focusing on complex carb (whole grains, legumes, vegetables) for slow release
  - *Proteins*: 15–20% for muscle repair; include lean sources (pulses, fish, poultry, low-fat dairy)
  - *Fats*: 20–30% from healthy sources (nuts, seeds, olive oil, and fatty fish) for hormone regulation and satiety
- *Glycemic management*:
  - Choose low-to-moderate glycemic index (GI) foods (e.g., oats, barley, sweet potatoes) to prevent rapid spikes.
  - Pair carbs with protein/fiber (e.g., chickpeas with rice, nuts with fruit) to blunt post-meal glucose rise.
- Meal timing and frequency **(Table 1)**
- Hydration and electrolytes for diabetics undertaking sports and exercises **(Table 2)**
- Sample diabetic (2,500 kcal) athlete meal plan **(Table 3)**

Adjust portions based on individual energy needs, activity level, and blood glucose response.

Practical Tips for Diabetic Indian Athletes

- Swap white rice for *red/brown rice, millets (bajra, jowar), or quinoa.*
- *Use ghee/cold-pressed oils* in moderation for flavor and sustained energy.
- *Incorporate regional superfoods*: Fenugreek seeds, amla, turmeric, and bitter gourd for their glucose-lowering properties.
- *Carry portable snacks*: Roasted makhana, dates, or murmura (puffed rice) with peanuts for quick carbs during training.
- *Monitor and log*: Keep a daily food + glucose diary; adjust carbs based on pre/postexercise readings.

Common Pitfalls and How to Avoid Them

- *Skipping meals*: Hypoglycemia, stick to scheduled timings
- *Overrelying on sugary drinks*: Opt for natural sources like fruit juice diluted with water.
- *Ignoring portion sizes*: Use standard measures (cup, fist-sized) to control carb intake.
- *Neglecting nighttime snacks*: A small protein + carb combo prevents nocturnal lows.[5-8]

EXERCISE AND DIABETES MELLITUS

Close collaboration between sports physicians and endocrinologists is essential when crafting an exercise regimen for individuals with diabetes mellitus. Adults should aim to perform a minimum of 30 minutes of continuous moderate physical activity—such as brisk walking—on most days of the week. Alternatively, shorter durations of high-intensity exercise may be beneficial, provided that underlying cardiovascular or hypertensive issues are considered. Due to autonomic neuropathy, heart rate monitoring may not reliably reflect exertion levels; instead, perceived exertion rating scales are recommended.

Exercise, combined with appropriate nutrition and medication, remains central to diabetes mellitus management. However, insulin users require special consideration. Both insulin and physical activity enhance glucose uptake through GLUT4 transporter activation. Their combined effects can significantly increase glucose transport into muscle cells. For individuals with type 1 diabetes mellitus, this often results in up to a 30% reduction in insulin requirements during periods of regular exercise. Nevertheless, exercise alone does not guarantee better glycemic control unless insulin dosage and dietary intake are properly adjusted. Insulin sensitivity tends to decline rapidly—even after short periods of physical inactivity.

It is crucial for individuals with diabetes mellitus to closely monitor their blood glucose levels before and after each workout. During prolonged activity or if symptoms present, midsession glucose testing is advisable. If glucose monitoring is unavailable prior to exercise, sessions should be kept short and low in intensity, with quick-access carbohydrate sources on hand.

Environmental factors such as high temperatures or strong winds may necessitate additional glucose intake during activity. Conversely, during illness or minor infections, elevated glucose levels may occur, warranting closer monitoring.

Diabetic individuals should always carry a form of medical identification. They should be taught to recognize early symptoms of hypoglycemia, especially during the 6–12 hours following physical activity. It is also essential to carry glucose tablets or alternative fast-acting carbohydrates at all times. Maintaining hydration is vital, and exercising with a partner is recommended when possible.[9]

BENEFITS OF EXERCISE

In people with type 1 diabetes mellitus, regular exercise enhances insulin sensitivity, improves lipid profiles, lowers resting heart rate and blood pressure, and helps with weight control—factors that contribute to a reduced risk of coronary heart disease. While improved glycemic control is not consistently observed, insulin needs may decrease slightly. Most of the benefits are cardiovascular in nature.

Engaging in consistent physical activity is associated with increased life expectancy in individuals with type 2 diabetes mellitus.[10] Regular exercise also significantly lowers the risk of developing type 2 diabetes mellitus. Those already diagnosed with type 2 diabetes mellitus may experience major metabolic improvements through sustained physical activity.[11] A structured exercise program can help reverse impairments in both lipid and glucose metabolism common in type 2 diabetes mellitus.[12]

Glycated hemoglobin, a marker for long-term glucose regulation, tends to decrease with long-term exercise in people with type 2 diabetes mellitus. However, evidence for this effect in type 1 diabetes mellitus remains less compelling.

EXERCISE AND TYPE 1 DIABETES MELLITUS

Managing blood glucose in type 1 diabetes mellitus relies on careful balancing of food intake, physical activity, and insulin dosing. Meal plans and insulin amounts must be tailored based on how each individual responds to exercise. This often involves a trial-and-error approach when beginning new physical activities. Frequent self-monitoring is critical until a personalized balance is achieved. Ideally, blood glucose should be maintained between 6.6 and 10 mmol/L (up to 180 mg/dL) before exercising.

Individuals with glucose levels above 11 mmol/L (200 mg/dL) or >16.5 mmol/L (300 mg/dL)—especially if ketones are present—should avoid exercise and take corrective insulin. Conversely, those with glucose levels below 5.5 mmol/L (100 mg/dL) should consume a carbohydrate-rich snack prior to exercising.

Low-intensity activities lasting 20–30 minutes (e.g., walking, golf) require minimal insulin adjustments, with a small carbohydrate intake of 15 g (about 60 calories). Moderate activities under 1 hour (e.g., jogging, swimming) usually necessitate a 25% reduction in pre-exercise insulin and 15–30 g of carbohydrate before and every 30 minutes during activity. High-intensity or prolonged exercise (e.g., triathlons) may demand a 30–80% reduction in insulin and double carbohydrate intake every 30 minutes.

Excess insulin heightens the risk of hypoglycemia, particularly during intense exercise. Morning exercise may require reducing the previous night's intermediate-acting insulin by 20–50% and adjusting or skipping the morning dose of short-acting insulin. Further reductions of 30–50% may be needed at subsequent meals based on exercise duration and intensity. Although hyperglycemia may follow exercise, insulin doses should still be reduced due to increased insulin sensitivity lasting up to 15 hours.

Post-exercise carbohydrate intake within 30 minutes can enhance muscle glycogen restoration and help prevent delayed hypoglycemia, which may occur up to 24 hours later.[13] If physical activity is unplanned, insulin adjustments may not be feasible; instead, consuming 20–30 g of carbohydrates at the start and every 30 minutes during exercise can reduce hypoglycemia risk.

Elite athletes often require greater reductions in insulin dosing during intense exercise. During rest periods—such as vacation or recovery from injury—higher insulin doses are typically needed.

TYPE 2 DIABETES MELLITUS, EXERCISE, AND SPORTS

Individuals with type 2 diabetes mellitus managed through diet alone usually do not need to adjust their routine for exercise. However, those on oral hypoglycemics might need to reduce or skip doses before prolonged activity, depending on glucose readings. Carrying fast-acting glucose and recognizing symptoms of hypoglycemia is essential.

Hypoglycemia poses a greater risk for those taking sulfonylureas due to their prolonged effects and increased insulin production. In contrast, medications like metformin (a biguanide) pose a lower risk as they do not enhance insulin secretion.

COMPETITION AND DIABETES MELLITUS

Athletes with diabetes mellitus involved in team sports must have a clear understanding of their typical glucose responses to exercise. Because competitions often involve interstate travel and changes in dietary habits, diabetic athletes should simulate game-day routines beforehand and keep

DIABETES MELLITUS AND MANIFESTATIONS OF MUSCULOSKELETAL DISORDERS

Several musculoskeletal disorders are more prevalent in diabetics. Common conditions include:

- Osteoarthritis—18% in diabetics versus 5% in nondiabetics
- Frozen shoulder—11–30% versus 2–10%
- Limited joint mobility—8–50% versus 0–26%
- Dupuytren's contracture—20–63% versus 13%
- Carpal tunnel syndrome—11–16% versus 0.125%
- Flexor tenosynovitis—11% versus <1%
- Diffuse idiopathic skeletal hyperostosis—13–49% versus 1.6–13%[15]

WORLD ANTI-DOPING AGENCY AND THE DIABETIC ATHLETE

To prevent Anti-Doping Rule Violations (ADRVs), physicians must understand World Anti-Doping Agency (WADA) regulations:

- Oral hypoglycemics are not prohibited.
- Insulin for type 1 diabetics mellitus is permitted and must be declared.
- IV infusions >100 mL/12 hours are prohibited unless administered in a clinical setting.
- Metformin, sodium-glucose cotransporter-2 (SGLT-2) inhibitors, glucagon-like peptide-1 (GLP-1) agonists are allowed. Stimulants with performance benefits are subject to WADA rules.
- Athlete biological passport (ABP) abnormalities may trigger testing, but insulin and necessary diabetic treatment are not penalized.[16-19]

Key takeaways:

- Secure a *therapeutic use exemption* (TUE) for insulin.
- Adhere to IV fluid limits outside of clinical settings.
- Review annual WADA updates for relevant changes.

RECENT ADVANCES AND LATEST TRENDS FOR DIABETIC ATHLETES

- *Continuous glucose monitors (CGM)*: Provide real-time glucose trends and alerts for insulin/carb adjustments.
- *Smart pumps and closed-loop systems*: Auto-adjust insulin delivery using CGM data.
- *Ultra-rapid insulin analogues*: Allow precise postexercise dosing.
- *CGM-driven adjustments*: Pair CGM with smart pens for insulin and carb precision.
- *Mini-dose glucagon and dual-hormone pumps*: Minimize hypoglycemia during long bouts.
- *Exercise-specific apps*: Offer dosing advice, snack timing, and recovery support.
- *High-intensity interval training (HIIT) guidance*: Use GLUT-4 activation; basal rate cuts and fast carbs aid performance.
- *Personalized strategies*: Exercise timing and snack planning optimize glycemia.
- *Nutrition tweaks*: Mediterranean diet, protein balance, and carb timing boost performance.
- *Mental conditioning*: Stress management and focus training help athletes maintain control under pressure.[20-24]

CONCLUSION

Diabetic athletes and their support staff must understand the interplay of exercise and glycemia. With consistent glucose monitoring and tailored insulin and carb strategies, diabetic athletes can safely and effectively engage in sports.

A combined aerobic and resistance training regimen offers optimal benefits. Thanks to new advancements in CGMs, insulin delivery, and AI-driven tools, even those with severe diabetes mellitus can aim for peak performance levels.

The synergy of real-time monitoring, smarter delivery systems, and data-driven decision-making empowers diabetic athletes to train smarter, compete safely, and recover efficiently.

REFERENCES

1. World Health Organization. Diabetes — Health topics. WHO Regional Office for Europe. [online] Available from https://www.who.int/europe/health-topics/diabetes [Last accessed December, 2025].
2. Hossain P, Kawar B, El Nahas M. Obesity and diabetes in the developing world: a growing challenge. N Engl J Med. 2007;356(3):213-5.
3. American Diabetes Association. Diagnosis and classification of diabetes mellitus. Diabetes Care. 2010;33(Suppl 1):S62-9.
4. Riebe D, Franklin BA, Thompson PD, Garber CE, Whitfield GP, Magal M, et al. Updating ACSM's recommendations for exercise preparticipation health screening. Med Sci Sports Exerc. 2015;47(11):2473-9.
5. Today's Dietitian. Fueled by technology — athletic performance and nutrition trends [online] Available from https://www.todaysdietitian.com [Last accessed October, 2025].
6. Thomas DT, Erdman KA, Burke LM. The competitive athlete with type 1 diabetes mellitus: nutritional strategies for optimal performance. Nutr Rev. 2016;74(2):101-14.
7. Burke LM, Hawley JA. Current trends and strategies in sports nutrition for performance enhancement. Curr Opin Clin Nutr Metab Care. 2018;21(6):452-8.
8. Mujika I, Burke LM. Nutritional therapy for athletes: practical applications and future perspectives. Nutrients. 2021;13(10):3456.
9. Brukner P, Khan K, Clarsen B, Cook J, Cools A, Crossley K, et al. Brukner & Khan's Clinical Sports Medicine: Injuries, Volume 1, 5th edition. North Ryde: McGraw-Hill Education; 2021.
10. Moy CS, Songer TJ, LaPorte RE, Dorman JS, Kriska AM, Orchard TJ, et al. Insulin-dependent diabetes mellitus, physical activity, and death. Am J Epidemiol. 1993;137(1):74-81.
11. Boule NG, Haddad E, Kenny GP, Wells GA, Sigal RJ. Effects of exercise on glycemic control and body mass in type 2 diabetes mellitus: a meta-analysis of controlled clinical trials. JAMA. 2001;286(10):1218-27.
12. Farrell PA. Diabetes, exercise and competitive sports. Gatorade Sports Sci Inst Sports Sci Exchange. 2003;16(1):1-6.
13. Colberg SR, Sigal RJ, Yardley JE, Riddell MC, Dunstan DW, Dempsey PC, et al. Physical activity/exercise and diabetes: a position statement of the American Diabetes Association. Diabetes Care. 2016;39(11):2065-79.
14. Draznin M. Type 1 diabetes and sports participation: strategies for training and competing safely. Physician Sportsmed. 2000;28(12):49-56.
15. Smith LL, Burnet SP, McNeil JD. Musculoskeletal manifestations of diabetes mellitus. Br J Sports Med. 2003;37(1):30-5.
16. Riddell MC, Gallen IW, Smart CE, Taplin CE, Adolfsson P, Lumb AN, et al. Exercise management in type 1 diabetes: a consensus statement. Lancet Diabetes Endocrinol. 2017;5(5):377-90.
17. Yardley JE, Sigal RJ. Exercise strategies for hypoglycemia prevention in individuals with type 1 diabetes. Diabetes Spectrum. 2022;35(1):38-47.
18. Bally L, Thabit H, Hartnell S, Andereggen E, Ruan Y, Wilinska ME, et al. Closed-loop insulin delivery for prevention of hypoglycemia during exercise in adults with type 1 diabetes. Diabetologia. 2021;64(3):597-606.
19. Jeukendrup AE. Periodized nutrition for athletes. Sports Med. 2017;47(Suppl 1):51-63.
20. International Diabetes Federation. Home | International Diabetes Federation. [online] Available from https://idf.org/[Last accessed December, 2025].
21. International Diabetes Federation. Type 1 diabetes. IDF – About diabetes: Types of diabetes. [online] Available from https://idf.org/about-diabetes/types-of-diabetes/type-1-diabetes/[Last accessed December, 2025].
22. World Anti-Doping Agency. Therapeutic Use Exemptions (TUEs). WADA. [online] Available from https://www.wada-ama.org/en/athletes-support-personnel/therapeutic-use-exemptions-tues [Last accessed December, 2025].
23. World Anti-Doping Agency. Athlete Biological Passport. WADA. [online] Available from https://www.wada-ama.org/en/athlete-biological-passport [Last accessed December, 2025].
24. World Anti-Doping Agency. 2025 List of Prohibited Substances and Methods . [online] Available from https://www.wada-ama.org/sites/default/files/2024-09/2025list_en_final_clean_12_september_2024.pdf [Last accessed Sptember, 2024 and December, 2025].

29

Obesity Management in Diabetes Mellitus Care: Integrative Approaches

Neeta Deshpande, Brij Mohan Makker

ABSTRACT

The global rise in type 2 diabetes mellitus (T2DM) and obesity represents an intertwined "twin pandemic", driven largely by an obesogenic environment characterized by caloric excess and physical inactivity. Increasing evidence identifies adipose tissue dysfunction (adiposopathy) as a central pathophysiological mechanism linking obesity to insulin resistance (IR), dysglycemia, and cardiometabolic disease. Visceral adiposity, in particular, contributes to metabolic derangements through lipotoxicity, chronic inflammation, oxidative stress, and hormonal dysregulation. These processes collectively impair insulin signaling and β-cell function, leading to progressive metabolic decline.

Therapeutic strategies that address the underlying adipocentric pathology rather than focusing solely on glucose lowering offer a more comprehensive and disease-modifying approach. Sustained weight loss of 5–15% improves insulin sensitivity, reduces medication burden, and, when substantial (>15%), may achieve diabetes mellitus remission. Management should integrate lifestyle intervention, including dietary modification, physical activity, and behavioral therapy, alongside pharmacological agents that simultaneously improve glycemia and reduce body weight, such as glucagon-like peptide-1 receptor agonists (GLP-1RAs), dual GIP (glucose-dependent insulinotropic polypeptide)/GLP-1 agonists, and sodium-glucose cotransporter-2 inhibitors (SGLT-2i). For selected patients, metabolic surgery (MS) provides the most durable remission rates and long-term cardiovascular (CV) and renal benefits.

An integrative, multidisciplinary, weight-centric approach targeting adipose tissue dysfunction represents the future of T2DM management. By focusing on the root cause—adiposopathy—clinicians can move toward not only optimizing metabolic control but also achieving remission, preventing complications, and improving long-term survival and quality of life (QoL).

Keywords: Type 2 diabetes mellitus, Obesity, Adiposopathy, Insulin resistance, Weight-centric management, GLP-1 receptor agonists, Metabolic surgery.

INTRODUCTION

The twin pandemic of type 2 diabetes mellitus (T2DM) and obesity and the increasing prevalence of both conditions pose a major healthcare challenge globally. In recent times, it has been seen that both conditions are rather heterogeneous in nature. The modern obesogenic environment, which mainly comprises excessive caloric intake and sedentary behaviors, has been very conducive to this increasing prevalence. The current estimated global numbers of people living with T2DM is in excess of 590 million. This number is expected to exceed 853 million by 2050. There is no doubt that obesity drives these numbers. There is a strong pathogenetic and causal correlation between the rise of obesity globally and the increasing prevalence of T2DM. Obesity, particularly the central obesity with excessive visceral adiposity, is the key driver of all metabolic disorders, particularly T2DM. Genetic predisposition adds to this pathogenetic mechanism. Historically, it is known that T2DM results from a varying combination of insulin resistance (IR) and relative insulin deficiency. However, it is now evident that there are other pathogenetic mechanisms that are responsible additionally, conferring considerable heterogeneity. Prominently, adipose tissue and its response to excessive caloric intake is increasingly being recognized as the major causative mechanism in T2DM. Hence the new term "diabesity".[1] The sick adipose tissue in this case has also been termed "adiposopathy". The accumulation of such fat in the viscera leads to metabolic dysfunction including dysglycemia, hypertension, and dyslipidemia, in susceptible individuals. Cardiovascular disease (CVD) is one of the major consequences of this dysfunction. From the viewpoint of therapeutics, glycemic control has been the major focus in the treatment of T2DM, and research has validated this approach. However, with emerging knowledge about the connection between adiposopathy and T2DM, in recent years, the focus has gradually been shifting toward a weight-centric approach, specifically adipose tissue. This approach, as a primary target, appears to be more focused and comprehensive in terms of treating the root cause. Besides, the weight-centric approach has a wider compass in terms of improving other cardiometabolic complications. Additionally, disease remission is a distinct possibility with this approach, improving quality of life (QoL) and ultimately impacting survival positively in the long run. Of course, adipose tissue reduction is expected with the weight-centric approach. This can be ensured by monitoring metrics such as waist circumference and fat mass. To this end, the pillars of therapy comprise therapeutic lifestyle changes, pharmacotherapy, and metabolic surgery (MS).

OBESITY AS A PATHOGENETIC FACTOR IN TYPE 2 DIABETES MELLITUS

Adipose tissue is a dynamic endocrine and immune organ that plays a central role in maintaining systemic energy homeostasis. It functions as the body's primary reservoir for excess energy; however, in the context of obesity, this storage system undergoes maladaptive changes. When fat tissue becomes metabolically impaired—a condition termed adiposopathy—it becomes a central contributor to metabolic dysfunction. Pathological adipose expansion in obesity tends to occur through hypertrophy (enlargement of existing adipocytes) rather than hyperplasia (generation of new adipocytes). Enlarged adipocytes develop local hypoxia, fibrosis, limited expandability, and inflammation, which in turn promote lipotoxicity and free fatty acid (FFA) overflow into nonadipose organs. The "adipose tissue expandability hypothesis" proposes that when adipose tissue can no longer accommodate excess lipids, triglycerides (TGs) accumulate ectopically in tissues such as the liver and skeletal muscle, impairing metabolic signaling. Among fat depots, visceral adipose tissue is particularly metabolically active. It releases higher amounts of FFAs that interfere with insulin signaling in hepatic and muscle tissues. Furthermore, dysfunctional fat depots exhibit altered secretion of adipokines, shifting the hormonal balance toward inflammation and IR, thereby linking adipose dysfunction directly to systemic metabolic disease.

Chronic low-grade inflammation is a defining feature of obesity and a key driver of T2DM. In obese adipose tissue, macrophages accumulate and shift from an anti-inflammatory M2 to a pro-inflammatory M1 phenotype. These cells release tumor necrosis factor alpha (TNF-α), interleukin 6 (IL-6), and MCP-1, which activate inflammatory kinases and impair insulin signaling. This inflammatory state extends systemically, reducing insulin sensitivity in the liver and muscle and inducing β-cell stress in the pancreas.

Insulin resistance is the key metabolic link between obesity and T2DM, arising when the liver, skeletal muscle, and adipose tissue fail to respond adequately to insulin. In the liver, IR drives excessive gluconeogenesis; in muscle, it reduces glucose uptake; and in adipose tissue, it reduces glucose uptake and promotes lipolysis and FFA release. The resulting lipid overload in liver and muscle generates toxic intermediates—diacylglycerol (DAG) and ceramides—that activate protein kinase C, leading to IRS-1 phosphorylation and impaired GLUT4-mediated glucose uptake. Inflammatory cytokines and oxidative stress further amplify this cycle of IR and hyperglycemia. Progression to overt T2DM occurs when β-cell compensation fails.

Cellular stress pathways form a vital link between overnutrition and metabolic dysfunction. In obesity, excess nutrients supply leads to increased production of reactive oxygen species (ROS), driving oxidative stress that triggers inflammation and disrupts insulin signaling. ROS damage cellular components and impair mitochondrial function, leading to reduced ATP production and defective fatty acid oxidation, which promotes ectopic fat accumulation. At the same time, endoplasmic reticulum (ER) stress activates inflammatory and apoptotic cascades, contributing to IR and β-cell loss. Together, these stresses accelerate metabolic decline in obesity and T2DM.

In obesity, dysfunctional adipose tissue disrupts adipokine secretion, promoting inflammation and IR. Leptin levels rise but are accompanied by leptin resistance, while adiponectin, a key insulin-sensitizing hormone, declines. Other adipokines—resistin, visfatin, and PAI-1—further impair glucose metabolism, with PAI-1 serving as a strong predictor of future T2DM. Obesity also alters sex hormone balance, as increased aromatase activity lowers testosterone in men and disturbs estrogen regulation in women. Elevated glucocorticoid activity further aggravates adipose dysfunction and IR.

WEIGHT LOSS IMPROVES GLYCEMIC CONTROL

Research has thrown light the outcomes of weight loss in terms of glycemic control. The modalities of weight loss may be varied. However, glycemic control is certain following weight loss in T2DM. Even modest weight loss of 5–15% has benefit in improving glycemic control.[2,3] This benefit occurs because weight loss improves insulin sensitivity by reducing glucotoxicity as well as the lipid burden. Consequently, there is a reduced need for antidiabetic medication.[4] During intensive weight loss, whether through diet or early after MS, rapid loss of ectopic fat from skeletal muscle and liver leads to significant improvements in hepatic and muscle insulin sensitivity, as well as pancreatic first-phase insulin secretion.[5,6] The primary reason for weight loss being efficacious as an antihyperglycemic measure is reversal of the diabetogenic process. This, in effect, is the proposed *twin cycle hypothesis*, which postulates that severe caloric restriction can move the fat depots out of the liver and pancreas, thereby reestablishing insulin sensitivity and insulin secretion, respectively.[6] If the severe caloric restriction leads to greater than 15% weight loss, the possibility of diabetes mellitus remission is very high, as it would lead to appropriate insulin secretion from the pancreas, the fat content of the pancreas having been reduced considerably. In fact, the achievement of diabetes mellitus remission is the best evidence of the efficacy of weight loss in treatment of hyperglycemia. Attempts at remission and the success thereof have the best outcomes; chronic kidney disease (CKD) incidence reduction of 33% and that of CVD by 40% have been seen in the long-term study LOOK-AHEAD.[7]

INTEGRATIVE APPROACHES IN OBESITY MANAGEMENT

Optimal management requires a comprehensive, multimodal approach that is overseen by a qualified, multidisciplinary team. Specialized dietary approaches, such as programs incorporating an initial hypocaloric formula "total diet replacement" (TDR) phase, have shown high efficacy in achieving T2DM remission in certain cohorts. Furthermore, combined exercise (aerobic and resistance training) significantly improves glycemic control, enhances insulin sensitivity, and aids in weight loss among patients with T2DM and concurrent overweight/obesity. When pharmacological agents are chosen, treatment intensification should prioritize agents that promote weight loss while simultaneously delivering CV and renal benefits. This includes SGLT-2 inhibitors (SGLT-2i) and glucagon-like peptide-1 receptor agonists (GLP-1RAs). Newer pharmacological breakthroughs, such as dual GLP-1/GIP (glucose-dependent insulinotropic polypeptide) receptor agonists (e.g., tirzepatide) or triple agonists, are emerging as highly effective options for lowering body weight and improving metabolic markers. For appropriate candidates, MS is a highly effective, though complementary, method to achieve significant and sustained weight loss and drive T2DM remission.

LIFESTYLE INTERVENTION FOR WEIGHT MANAGEMENT IN DIABETES MELLITUS

The various studies cited above are proof enough that weight loss strategies work very well to treat hyperglycemia. Lifestyle intervention, primarily diet and physical activity, are of prime importance. Sustained weight loss is even more effective. Behavioral therapy is also an integral part of lifestyle intervention. This multimodal approach provides benefits beyond weight reduction, including improvements in sexual and motor functions, enhanced QoL, and a reduction in overall CV mortality. Apart from overall weight loss, targeting visceral adiposity is vital. The initial goal can be modest; a weight reduction of 3-5% will yield health benefits. However, greater weight loss must be attempted, to get optimal and increasing benefits. The goal of lifestyle intervention is generally to achieve weight reduction of at least 3-5% from baseline for apparent health benefits, although greater weight loss yields greater advantages.[8]

Dietary Intervention

The caloric restriction that is required for greater metabolic benefit is larger than that recommended in the medical nutrition therapy (MNT) guidelines of most associations. The American Diabetes Association (ADA) generally recommends an overall energy deficit of 500–750 kcal/day. This deficit translates roughly to a daily caloric content of 1,200–1,500 kcal/day for women and 1,500–1,800 kcal/day for men. Although most guidelines advocate personalized goals and therapies for weight loss, no specific diet pattern is recommended, although there is evidence for benefit for certain patterns such as the Mediterranean diet.[9] The DASH (Dietary Approaches to Stop Hypertension) diet and the low-carbohydrate diet are also considered beneficial.[10] The macronutrient composition must be computed sensibly to include 40–45% carbohydrates, 30–40% fats, and 20–30% proteins, regardless of any specific pattern. However, in certain ethnic groups such as in India, the carbohydrates tend to be higher than this. While reducing caloric intake, adequate or higher protein and sufficient micronutrient intake should be ensured. Intensive caloric restriction has gained evidence in recent times for its efficacy in achieving remission of T2DM. Typically, such very low-calorie diets (VLCDs) consist of 600–800 kcals, administered generally for not more than 4-6 months. The weight loss with such diets is much greater than the standard low-calorie diets. Another way of achieving this is by using TDR, an initial hypocaloric liquid formula. Such programs have been found to be most effective for T2DM remission.[4] Of course, all such programs need to be administered under close supervision of a registered dietitian. Patients should reduce consumption of products rich in saturated and trans-unsaturated fats. Adequate hydration is crucial for metabolic processes supporting weight loss, and the consumption of sweetened drinks should be reduced. Alcohol consumption should be minimized due to its high energy content and lack of nutritional value.

Exercise and Physical Activity

Regular physical activity is indispensable for T2DM and obesity management, improving diabetes mellitus control, metabolic function, and CV risk factors. The most beneficial effects are produced when aerobic and resistance exercises are combined. Guidelines recommend a minimum of 150 minutes per week of moderate-intensity aerobic exercise. Additional benefits can be achieved by increasing activity to 300 minutes of moderate-intensity or 150 minutes of high-intensity exercise weekly.[11] At least two weekly sessions of resistance training (e.g., 8–12 repetitions 3 sets per muscle group) are recommended. Resistance training is particularly advantageous because it can be safely performed by patients who must refrain from aerobic activity. A meta-analysis showed that combined exercise significantly reduced glycated hemoglobin (HbA1c) and BMI.[12] The synergistic effect arises because aerobic training reduces visceral fat mass, while resistance exercise enhances insulin sensitivity by increasing glucose expenditure in hypertrophied muscles.

Behavioral Therapy

Behavioral interventions, often delivered through structured programs, are vital for weight management induction and long-term maintenance. Behavioral programs help patients sustain new behaviors, relationships with foods, and adherence to dietary advice. Optimal outcomes are attained when weight management is overseen by a qualified, multidisciplinary team of specialists (e.g., physicians, registered dietitians, diabetes mellitus counselors). Patients should be enrolled in a structured program that integrates a healthy eating plan, physical activity, and behavioral intervention. Such interventions have been shown to lead to a significant improvement in serum HbA1c levels [standardized mean difference (SMD) = 0.272] and body weight (SMD = 0.526) in the intervention group.[13]

PHARMACOTHERAPY OF OBESITY TO TREAT DIABETES MELLITUS

Majority of people living with T2DM are overweight or obese. Pharmacological interventions are crucial for achieving the intensive weight loss necessary in the management of T2DM that is a consequence of excessive adipose tissue. The goal of drug therapy within the adipocentric treatment paradigm is to prioritize weight loss, preferably targeting a reduction of at least 10%, and optimally 15%, along with reduced waist circumference and body fat percentage, to achieve disease remission or optimal metabolic control. Current international guidelines recommend incorporating pharmacologic agents that promote weight loss into the therapeutic strategy for patients with T2DM and concurrent overweight or obesity.

The pharmacological landscape for obesity management in T2DM involves two main categories:

1. *Antihyperglycemic agents with proven weight loss and cardiorenal benefits*: This category includes GLP-1RAs, dual GLP-1/GIP receptor agonists (e.g., tirzepatide), and SGLT-2i. These agents are often prioritized, especially in patients with established CVD, heart failure (HF), or CKD, due to their benefits beyond glucose control.
2. *Dedicated weight loss medications*: These agents are specifically approved for chronic weight management in eligible patients (BMI

30 kg/m^2 or BMI 27 kg/m^2 with comorbidities) and include orlistat, naltrexone/bupropion, phentermine/topiramate, and short-term use phentermine. In this category, currently, only orlistat is available.

Glucagon-like Peptide 1 Receptor Agonist-based Therapies

The GLP-1RAs and the newer dual (GLP-1/GIP) and triple agonists are prioritized in the adipocentric paradigm due to their potent effects on weight reduction, glycemic control, and cardiorenal protection. GLP-1RAs are pharmacological peptides that activate the human GLP-1 receptor. Their mechanism of action is multifaceted: They stimulate glucose-dependent insulin secretion from β cells while reducing glucagon secretion, which limits the risk of hypoglycemia. Their primary role in weight loss stems from their anorexigenic effects, mediated by activation of GLP-1 receptors in the central nervous system (CNS). They also slow postprandial gastric emptying, contributing to satiety and reduced caloric intake. The newer dual GLP-1/GIP agonist, tirzepatide, and emerging triple agonists (such as retatrutide) display overall better efficacy in reducing HbA1c, fasting blood glucose, and body weight compared to traditional GLP-1RA drugs. GIP and GLP-1 regulate food intake and metabolic homeostasis by stimulating insulin secretion, maintaining healthy adipocytes, reducing ectopic fat distribution, and increasing adiponectin production. GLP-1RA-based therapies demonstrate a strong dose-dependent effect on efficacy, meaning higher doses often lead to greater reductions in HbA1c, fasting blood glucose, body weight, and waist circumference, as notably observed with tirzepatide.[14] GLP-1RAs deliver substantial CV and renal benefits, reducing major adverse cardiovascular events (MACE) by 14% and CKD progression by 21%. This dual benefit makes them a priority, especially for patients with established CVD, HF, or CKD. The most common adverse effects are gastrointestinal ailments, including nausea, vomiting, and diarrhea. These effects are generally most pronounced early in therapy. Agents like lixisenatide, semaglutide, exenatide, tirzepatide, and liraglutide have a significantly higher odds ratio of discontinuation due to adverse events compared with placebo. Notably, the odds ratios of gastrointestinal side effects are observed to increase with increasing doses of drugs like tirzepatide, semaglutide, and dulaglutide. GLP-1RAs are contraindicated in women of childbearing potential due to lack of safety data during pregnancy and breastfeeding.

Orlistat

Orlistat is a dedicated medication approved for chronic weight management in eligible patients. Orlistat acts locally in the gastrointestinal tract as a strong, selective inhibitor of pancreatic and gastric lipase. This action prevents the hydrolysis of TGs consumed in food, leading to the excretion of approximately 30% of dietary TGs in feces. Uniquely, orlistat is the only weight management drug that does not affect the hypothalamic satiety nuclei in the CNS. Compared to the highly effective GLP-1-based therapies, orlistat offers modest weight loss, ranging from −2.9% to −4.0% (or to kg) versus placebo.[15] However, studies show that orlistat reduces the risk of progression from prediabetes to overt T2DM by 37.3%.

Adverse effects are primarily gastrointestinal, including fatty stools, steatorrhea, and flatulence. Orlistat can affect the absorption of certain drugs (e.g., levothyroxine, cyclosporine) and fat-soluble vitamins (A, D, E, K), necessitating supplementation of these vitamins and careful monitoring of patients (e.g., those on oral anticoagulants due to vitamin K dependence). Orlistat is contraindicated in patients with chronic malabsorption syndrome and cholestasis, as well as in pregnant or breastfeeding women.

Table 1 summarizes the comparative efficacy and safety profile of orlistat and individual GLP-1RA-based therapies against placebo in adults with T2DM, based on pooled data from systematic reviews and network meta-analyses (NMA) and **Table 2** is a practical guide to the use of these medications.

TABLE 1: Summary of key pharmacotherapy options in T2DM and obesity.[14]

Feature	*Orlistat*	*Liraglutide*	*Dulaglutide*	*Semaglutide*	*Tirzepatide*	*CagriSema*	*Retatrutide*
Drug class/type	Lipase inhibitor	GLP-1RA	GLP-1RA	GLP-1RA	Dual GIP/GLP-1 agonist	Dual (semaglutide + cagrilintide)	Triple agonist (GIP + GLP-1 + glucagon)
Primary mechanism	Blocks ~30% of dietary fat absorption	Enhances satiety and insulin secretion via GLP-1 pathway	Enhances satiety and insulin secretion	Enhances satiety, slows gastric emptying, increases insulin release	Activates both GIP and GLP-1 receptors for enhanced insulin response	Combines GLP-1 and amylin analog for stronger appetite suppression	Activates GIP, GLP-1 and glucagon receptors to boost metabolism
Route/frequency	Oral, three times daily	Subcutaneous (daily)	Subcutaneous (weekly)	Subcutaneous (weekly) or oral	Subcutaneous (weekly)	Subcutaneous (weekly)	Subcutaneous (weekly)
Mean weight loss (vs. placebo)	−2.9% to −4% (~−3 kg)	−1.33 kg (95% CI −2.08 to −0.59)	−0.73 kg (95% CI −1.56 to 0.10)	−3.13 kg (95% CI −3.95 to −2.31)	−8.47 kg (95% CI −9.68 to −7.26)	−14.03 kg (95% CI −17.05 to −11.00)	−7.87 kg (95% CI −9.95 to −5.79)
HbA1c reduction (vs. placebo)	≈−0.4%	≈−1.0%	≈−1.1%	≈−1.4%	≈−2.1%	≈−1.8%	≈−1.3%
CV/renal benefit	No	Yes (LEADER trial)	Yes (REWIND trial)	Yes (SUSTAIN-6, SOUL)	Yes (SURPASS/ class effect)	Yes (class effect)	Yes (class effect)
Other key considerations	Requires vitamin supplementation; avoid in malabsorption	Approved for obesity; monitor gallbladder	Dose-dependent efficacy; weekly injection	Approved for obesity; strong CV benefit	Most effective for glycemic and weight reduction	Strongest weight-loss effect; under evaluation	Triple agonist; superior efficacy under study

(CI: confidence interval; CV: cardiovascular; GIP: glucose-dependent insulinotropic polypeptide; GLP-1RA: glucagon-like peptide-1 receptor agonist; HbA1C: glycated hemoglobin)

TABLE 2: Practical guide to common anti-obesity medications.

Drug/class	*Mode of administration*	*Frequency*	*Typical dose range*	*Titration/ initiation*	*Key practical points*
Orlistat (lipase inhibitor)	Oral capsule (120 mg)	With each main meal (TDS)	120 mg with meals containing fat	Start 1 capsule with largest meal; skip if meal skipped or fat-free	Oily stools, urgency; advise low-fat diet (<30% calories from fat); supplement fat-soluble vitamins if long-term use
Liraglutide 3.0 mg (GLP-1RA)	Subcutaneous injection (pen)	Once daily	0.6 mg → increase weekly by 0.6 mg → 3.0 mg daily	Gradual uptitration over 5 weeks reduces nausea	Improves satiety, glycemia and CV profile; inject consistently; monitor for pancreatitis or gallstones
Semaglutide 2.4 mg (GLP-1 RA)	Subcutaneous injection (pen)	Once weekly	0.25 → 0.5 → 1.0 → 1.7 → 2.4 mg weekly (every 4 weeks)	Titrate every 4 weeks; inject same day each week	Highest average % weight loss; counsel on nausea/constipation; avoid abrupt discontinuation
Tirzepatide (dual GIP/GLP-1 RA)	Subcutaneous injection (pen)	Once weekly	2.5 → 5 → 7.5 → 10 → 12.5 → 15 mg weekly (every 4 weeks)	Start 2.5 mg for 4 weeks then escalate stepwise	Dual-pathway action; strong efficacy in T2DM; avoid in medullary thyroid CA or MEN-2

(CA: cancer; CI: confidence interval; CV: cardiovascular; GIP: glucose-dependent insulinotropic polypeptide; GLP-1RA: glucagon-like peptide-1 receptor agonist; MEN-2: multiple endocrine neoplasia type 2)

METABOLIC SURGERY

Metabolic surgery, often referred to as bariatric surgery, represents the most aggressive and highly effective intervention for achieving significant weight loss and subsequent improvement or remission of T2DM. In T2DM with obesity, MS is prioritized alongside intensive lifestyle modifications and potent pharmacological agents that promote weight loss. International guidelines recommend MS for patients with T2DM and a BMI above 30 kg/m^2 who have failed to meet their glycemic control or weight loss goals despite adhering to lifestyle and pharmacological interventions.[2] The integration of MS into the T2DM treatment algorithm is supported by major international diabetes mellitus organizations.

Metabolic surgery has demonstrated superior results compared to standard medical care in achieving T2DM remission.[16] Randomized controlled trials consistently show higher remission rates following MS. While remission rates decline over time, MS provides durable benefits. Data from the Swedish Obese Subjects (SOS) study and other meta-analyses suggest long-term remission rates are sustained at approximately 30%.[17] The likelihood of achieving remission postsurgery is associated with markers of β-cell health, including a shorter duration of T2DM, younger age, lack of insulin use, and favorable baseline C-peptide and HbA1c levels.

While significant weight loss is a core driver of improvement, the benefits of MS extend beyond caloric restriction alone. The efficacy of MS relies on multifactorial mechanisms. Weight loss achieved through surgery reduces fat deposits in the liver and pancreas, resolving hepatic and pancreatic steatosis. MS enhances nutrient delivery to the distal intestine and increases the secretion of anorexigenic gut hormones.

INDEX

Page numbers followed by *f* refer to figure, *fc* refer to flowchart, and *t* refer to table.

A

B

C

E